# SIGNS & SYMPTOMS

D1455042

Springhouse Corporation
Springhouse, Pennsylvania

# Staff

**Executive Director, Editorial:** Stanley Loeb

**Editorial Director:** Matthew Cahill

**Clinical Director:** Barbara McVan, RN

**Art Director:** John Hubbard

**Drug Information Editor:** George J. Blake, RPh, MS

**Editors:** Stephen Daly (senior editor), Catherine E. Harold, Peter H. Johnson, Michael Shaw, Gale A. Sloan

**Copy Editors:** Jane V. Cray (supervisor), Terri Goshko, Nancy Papsin, Doris Weinstock

**Designers:** Stephanie Peters (associate art director), Matie Patterson (senior designer)

**Cover Art:** Robert Jackson

**Art Production:** Robert Perry (manager), Anna Brindisi, Donald Knauss, Tom Robbins, Robert Wieder

**Typography:** David Kosten (director), Diane Paluba (manager), Elizabeth Bergman, Joyce Rossi Biletz, Phyllis Marron, Robin Rantz, Valerie Rosenberger

**Manufacturing:** Deborah Meiris (manager), T.A. Landis, Jennifer Suter

**Production Coordination:** Colleen M. Hayman

**Indexer:** Janet Hodgson

**Editorial Assistants:** Maree DeRosa, Beverly Lane, Mary Madden

RRDIA-051195

℞ A member of the Reed Elsevier plc group

---

**Library of Congress Cataloging-in-Publication Data**

Signs and symptoms.
    p.    cm. — (Nurse's Ready Reference™)
    Includes bibliographical references and index.
    1. Nursing diagnosis — Handbooks, manuals, etc.   I. Springhouse Corporation.  II. Series.
    [DNLM:  1. Nursing Diagnosis — handbooks.  WY 39 S5775]
RT48.6.S54    1991
616.075 — dc20
DNLM/DLC
ISBN 0-87434-366-6           91-4608

# Contents

Keeping up-to-date with the latest developments in health care is a daunting task. Treatments and procedures change frequently. Cost constraints have put time and staffing pressures on all health care providers. And nurses are expected to know and do more—to recognize and interpret the subtlest indications of a patient's illness. To deliver quality care under these circumstances, you need dependable, accessible information at your fingertips. Fortunately, *Signs & Symptoms*, the latest book in the Nurse's Ready Reference series, provides just that.

Nearly 300 signs and symptoms packaged in a spiral-bound book that's compact and flexible, *Signs & Symptoms* is designed for use in any clinical or academic setting. You can lay the book flat or, with its fold-out easel back, prop it upright, using the book flipchart-style while caring for a patient or reviewing information. Arranged alphabetically, the entries are printed on both sides of the pages with a convenient letter guide at the bottom.

All of the entries have been reviewed for clinical accuracy and streamlined to provide the information most relevant to nurses, saving you from a time-consuming search through the literature to find what you need. Each entry begins with a concise definition and description of the sign or symptom. This is followed in many entries by *Emergency interventions*, a highlighted section that explains what to do if the sign or symptom is life-threatening.

The next section, *History,* summarizes the information you need to gather from the patient or, in some cases, his family. The *Physical exam* section describes how to examine the patient and explains what you may learn from your observations. The *Causes* section lists all of the major causes of the sign or symptom, detailing the most important of these and describing other clinical features a patient with that disorder is likely to have. Finally, *Nursing considerations* explains your additional responsibilities in caring for the patient.

In a time of expanding responsibilities for nurses, when the amount of information you need to know can seem overwhelming, Nurse's Ready Reference *Signs & Symptoms* will prove a welcome addition to your working library. A useful tool for both the practicing nurse and student nurse, it will save you time and energy and help ensure that you're providing the best possible care for your patients.

Generalized abdominal distention results from the accumulation of fluid or gas (or both) within the GI tract or peritoneal cavity. In the peritoneal cavity, distention may reflect acute bleeding, accumulation of ascitic fluid, or air from perforation of an abdominal organ.

## ▶ Emergency interventions

If you detect abdominal distention, check for signs of hypovolemia. Is the patient experiencing severe abdominal pain or having difficulty breathing? Ask about any recent accidents and look for signs of trauma. Then auscultate bowel sounds in all abdominal quadrants. Gently palpate the abdomen for rigidity.

If you detect abdominal distention, pain and rigidity, and abnormal bowel sounds, have another nurse notify the doctor immediately. Place the patient supine, give oxygen, and insert an I.V. line, as ordered. Prepare to insert a nasogastric tube.

## History

If the patient's abdominal distention isn't acute, ask him about onset and duration. The patient with generalized distention may report a bloated feeling, a pounding heart, and difficulty breathing deeply or when lying flat. He may also feel unable to bend at his waist. Be sure to ask about abdominal pain, fever, nausea, vomiting, anorexia, altered bowel habits, and weight changes.

Obtain a medical history, noting GI or biliary disorders. Note chronic constipation. Ask about recent abdominal surgery or trauma.

## Physical exam

Assess the patient for abdominal asymmetry and contour. Taut skin and bulging flanks may indicate ascites. Note the umbilicus. An everted umbilicus may indicate ascites or umbilical hernia. An inverted umbilicus may indicate gas distention. Look for signs of inguinal or femoral hernia, and for incisions that may indicate adhesions. Then auscultate for bowel sounds, abdominal friction rubs, and bruits.

Next, percuss and palpate the abdomen to determine if distention results from air, fluid, or both. A tympanic note heard throughout suggests an air-filled peritoneal cavity. A dull percussion note throughout a generally distended abdomen suggests a fluid-filled peritoneal cavity. Remember that obesity also causes a dull note throughout the abdomen.

Palpate the abdomen for generalized tenderness. Finally, measure abdominal girth.

## Causes

*Cirrhosis.* Ascites causes generalized distention and is confirmed by a fluid wave and shifting dullness. Umbilical eversion and dilated veins around the umbilicus are common. Other findings include a feeling of fullness or weight gain, anorexia, constipation or diarrhea, bleeding tendencies, and spider angiomas.

*Congestive heart failure.* Abdominal distention caused by ascites is confirmed by shifting dullness and a fluid wave. Other findings include peripheral edema, jugular vein distention, dyspnea, and tachycardia.

*Nephrotic syndrome.* This syndrome may produce massive edema, causing generalized abdominal distention with a fluid wave and shifting dullness.

*Paralytic ileus.* Generalized distention is marked by a tympanic percussion note accompanied by absent or hypoactive bowel sounds.

*Peritonitis.* In this life-threatening disorder, fluid accumulation causes a fluid wave and shifting dullness. Other findings include sudden and severe abdominal pain that worsens with movement, rebound tenderness, and abdominal rigidity.

*Other causes.* Abdominal cancer, abdominal trauma, and acute toxic megacolon.

## Nursing considerations

• If the patient has ascites, elevate the head of the bed to ease his breathing. Advise the anxious patient to breathe slowly.

**A**

Localized abdominal distention results from the accumulation of fluid or gas (or both) within the lumen of the GI tract or peritoneal cavity. In the peritoneal cavity, distention may reflect acute bleeding, accumulation of ascitic fluid, or air from perforation of an abdominal organ.

## ▶ Emergency interventions

If you detect abdominal distention, check for signs of hypovolemia. Is the patient in severe abdominal pain or having difficulty breathing? Ask about any recent accidents and look for signs of trauma. Then auscultate bowel sounds in all abdominal quadrants. Gently palpate the abdomen for rigidity.

If you detect abdominal distention, pain, and rigidity along with abnormal bowel sounds, have another nurse notify the doctor immediately. Position the patient supine, give oxygen, and insert an I.V. line, as ordered. Prepare to insert a nasogastric tube.

## History

If the patient's abdominal distention isn't acute, ask him about onset and duration. A patient with localized distention may report a feeling of pressure, fullness, or tenderness in the affected area. Be sure to ask about abdominal pain, fever, nausea, vomiting, anorexia, constipation, and weight changes.

Obtain a medical history, noting GI or biliary disorders. Ask about recent abdominal surgery or trauma.

## Physical exam

Look for signs of inguinal or femoral hernia and for incisions that may indicate adhesions. Then auscultate for bowel sounds, abdominal friction rubs, and bruits.

Next, percuss and palpate the abdomen to determine if distention results from air, fluid, or both. A tympanic note in the left lower quadrant suggests an air-filled descending or sigmoid colon.

Palpate the abdomen for localized tenderness. Finally, measure and mark abdominal girth.

## Causes

*Bladder distention.* Slight dullness on percussion above the symphysis pubis indicates mild bladder distention. A palpable, fluctuant suprapubic mass suggests severe distention.

*Gastric dilatation (acute).* Left upper quadrant distention is accompanied by persistent vomiting and, possibly, epigastric pain. Other findings include tympany and gastric tenderness.

*Irritable bowel syndrome.* Intermittent, localized distention results from periodic intestinal spasms, which occur with lower abdominal pain or cramping. Other findings include diarrhea, mu-

cus-streaked stool, and dyspepsia.

*Large-bowel obstruction.* Dramatic abdominal distention marks this life-threatening disorder; loops of the large bowel may become visible on the abdomen. Constipation precedes the distention.

*Mesenteric artery occlusion (acute).* In this life-threatening disorder, abdominal distention usually occurs several hours after sudden onset of severe, colicky periumbilical pain that later becomes constant and diffuse. Other signs include severe abdominal tenderness with guarding and rigidity, and absent bowel sounds.

*Ovarian cysts.* Typically, large ovarian cysts produce lower abdominal distention. Lower abdominal pain and a palpable mass may be present.

*Small-bowel obstruction.* Abdominal distention marks this life-threatening disorder. Auscultation reveals hyperactive bowel sounds. Percussion produces a tympanic note. Other findings include colicky periumbilical pain, constipation, nausea, vomiting, and rebound tenderness.

## Nursing considerations

• Advise the anxious patient to breathe slowly.
• Give drugs to relieve pain, as ordered.

An abdominal mass is a localized swelling in one of the abdominal quadrants. Typically, this sign develops insidiously and may represent an enlarged organ, tumor, abscess, vascular defect, or a fecal mass.

## History

Ask the patient to show you where he feels the mass. Ask him how long he has had the mass and if he has noticed any change in its size or location. Ask him if the mass is painful. If so, is the pain constant, or does it occur only on palpation? Ask about GI signs and symptoms. Ask the female patient about her menstrual pattern.

## Physical exam

Auscultate for bowel sounds in each lower quadrant. Listen for bruits or friction rubs, and check for enlarged veins. Palpate the abdomen lightly, then deeply, assessing any painful or suspicious areas last. (With a suspected abdominal tumor, do *not* perform deep palpation.) Note the patient's position when you locate the mass. Some masses can only be detected with the patient supine; others require a side-lying position.

Estimate the size of the mass. Is it smooth, rough, sharply defined, nodular, or irregular? Does it feel doughy, soft, solid, or hard? A dull sound on percussion indicates a fluid-filled mass; a tympanic sound indicates an air-filled mass.

Next, evaluate the mass's mobility. Does it move with your hand or with respiration? Is it free-floating or attached to intra-abdominal structures? Ask the patient to lift his head and shoulders off the examination table, thereby contracting his abdominal muscles. As he does so, try to palpate the mass. If you can, the mass is in the abdominal wall; if you can't, it's within the abdominal cavity.

## Causes

*Bladder distention.* A smooth, rounded, fluctuant suprapubic mass is characteristic. Severe suprapubic pain and urinary frequency and urgency may also occur.

*Colonic cancer.* A right lower quadrant mass may occur in cancer of the right colon, which may also cause black, tarry stools and abdominal aching, pressure, or dull cramps.

*Crohn's disease.* Tender, sausage-shaped masses are usually palpable in the right lower quadrant and, sometimes, in the left lower quadrant. Colicky right lower quadrant pain and diarrhea are common. Other findings include fever, anorexia, weight loss, hyperactive bowel sounds, nausea, and abdominal tenderness with guarding.

*Diverticulitis.* This disorder may produce a left lower quadrant mass. Other findings include intermittent abdominal pain that's relieved by defecation or passage of flatus, alternating diarrhea and constipation, nausea, and low-grade fever.

*Ovarian cyst.* A large cyst may produce a smooth, fluctuant mass in the suprapubic region. Other findings may include pelvic discomfort, low back pain, and menstrual irregularities.

*Uterine leiomyomas (fibroids).* These benign tumors may produce a round, multinodular, suprapubic mass. The patient usually reports menorrhagia. Other findings may include a feeling of heaviness in the abdomen, back pain, constipation, and urinary frequency or urgency.

*Other causes.* Abdominal abscess, Hirschsprung's disease, intussusception, and volvulus.

## Nursing considerations

- Position the patient comfortably.
- If the mass causes bowel obstruction, watch for signs of peritonitis and shock.

# Index

# Abdominal mass, upper quadrants

An abdominal mass is a localized swelling in one of the abdominal quadrants. Typically, this sign develops insidiously and may represent an enlarged organ, a tumor, an abscess, a vascular defect, or a fecal mass.

▶ **Emergency interventions**
If the patient has a pulsating midabdominal mass and severe abdominal pain, suspect an aortic aneurysm. Have another nurse notify the doctor immediately. Withhold food or fluids until the doctor can examine the patient, start an I.V. line, and administer oxygen.

**History**
Ask the patient to show you where he feels the mass. Ask him how long he has had the mass and if he has noticed any changes in its size or location. If the mass is painful, ask if it hurts constantly or only when he presses on it. Ask about GI signs and symptoms.

**Physical exam**
First, auscultate for bowel sounds in each upper quadrant. Listen for bruits or friction rubs, and check for enlarged veins. Palpate the abdomen lightly, then deeply, assessing any painful or suspicious areas last. (With a suspected abdominal tumor, do *not* perform deep palpation.) Note the patient's position when you locate the mass. Some masses can only be detected with the patient supine; others require a side-lying position.

Estimate the size of the mass in centimeters. Is it smooth, rough, sharply defined, nodular, or irregular? Does it feel doughy, soft, solid, or hard? A dull sound on percussion means it's fluid-filled; a tympanic sound means it's air-filled.

Next, evaluate the mass's mobility. Does it move with your hand or with respiration? Is it free-floating or attached to intra-abdominal structures? Ask the patient to lift his head and shoulders off the examination table, thereby contracting his abdominal muscles. As he does so, try to palpate the mass. If you can, the mass is in the abdominal wall; if you can't, it's within the abdominal cavity.

**Causes**
*Abdominal aortic aneurysm.* Upon expanding, this vascular defect produces constant severe upper abdominal and back pain. If ruptured, it no longer pulsates. Other findings: absent femoral and pedal pulses, mottled skin below the waist, and lower blood pressure in the legs than in the arms.

*Cholecystitis.* Deep palpation below the liver border may detect a smooth, firm, sausage-shaped mass. But an acutely inflamed gallbladder is usually too tender to palpate. Other findings include severe right upper quadrant pain that radiates to the shoulder, chest, or back; abdominal rigidity and tenderness; and nausea and vomiting.

*Cholelithiasis.* Passage of a stone through the bile or cystic duct may cause severe right upper quadrant pain radiating to the epigastrium, back, or shoulder blades.

*Hepatomegaly.* This produces a firm, blunt, irregular mass in the epigastric region or below the right costal margin. Other signs may include ascites and right upper quadrant pain and tenderness.

*Hydronephrosis.* This disorder produces a smooth, boggy mass in one or both flanks. Other findings may include renal pain or dull flank pain.

*Splenomegaly.* The smooth edge of the enlarged spleen is palpable in the left upper quadrant. Other findings may include abdominal pain, splenic friction rub, and splenic bruits.

*Other causes.* Abdominal abscess, gallbladder carcinoma, gastric carcinoma, hepatic carcinoma, Hirschsprung's disease, intussusception, neuroblastoma, pancreatic abscess or pseudocysts (in epigastric area), pyloric stenosis, volvulus, and Wilms' tumor.

**Nursing considerations**
• Position the patient comfortably.
• If the mass causes bowel obstruction, watch for signs of peritonitis and shock.

Also known as sibilant rhonchi, wheezes are adventitious breath sounds with a high-pitched, musical, squealing, creaking, or groaning quality. They can be heard by placing an unaided ear over the chest wall or mouth or by placing a stethoscope over the anterior or posterior chest. Unlike crackles and rhonchi, wheezes can't be cleared by coughing.

### ▶ Emergency interventions

Assess the patient's respiratory distress. Is he responsive? Is he restless, confused, or anxious? Are respirations fast, slow, shallow, or deep? Are they irregular? Does he have increased use of accessory muscles; increased chest wall motion; retractions; stridor; or nasal flaring? Help him relax, and administer humidified oxygen. Suction him, and encourage coughing and slow, deep breathing. Keep emergency resuscitation equipment nearby.

### History

Find out what provokes the patient's wheezing. Does he have a history of asthma, allergies or pulmonary, cardiac, or circulatory disorders? Does he smoke? Ask about recent surgery, illness, or trauma, and obtain a drug history. Ask about changes in appetite, exercise tolerance, or sleep patterns. If he has a cough, ask how it sounds, when it starts, and how often it occurs. Does he have paroxysms of coughing? Is his cough dry, sputum-producing, or bloody?

### Physical exam

Examine the patient's nose and mouth for congestion, drainage, and signs of infection. Obtain a sputum sample. Check for cyanosis, pallor, masses, chest wall tenderness, distended neck veins, and enlarged lymph nodes. Inspect his chest for abnormal configuration and asymmetrical motion, and determine if the trachea is in position. Percuss for dullness or hyperresonance, and auscultate for crackles, rhonchi, and pleural friction rubs. Note absent or hypoactive breath sounds, or abnormal heart sounds.

### Causes

*Anaphylaxis.* Besides severe wheezing and stridor, findings may include congestion, rhinorrhea, chest or throat tightness, and dysphagia.

*Aspiration of a foreign body.* Sudden wheezing, stridor, and a dry, paroxysmal cough may occur.

*Aspiration pneumonitis.* Wheezing may accompany tachypnea, dyspnea, cyanosis, tachycardia, fever, productive cough, and pink, frothy sputum.

*Asthma.* Wheezing occurs during expiration. Other findings include apprehension, prolonged expiration, retractions, rhonchi, accessory muscle use, nasal flaring, and tachypnea.

*Bronchiectasis.* Excessive mucus commonly causes intermittent wheezing. A cough may be accompanied by hemoptysis and coarse crackles.

*Bronchitis (chronic).* Besides wheezing, findings may include prolonged expiration, coarse crackles, and a cough that later becomes productive.

*Chemical pneumonitis (acute).* Mucosal injury leads to wheezing, dyspnea, orthopnea, and crackles.

*Emphysema.* Mild to moderate wheezing may occur with dyspnea, diminished breath sounds, peripheral cyanosis, and pursed-lip breathing.

*Pneumothorax (tension).* Besides wheezing, possible findings include dyspnea, tachycardia, tachypnea, and sudden, severe, sharp chest pain.

*Pulmonary edema.* Wheezing may occur along with coughing, exertional and paroxysmal nocturnal dyspnea, and orthopnea.

*Tracheobronchitis.* Auscultation may reveal wheezing, rhonchi, and crackles. The patient also has a cough, slight fever, and substernal tightness.

*Other causes.* Bronchial adenoma, bronchogenic carcinoma, inhalation injury, pulmonary coccidioidomycosis, pulmonary embolus, pulmonary tuberculosis, thyroid goiter, and Wegener's granulomatosis.

### Nursing considerations

• Provide humidification and perform pulmonary physiotherapy as needed.
• Encourage the patient to drink plenty of fluids.

# Abdominal pain, generalized

Usually, abdominal pain results from GI disorders. However, it can also result from cardiovascular, reproductive, respiratory, genitourinary (GU), and musculoskeletal disorders; drug use; and the effects of toxins. At times, it signals life-threatening complications.

## ▶ Emergency interventions

In sudden and severe abdominal pain, take the patient's vital signs. If you suspect hypovolemic shock, dissecting abdominal aortic aneurysm, or bowel rupture, have another nurse notify the doctor. Prepare to give oxygen and I.V. fluids or volume expanders. As ordered, insert an indwelling urinary catheter and a nasogastric tube. Prepare the patient for surgery, if required.

## History

If the patient is not in immediate danger, ask him if the pain is constant or intermittent and when it began. Ask about its location and about precipitating and mitigating factors. Ask about appetite changes, nausea or vomiting, changes in bowel habits, and urinary frequency or urgency. Ask about drug and alcohol use, and past vascular, GI, GU, or reproductive disorders. Ask the female patient about her menstrual pattern.

## Physical exam

Take vital signs. Assess skin turgor and mucous membranes. Inspect the abdomen for distention or visible peristaltic waves; if indicated, measure abdominal girth. Auscultate for bowel sounds. Percuss all quadrants. Palpate the entire abdomen for masses, rigidity, and tenderness. Note costovertebral angle tenderness, abdominal tenderness with guarding, and rebound tenderness.

## Causes

*Abdominal trauma.* Generalized or localized abdominal pain occurs with possible ecchymoses on the abdomen; abdominal tenderness; vomiting; and, with hemorrhage into the peritoneal cavity, abdominal rigidity.

*Intestinal obstruction.* Short episodes of colicky, cramping pain alternate with pain-free intervals in this life-threatening disorder. Other findings may include abdominal distention, tenderness, and guarding; visible peristaltic waves; hyperactive sounds proximal to obstruction and hypoactive or absent sounds distally.

*Mesenteric artery ischemia.* Severe, diffuse abdominal pain is preceded by 2 to 3 days of colicky periumbilical pain and diarrhea. Associated findings include vomiting, anorexia, and diarrhea alternating with constipation.

*Peritonitis.* Sudden, severe pain can be diffuse or localized, and it worsens with movement. Typical findings include fever; chills; nausea; vomiting; hypoactive or absent bowel sounds; abdominal tenderness, distention, and rigidity; rebound tenderness and guarding.

*Sickle cell crisis.* Sudden, severe abdominal pain may accompany chest, back, hand, or foot pain. Other findings may include weakness, aching joints, dyspnea, and scleral jaundice.

*Uremia.* Marked by generalized or periumbilical pain that shifts and varies in intensity, this disorder causes diverse GI symptoms, such as nausea, anorexia, vomiting, and diarrhea. Abdominal tenderness, visual disturbances, bleeding, headache, decreased level of consciousness, vertigo, and oliguria or anuria may occur.

*Other causes.* Abdominal cancer, adrenal crisis, heavy metal poisoning, herpes zoster, insect toxins, lactose intolerance, Meckel's diverticulum, mesenteric adenitis, nonsteroidal anti-inflammatory drugs, renal calculi, salicylates, systemic lupus erythematosus, and volvulus.

## Nursing considerations

• Before diagnosis, withhold analgesics, food, and fluids, and prepare for I.V. infusion. If ordered, prepare to insert a nasogastric tube and to assist with peritoneal lavage or paracentesis.

**A**

# Weight loss

Weight loss may reflect decreased food intake, increased metabolism, or a combination of the two.

## History
Begin with a thorough diet history. If your patient eats poorly, try to determine why. Ask about his previous weight and about recent changes in bowel habits. Ask about excessive thirst, excessive urination, and heat intolerance. Take a careful drug history, noting use of diet pills and laxatives.

## Physical exam
Carefully check the patient's height and weight. Take his vital signs and note his general appearance. Is he well nourished? Do his clothes fit? Is muscle wasting evident? Now examine the patient's skin for turgor and abnormal pigmentation, especially around the joints. Does he have pallor or jaundice? Examine his mouth, including the condition of his teeth or dentures. Also check the patient's eyes for exophthalmos and his neck for swelling. Palpate his abdomen for masses, tenderness, and an enlarged liver.

## Causes
*Adrenal insufficiency.* Weight loss may occur along with anorexia, weakness, fatigue, irritability, syncope, nausea, vomiting, abdominal pain, and diarrhea or constipation. Hyperpigmentation may appear over the joints.

*Anorexia nervosa.* Self-imposed weight loss may be accompanied by skeletal muscle atrophy, loss of fatty tissue, constipation, frequent infection, blotchy or sallow skin, cold intolerance, loss of scalp hair, and amenorrhea.

*Cancer.* Weight loss typically occurs. Other findings include fatigue, pain, nausea, vomiting, anorexia, abnormal bleeding, and a palpable mass.

*Crohn's disease.* Weight loss occurs with chronic cramping, abdominal pain, and anorexia. Other findings include diarrhea, tachycardia, abdominal tenderness and guarding, hyperactive bowel sounds, abdominal distention, and pain.

*Diabetes mellitus.* Weight loss may accompany polydipsia, weakness, fatigue, and polyuria.

*Esophagitis.* Inflammation of the esophagus leads to weight loss. Other findings may include mouth pain, dysphagia, and hematemesis.

*Gastroenteritis.* Malabsorption and dehydration cause weight loss. Other findings include abdominal pain and tenderness, poor skin turgor, dry mucous membranes, tachycardia, hypotension, diarrhea, hyperactive bowel sounds, vomiting, and fever.

*Leukemia. Acute leukemia* causes progressive weight loss accompanied by severe prostration, high fever, and bleeding tendencies. *Chronic leukemia* causes progressive weight loss with fatigue, pallor, an enlarged spleen, bleeding tendencies, anemia, skin eruptions, anorexia, and fever.

*Lymphoma. Hodgkin's disease* and *non-Hodgkin's lymphoma* cause gradual weight loss. Associated findings include fever, fatigue, night sweats, hepatosplenomegaly, and lymphadenopathy.

*Pulmonary tuberculosis.* Gradual weight loss may accompany fatigue, weakness, anorexia, night sweats, and low-grade fever. Other findings include a cough with bloody or mucopurulent sputum.

*Stomatitis.* Weight loss may result from inflammation of the oral mucosa. Other findings may include fever, increased salivation, malaise, mouth pain, anorexia, and swollen, bleeding gums.

*Thyrotoxicosis.* Increased metabolism causes weight loss. Other findings: nervousness, heat intolerance, diarrhea, increased appetite, palpitations, tachycardia, diaphoresis, fine tremors and, possibly, an enlarged thyroid and exophthalmos.

*Ulcerative colitis.* Besides weight loss, findings include bloody diarrhea with pus or mucus; weakness; crampy lower abdominal pain; and tenesmus.

*Other causes.* Depression; drugs, such as amphetamines, chemotherapeutic agents, laxatives, and thyroid preparations; and Whipple's disease.

## Nursing considerations
• If the patient has a chronic disease, administer total parenteral nutrition or tube feedings, as ordered. Count calories daily and weigh him weekly.

Although abdominal pain usually results from GI disorders, it can also result from respiratory, reproductive, genitourinary (GU), musculoskeletal, and cardiovascular disorders; drug use; and the effects of toxins. At times, it signals life-threatening complications.

▶ **Emergency interventions**
In sudden and severe abdominal pain, quickly take the patient's vital signs, and have another nurse notify the doctor—especially if you suspect hypovolemic shock, dissecting abdominal aortic aneurysm, or bowel rupture. Prepare to give oxygen and I.V. fluids or volume expanders. As ordered, insert an indwelling urinary catheter and a nasogastric tube.

## History
If the patient is not in immediate danger, ask him if the pain is constant or intermittent and when it began. Ask about the pain's location and about precipitating and mitigating factors, appetite changes, nausea or vomiting, changes in bowel habits, and urinary frequency or urgency. Ask about drug and alcohol use, and obtain a history of vascular, GI, GU, and reproductive disorders. Ask the female patient about menstrual patterns.

## Physical exam
Take vital signs and assess skin turgor and mucous membranes. Inspect the abdomen for distention or visible peristaltic waves. Auscultate for bowel sounds. Percuss all quadrants and note sounds. Palpate for masses, rigidity, and tenderness—specifically for costovertebral angle (CVA) tenderness, abdominal tenderness with guarding, and rebound tenderness.

## Causes
*Abdominal aortic aneurysm (dissecting).* This produces constant abdominal pain, which may worsen when the patient lies down and abate when he leans forward or sits up. It also produces mottled skin below the waist. Palpation may reveal a pulsating epigastric mass before rupture.

*Appendicitis.* Dull discomfort in the epigastric or umbilical region typically precedes anorexia, nausea, and vomiting. Pain localizes at McBurney's point in the right lower quadrant.

*Crohn's disease (acute).* Severe, cramping pain may occur in the lower abdomen and cause diarrhea, bloody stools, and hyperactive bowel sounds.

*Diverticulitis.* Mild diverticulitis usually produces intermittent abdominal pain, which may be relieved by defecation or passage of flatus.

*Ectopic pregnancy.* Lower abdominal pain may be sharp, dull, or cramping, constant or intermittent. Vaginal bleeding may occur, along with a tender adnexal mass, and amenorrhea.

*Irritable bowel syndrome.* Lower abdominal cramping or pain is aggravated by eating coarse or raw foods and may be alleviated by defecation or passage of flatus.

*Pelvic inflammatory disease.* Vague to severe pain in the right or left lower quadrant is typical. Pain accompanies cervical or adnexal palpation.

*Pyelonephritis (acute).* This is marked by progressive lower quadrant pain in one or both sides, flank pain, and CVA tenderness. Pain may radiate to the lower midabdomen or to the groin.

*Ulcerative colitis.* Vague abdominal discomfort leads to cramping lower abdominal pain. Recurrent and possibly severe diarrhea with blood, pus, and mucus may relieve the pain.

*Other causes.* Cystitis, endometriosis, heavy metal poisoning, hepatic amebiasis, intussusception, juvenile rheumatoid arthritis, lactose intolerance, Meckel's diverticulum, mesenteric adenitis, nonsteroidal anti-inflammatory drugs, ovarian cyst, prostatitis, salicylates, and volvulus.

## Nursing considerations
• Before diagnosis, withhold analgesics, food and fluids, and prepare for I.V. infusion. If ordered, prepare to assist with peritoneal lavage or paracentesis.

**A**

Weight gain occurs when ingested calories exceed body requirements for energy, causing increased adipose tissue storage. Fluid retention leading to edema may also cause weight gain.

## History

Discuss previous patterns of weight gain and loss. Does the patient's family have a history of obesity, thyroid disease, or diabetes mellitus? Assess eating and activity patterns. Has his appetite increased? Does he exercise regularly? Ask about related symptoms, such as impotence, visual disturbances, hoarseness, paresthesia, and increased urination and thirst. Ask a female patient about irregularities or weight gain during menstruation.

Assess mental status, noting any signs of anxiety or depression. Does the patient respond slowly? Is his memory poor? What medications is he currently using?

## Physical exam

Measure skinfold thickness to estimate fat reserves. Note fat distribution and the presence of localized or generalized edema. Inspect for abnormal body hair distribution, hair loss, dry skin, and other abnormalities. Measure vital signs.

## Causes

*Acromegaly.* Besides moderate weight gain, findings may include coarsened facial features, prognathism, enlarged hands and feet, increased sweating, oily skin, deep voice, back and joint pain, lethargy, sleepiness, and heat intolerance.

*Congestive heart failure.* Despite anorexia, weight gain may result from edema. Other findings include paroxysmal nocturnal dyspnea, orthopnea, and fatigue.

*Diabetes mellitus.* Weight gain or loss is possible. Other findings may include fatigue, polydipsia, polyuria, nocturia, weakness, polyphagia, and somnolence.

*Hypercortisolism.* Marked weight gain usually occurs along the trunk and the back of the neck. Other findings include slender extremities, moon face, weakness, purple striae, emotional lability, and increased susceptibility to infection.

*Hyperinsulinism.* The patient may develop an increased appetite along with indigestion, weakness, diaphoresis, tachycardia, visual disturbances, and syncope.

*Hypogonadism.* Weight gain is common. *Prepubertal hypogonadism* causes eunuchoid body proportions with relatively sparse facial and body hair and a high-pitched voice. *Postpubertal hypogonadism* causes impotence, infertility, and loss of libido.

*Hypothalamic dysfunction.* A voracious appetite may lead to weight gain. Other findings include altered body temperature and sleep rhythms.

*Hypothyroidism.* Weight gain occurs despite anorexia. Other findings include fatigue; cold intolerance; constipation; menorrhagia; slowed motor and intellectual activity; dry, pale, cool skin; dry, sparse hair; and thick, brittle nails.

*Nephrotic syndrome.* Weight gain results from edema. Anasarca may develop in severe cases. Related effects include abdominal distention, orthostatic hypotension, and lethargy.

*Pancreatic islet cell tumor.* Excessive hunger leads to weight gain. Other findings include emotional lability, weakness, malaise, fatigue, restlessness, diaphoresis, palpitations, tachycardia, visual disturbances, and syncope.

*Preeclampsia.* Abnormally rapid weight gain may accompany nausea and vomiting, epigastric pain, hypertension, and blurred or double vision.

*Other causes.* Drugs, such as corticosteroids, cyproheptadine, lithium, oral contraceptives, phenothiazines, and tricyclic antidepressants; and Sheehan's syndrome.

## Nursing considerations

• Assess whether the patient with weight gain could benefit from psychological counseling.
• If the patient is obese or has a cardiopulmonary disorder, seek a doctor's advice before recommending exercise.

Typically a result of GI disorders, abdominal pain can also result from cardiovascular, reproductive, respiratory, genitourinary (GU), and musculo-skeletal disorders; drug use; and the effects of toxins. It may signal life-threatening complications.

▶ **Emergency interventions**
In sudden and severe abdominal pain, quickly take the patient's vital signs. If you suspect hypovolemic shock, dissecting abdominal aortic aneurysm, or bowel rupture, have another nurse notify the doctor. Prepare to give oxygen and I.V. fluids or volume expanders. As ordered, insert an indwelling urinary catheter and a nasogastric tube. Prepare the patient for surgery, if required.

## History

If the patient is not in immediate danger, ask him if the pain is constant or intermittent and when it began. Then ask about its location, and get details about precipitating and mitigating factors.

Ask about appetite changes; onset and frequency of any nausea or vomiting; changes in bowel habits; and urinary frequency or urgency. Also ask about drug and alcohol use, and obtain a history of vascular, GI, GU, and reproductive disorders. Ask the female patient about menstrual patterns.

## Physical exam

Take vital signs and assess skin turgor and mucous membranes. Inspect the abdomen for distention or visible peristaltic waves. Auscultate for bowel sounds. Percuss upper quadrants. Palpate for masses, rigidity, costovertebral angle tenderness, abdominal tenderness with guarding, and rebound tenderness.

## Causes

*Abdominal aortic aneurysm (dissecting).* This produces constant upper abdominal pain, which may worsen when the patient lies down and abate when he leans forward or sits up. It also produces mottled skin below the waist. Palpation may reveal an epigastric mass that pulsates before rupture but not after it.

*Cholecystitis.* Severe right upper quadrant pain may be sudden or gradual and may radiate to the right shoulder, chest, or back. Accompanying it are nausea, vomiting, and abdominal rigidity.

*Cholelithiasis.* Sudden, severe, and paroxysmal pain in the right upper quadrant may last several minutes to several hours and may radiate to the epigastrium, back, or shoulder blades.

*Duodenal ulcer.* Localized abdominal pain may occur high in the midepigastrium or slightly to the right. Commonly, pain begins 2 to 4 hours after meals and may cause nocturnal awakening.

*Gastric ulcer.* Diffuse, gnawing pain in the left upper quadrant or epigastric area often occurs after meals. It may be relieved by food or antacids.

*Gastritis (acute).* Abdominal pain can range from mild epigastric discomfort to burning pain in the left upper quadrant.

*Gastroenteritis.* Cramping or colicky abdominal pain originates in the left upper quadrant and radiates to other quadrants. It's accompanied by diarrhea and hyperactive bowel sounds.

*Pancreatitis (acute).* This produces fulminating, continuous upper abdominal pain that may radiate to both flanks and to the back.

*Perforated ulcer.* Sudden, severe epigastric pain may radiate through the abdomen to the back. Other features: rigidity, tenderness with guarding, rebound tenderness, and absent bowel sounds.

*Other causes.* Cirrhosis, congestive heart failure, heavy metal poisoning, hepatic abscess, hepatic amebiasis, hepatitis, intussusception, juvenile rheumatoid arthritis, lactose intolerance, Meckel's diverticulum, mesenteric adenitis, myocardial infarction, nonsteroidal anti-inflammatory drugs, pleurisy, pneumonia, pneumothorax, salicylates, splenic infarction, and volvulus.

## Nursing considerations

• Before diagnosis, withhold analgesics, food, and fluids, and prepare for I.V. infusion.

**A**

# Vulvar lesions

Lesions—cutaneous lumps, nodules, papules, vesicles, or ulcers—may appear anywhere on the vulva. They result from benign or malignant tumors, dystrophies, dermatoses, or infection.

## History

Ask the patient when she first noticed a vulvar lesion. Find out about associated features, such as swelling, pain, tenderness, itching, or discharge. Does she have lesions elsewhere on her body? Has she experienced any signs of systemic illness? Also ask the patient if she is sexually active.

## Physical exam

Examine the lesion and assist the doctor during the pelvic examination and collection of specimens for culture.

## Causes

*Basal cell carcinoma.* Usually occurring in postmenopausal women, this nodular tumor has a central ulcer and a raised, rolled border. It may cause pruritus, bleeding, discharge, and burning.

*Benign cysts.* Usually round and producing no symptoms, *epidermal inclusion cysts* appear primarily on the labia majora. *Bartholin's cysts* are usually tense, nontender, and palpable. Infection of a Bartholin's cyst may cause pain and tenderness, vulvar swelling, redness, and deformity.

*Benign vulvar tumors.* Cystic or solid benign vulvar tumors usually produce no symptoms.

*Genital warts.* Painless warts appear on the vulva, vagina, and cervix. Warts start as tiny red or pink swellings, then enlarge (up to 10 cm) and become pedunculated.

*Gonorrhea.* Vulvar lesions may develop along with pruritus, a burning sensation, pain, and a greenish yellow vaginal discharge, but most patients are asymptomatic.

*Granuloma inguinale.* A single painless macule or papule appears on the vulva, ulcerating into a raised, beefy-red lesion with a granulated, friable border.

*Herpes simplex (genital).* Fluid-filled vesicles may appear on the cervix, vulva, labia, perianal skin, vagina, or mouth. Initially painless, vesicles may rupture and develop into extensive, shallow, painful ulcers with redness, marked edema, and tender inguinal lymph nodes.

*Lymphogranuloma venereum.* A single, painless papule or ulcer appears on the posterior vulva and heals in a few days. Inguinal lymphadenopathy develops about 2 weeks later.

*Malignant melanoma.* Irregular, pigmented vulvar lesions enlarge rapidly and may ulcerate and bleed.

*Molluscum contagiosum.* Vulvar papules, about 1 to 2 mm in diameter with a white core, appear.

Pruritic lesions may also appear on the face, eyelids, breasts, and inner thighs.

*Pediculosis pubis.* Erythematous vulvar papules accompany pruritus and skin irritation. Magnification reveals pubic lice nits.

*Squamous cell carcinoma.* Usually occurring in postmenopausal women, *invasive carcinoma* may produce vulvar pruritus and a vulvar lump. *Carcinoma in situ* usually occurs in premenopausal women, producing a white or red vulvar lesion that is raised, well defined, moist, crusted, and isolated.

*Syphilis.* Chancres may appear on the vulva, vagina, or cervix. Usually painless, they start as papules and then erode, with indurated, raised edges and clear bases.

*Other causes.* Chancroid, dermatoses (systemic), herpes zoster, hyperplastic dystrophy, and viral disease.

## Nursing considerations

- Expect to administer systemic antibiotics, antiviral agents, topical corticosteroids, topical testosterone, or an antipruritic agent, as ordered.
- If ordered, show the patient how to give herself a sitz bath.
- If the patient has a sexually transmitted disease, encourage her to inform her sexual partners. Advise her to avoid sexual contact until lesions are no longer contagious.

# Abdominal rigidity

Also called abdominal muscle spasm or involuntary guarding, abdominal rigidity refers to abnormal muscle tension or inflexibility of the abdomen.

Rigidity may be voluntary or involuntary. Voluntary rigidity may reflect the patient's nervousness upon palpation. Involuntary rigidity signals potentially life-threatening peritoneal irritation or inflammation. It's usually caused by GI disorders and marked by nausea, vomiting, and abdominal tenderness, distention, and pain.

## ▶ Emergency interventions

After palpating the rigid abdomen, quickly take the patient's vital signs and have another nurse notify the doctor. Even though the patient may not appear gravely ill or have markedly abnormal vital signs, his abdominal rigidity calls for emergency intervention. Prepare to administer oxygen and to insert an I.V. line for fluid and blood replacement. The doctor may also order drugs to support blood pressure. Prepare to catheterize the patient, as ordered, and monitor fluid intake and output. Be ready to assist with insertion of an intestinal tube to relieve abdominal distention. Because emergency surgery may be necessary, prepare the patient for laboratory tests and X-rays, as ordered.

## History

Find out when the abdominal rigidity began. Is it associated with abdominal pain? If so, did the pain begin at the same time? Determine whether abdominal rigidity is localized or generalized. Is it always present? Has its site changed or remained constant? Next, ask about aggravating or alleviating factors, such as position changes, coughing, vomiting, elimination, and walking.

## Physical exam

Inspect the abdomen for peristaltic waves, which may be visible in very thin patients. Also check for a visible distended bowel loop. Next, auscultate bowel sounds. Perform light palpation to locate the rigidity and determine its severity. Avoid deep palpation, which may exacerbate abdominal pain. Finally, check for poor skin turgor and dry mucous membranes, indicating dehydration.

## Causes

*Dissecting abdominal aortic aneurysm.* Mild-to-moderate abdominal rigidity occurs in this life-threatening disorder. Typically, it's accompanied by constant upper abdominal pain.

*Insect toxins.* Insect stings and bites, especially black widow spider bites, release toxins that can produce generalized, cramping abdominal pain usually accompanied by rigidity.

*Mesenteric artery ischemia.* Two to three days of persistent, low-grade abdominal pain and diarrhea precede abdominal rigidity in this life-threatening disorder. Rigidity in the central or periumbilical region is accompanied by severe abdominal tenderness, fever, and signs of shock, such as tachycardia and hypotension.

*Peritonitis.* Depending on the cause of peritonitis, abdominal rigidity may be localized or generalized. Peritonitis causes sudden and severe abdominal pain, tenderness, and distention.

*Pneumonia.* In lower lobe pneumonia, severe upper abdominal pain and tenderness accompany rigidity that diminishes with inspiration. Other findings include a hacking cough, blood-tinged or rusty sputum, dyspnea, achiness, headache, fever, and chills.

## Nursing considerations

• Continue to monitor the patient closely for signs of shock. Position him as comfortably as possible. Until the doctor makes a tentative diagnosis, withhold analgesics because they may mask symptoms.

• Emergency surgery may be required, so withhold food and fluids. Administer I.V. antibiotics, if ordered.

• Prepare the patient for diagnostic tests, which may include blood, urine, and stool studies; chest and abdominal X-rays; peritoneal lavage; and gastroscopy or colonoscopy. A pelvic or rectal examination may also be done.

**A**

The forceful expulsion of gastric contents through the mouth, vomiting is usually preceded by nausea. It results from a coordinated sequence of abdominal muscle contractions and reverse esophageal peristalsis.

### ▶ Emergency interventions
Projectile vomiting *unaccompanied* by nausea may indicate increased intracranial pressure (ICP), a life-threatening emergency. Check the patient's vital signs. Immediately call the doctor and elevate the patient's head 30 degrees if you detect widened pulse pressure or bradycardia.

### History
If the patient isn't in acute distress, ask him to describe the onset, duration, and intensity of his vomiting. If possible, collect and measure vomitus. Ask about nausea, abdominal pain, anorexia and weight loss, changes in bowel habits, and excessive belching or flatus. Ask him about GI, endocrine, and metabolic disorders; recent infections; and cancer, including any treatment. Also ask about medication use and alcohol consumption. Ask the female patient if she is or could be pregnant.

### Physical exam
Inspect the abdomen for distention, and auscultate for bowel sounds and bruits. Palpate for rigidity and tenderness, and test for rebound tenderness. Palpate and percuss the liver for enlargement.

### Causes
*Appendicitis.* Vomiting and nausea accompany vague epigastric or periumbilical discomfort that localizes in the right lower quadrant.

*Cholecystitis and cholelithiasis.* Nausea, vomiting, and severe right upper quadrant or epigastric pain occur after ingestion of fatty foods.

*Gastroenteritis.* Nausea, vomiting, diarrhea, abdominal cramping, and hyperactive bowel sounds are common.

*Increased ICP.* Features include projectile vomiting that *is not* preceded by nausea, as well as decreased level of consciousness, bradycardia, hypertension, and respiratory pattern changes.

*Intestinal obstruction.* Nausea occurs with high small intestinal obstruction. Vomiting may be bilious or fecal, and abdominal pain is usually episodic and colicky.

*Pancreatitis (acute).* Nausea — usually followed by vomiting — occurs early, along with steady, severe pain in the epigastrium or left upper quadrant that may radiate to the back.

*Peptic ulcer.* Nausea, vomiting, and epigastric pain occur when the stomach is empty or after ingestion of alcohol, caffeine, or aspirin.

*Peritonitis.* Nausea and vomiting usually accompany acute abdominal pain localized to the area of inflammation. Other findings may include high fever with chills, hypoactive or absent bowel sounds, and abdominal distention.

*Other causes.* Adrenal insufficiency; cirrhosis; congestive heart failure; diverticulitis; drugs, such as antibiotics, anesthetics, antineoplastic agents, chloride replacements, digitalis (overdose), estrogens, ferrous sulfate, levodopa, opiates, oral potassium, sulfasalazine, quinidine, and theophylline (overdose); ectopic pregnancy; electrolyte imbalance; gastric cancer; gastritis; hepatitis; hyperemesis gravidarum; infection; irritable bowel syndrome; labyrinthitis; Ménière's disease; mesenteric artery ischemia; mesenteric venous thrombosis; metabolic acidosis; migraine headache; motion sickness; myocardial infarction; preeclampsia; radiation therapy; renal and urologic disorders; surgery; thyrotoxicosis; and ulcerative colitis.

### Nursing considerations
• Have the patient breathe deeply to ease his nausea and help prevent further vomiting. Elevate his head or position him on his side to prevent aspiration of vomitus. Give I.V. fluids or have the patient sip clear liquids to maintain hydration.

# Accessory muscle use

The accessory muscles—the sternocleidomastoid, scalene, greater pectoral, trapezius, internal intercostals, and abdominal muscles—help the diaphragm maintain respiration when breathing requires extra effort. Some accessory muscle use normally takes place while singing, talking, coughing, defecating, or exercising. More pronounced use may signal acute respiratory distress.

## ▶ Emergency interventions

Signs of acute respiratory distress include decreased level of consciousness, shortness of breath, tachypnea, intercostal and sternal retractions, cyanosis, wheezing or stridor, diaphoresis, nasal flaring, and agitation. If these signs are present, auscultate for abnormal, diminished, or absent breath sounds; have another nurse notify the doctor immediately. If the airway is obstructed, try to restore patency. Insert an airway or assist with intubation. Begin suctioning and manual or mechanical ventilation. Administer oxygen; if the patient has chronic obstructive pulmonary disease, use a low flow rate. Insert an I.V. line, if ordered.

## History

Ask about onset, duration, and severity of symptoms. Focus on respiratory, cardiac, and neuromuscular disorders. Note allergies, asthma, rheumatoid arthritis, lupus erythematosus, and recent trauma (especially to the spine or chest). Note recent pulmonary function tests or respiratory therapy, smoking, exposure to chemical fumes or mineral dusts such as asbestos, and a family history of cystic fibrosis or neurofibromatosis.

## Physical exam

Perform a detailed chest examination, noting abnormal respiratory rate, rhythm, or depth. Assess the color, temperature, and turgor of the patient's skin, and check for fingernail clubbing.

## Causes

*Adult respiratory distress syndrome.* In this life-threatening disorder, accessory muscle use increases in response to hypoxia. Intercostal, supracostal, and sternal retractions occur on inspiration; grunting on expiration. Other findings include tachypnea, dyspnea, diaphoresis, diffuse crackles, and a cough with pink, frothy sputum.

*Airway obstruction.* Accessory muscle use typically increases. Airway obstruction's most telling sign is inspiratory stridor. Other findings include dyspnea, tachypnea, gasping, wheezing, coughing, intercostal retractions, cyanosis, and tachycardia.

*Amyotrophic lateral sclerosis.* This disorder typically affects the diaphragm, increasing accessory muscle use and involving fasciculations, muscle atrophy and weakness, spasticity, bilateral Babinski's reflex, hyperactive deep tendon reflexes, and incoordination. Other findings include impaired speech; difficulty chewing, swallowing, and breathing; urinary frequency and urgency.

*Pulmonary embolism.* This life-threatening disorder may cause increased accessory muscle use. It commonly produces dyspnea and tachypnea. Other signs include restlessness, tachycardia, productive cough, and low-grade fever.

*Spinal cord injury.* Increased accessory muscle use may occur. Other findings include Babinski's reflex; hyperactive deep tendon reflexes; spasticity; loss of pain and temperature sensation, proprioception, motor function; Horner's syndrome.

*Thoracic injury.* Increased accessory muscle use may occur. Other findings may include a chest wound or pain, dyspnea, cyanosis, and agitation.

*Other causes.* Asthma, chronic bronchitis, diffuse infiltrative (or fibrotic) lung disease, emphysema, pneumonia, pulmonary edema, tests and treatments.

## Nursing considerations

• If the patient is alert, elevate the head of the bed to ease breathing. Encourage fluid intake. Administer oxygen, as ordered. Prepare him for such tests as pulmonary function studies, chest X-rays, lung scans, arterial blood gas analysis, complete blood count, and sputum culture.

# Visual floaters

Visual floaters are particles of blood or cellular debris that move about in the vitreous. As these enter the visual field, they appear as spots or dots. Chronic floaters may occur normally in elderly or myopic patients. However, visual floaters may also be a symptom of retinal detachment.

## ▶ Emergency interventions

If onset of visual floaters is dramatic and sudden, suspect retinal detachment. Ask the patient if he also sees flashing lights or spots in the affected eye, and if he's experiencing a curtainlike loss of vision. If so, notify an ophthalmologist immediately. Restrict the patient's eye movements until the diagnosis is made.

## History

Obtain a drug and allergy history. Ask about any nearsightedness (a predisposing factor), use of corrective lenses, eye trauma, or other eye disorders. Also ask about a history of granulomatous disease, diabetes mellitus, or hypertension, which may predispose the patient to retinal detachment, vitreous hemorrhage, or uveitis.

## Physical exam

Inspect the patient's eyes for signs of injury, such as bruising or edema, and assess his visual acuity using the Snellen letter or symbol chart.

## Causes

*Retinal detachment.* Floaters and light flashes appear suddenly in the portion of the visual field where the retina is detached. As the retina detaches further (a painless process), gradual vision loss occurs, likened to a cloud or curtain falling in front of the eyes. Ophthalmoscopic examination reveals a gray, opaque, detached retina with an indefinite margin. Retinal vessels appear almost black.

*Uveitis (posterior).* Visual floaters may be accompanied by gradual eye pain, photophobia, blurred vision, and conjunctival injection.

*Vitreous hemorrhage.* Rupture of retinal vessels produces a shower of red or black dots or a red haze across the visual field. Vision is suddenly blurred in the affected eye, and visual acuity may be greatly reduced.

## Nursing considerations

• Encourage bed rest and provide a calm environment.
• The patient may require eye patches, surgery, and corticosteroids or other drug therapy. If bilateral eye patches are necessary, ensure the patient's safety. Identify yourself when you approach him, and orient him to time frequently. Provide sensory stimulation, such as a radio or tape player. Check the doctor's orders to determine the appropriate patient position, and place pillows or towels behind the patient's head to maintain it.
• Warn the patient to avoid touching or rubbing his eyes and to avoid straining or making sudden movements.

# Agitation

A state of increased tension and irritability, agitation can lead to confusion, hyperactivity, and overt hostility. It can result from various disorders, pain, fever, anxiety, drug use and withdrawal, and hypersensitivity reactions. Agitation arises gradually or suddenly, can last minutes or months, and worsens with increased fever, pain, and stress. It may indicate a developing disorder.

## History
Assess the patient's emotional lability, confusion, memory loss, hyperactivity, and hostility. Obtain a history from the patient or a family member, noting diet and known allergies. Find out if the patient is being treated for any illnesses or has had a recent infection, trauma, stress, or changes in sleep patterns. Ask about the use of prescribed or over-the-counter drugs and alcohol intake.

## Physical exam
Check for signs of drug abuse — needle tracks, dilated pupils. Check and record the patient's vital signs and neurologic status.

## Causes
*Alcohol withdrawal syndrome.* This syndrome causes mild to severe agitation marked by hyperactivity, tremors, and anxiety. In *delirium tremens*, which can be life-threatening, severe agitation occurs with visual hallucinations, insomnia, diaphoresis, and depression. Pulse rate and temperature rise as withdrawal progresses; status epilepticus, cardiac exhaustion, and shock can occur.

*Anxiety.* This state commonly produces agitation. The patient may be unaware of his anxiety or its cause. Other findings include nausea, vomiting, diarrhea, cool and clammy skin, frontal headache, back pain, insomnia, and tremors.

*Chronic renal failure.* Moderate to severe agitation occurs, marked by confusion and memory loss. It's accompanied by nausea, vomiting, anorexia, mouth ulcers, ammonia breath odor, GI bleeding, pallor, edema, dry skin, and uremic frost.

*Dementia.* Mild to severe agitation can result from common syndromes, such as Alzheimer's disease and Huntington's chorea. The patient may display a decrease in memory, attention span, problem-solving ability, and alertness.

*Drug withdrawal syndrome.* Mild to severe agitation commonly occurs. Related findings may include anxiety, abdominal cramps, diaphoresis, and anorexia.

*Hypersensitivity reaction.* Moderate to severe agitation appears and may be accompanied by urticaria, pruritus, and facial and dependent edema.

*Hypoxemia.* Agitation begins as restlessness but rapidly worsens. The patient may be confused and have impaired judgment and motor coordination, tachycardia, tachypnea, dyspnea, and cyanosis.

*Increased intracranial pressure.* Agitation usually precedes other symptoms. Findings may include headache; nausea; vomiting; respiratory changes; sluggish, nonreactive pupils; widening pulse pressure; tachycardia; decreased level of consciousness; seizures; and motor changes.

*Organic brain syndrome.* The patient's agitation is manifested as hyperactivity, emotional lability, confusion, and memory loss. He may display slurred or incoherent speech and paranoia.

*Post-head-trauma syndrome.* Shortly after or even years after injury, agitation develops, characterized by disorientation, loss of concentration, angry outbursts, and emotional lability. Other findings include fatigue, wandering behavior, and poor judgment.

*Other causes.* Central nervous system stimulants, contrast media, drug abuse, hepatic encephalopathy, and vitamin $B_6$ deficiency.

## Nursing considerations
• Monitor vital signs and neurologic status.
• Eliminate stressors. Ensure a balanced diet, and provide vitamin supplements as ordered.
• If appropriate, prepare the patient for diagnostic tests, such as computed tomography scanning, skull X-rays, magnetic resonance imaging, and blood studies.

# Visual blurring

Visual blurring refers to the loss of visual acuity with indistinct visual details.

## ▶ Emergency interventions

If your patient has visual blurring accompanied by sudden, severe eye pain, a history of trauma, or sudden vision loss, call the doctor immediately. (For further information, see the emergency interventions in *Vision loss*, page 286.)

## History

Ask the patient how long he has had visual blurring. Did blurring occur suddenly? Does it occur at specific times? Ask about associated symptoms. If visual impairment followed injury, obtain details. Obtain a medical and drug history.

## Physical exam

Inspect the patient's eye. Note an irregularly shaped iris (a sign of previous trauma) or excessive blinking (a sign of corneal damage). Assess for pupillary changes and test visual acuity.

## Causes

*Acute closed-angle glaucoma.* Unilateral visual blurring and severe pain begin suddenly. Other findings include halo vision; a moderately dilated, nonreactive pupil; and conjunctival injection.

*Brain tumor.* Visual blurring may accompany decreased level of consciousness (LOC), headache, behavioral changes, memory loss, and dizziness.

*Cataract.* Gradual blurring may accompany halo vision and progressive vision loss. The pupil may turn milky white.

*Cerebrovascular accident.* Brief attacks of bilateral visual blurring may occur. Other findings may include hemiplegia, dysarthria, dysphagia, ataxia, sensory loss, and apraxia.

*Concussion.* Vision may be blurred, double, or temporarily lost. Other findings include changes in LOC and behavior.

*Conjunctivitis.* Visual blurring may accompany photophobia, pain, burning, tearing, itching, and a feeling of fullness around the eyes.

*Corneal abrasions.* Visual blurring may occur with severe eye pain, photophobia, redness, and excessive tearing.

*Corneal foreign bodies.* Visual blurring may accompany a foreign-body sensation, excessive tearing, photophobia, and eye pain.

*Eye tumor.* Possible findings include visual blurring and varying visual field losses.

*Hypertension.* Visual blurring may accompany a recurring morning headache that decreases in severity during the day.

*Hyphema.* Besides visual blurring, effects include pain and diffuse conjunctival injection.

*Iritis.* Acute iritis causes sudden visual blurring, moderate to severe eye pain, photophobia, conjunctival injection, and a constricted pupil.

*Migraine headache.* Visual blurring may occur with paroxysmal headaches.

*Multiple sclerosis.* Blurred vision, diplopia, and paresthesia may occur.

*Optic neuritis.* The patient may experience an acute attack of visual blurring and vision loss.

*Retinal detachment.* Visual blurring occurs suddenly and grows worse, accompanied by visual floaters and recurring flashes of light.

*Retinal vein occlusion (central).* Gradual unilateral blurring occurs with vision loss.

*Temporal arteritis.* Sudden blurred vision may accompany vision loss and a throbbing unilateral headache in the temporal or frontotemporal region.

*Vitreous hemorrhage.* Sudden unilateral visual blurring, vision loss, and visual floaters may occur.

*Other causes.* Corneal dystrophies; diabetic retinopathy; dislocated lens; drugs, such as cycloplegics, guanethidine, reserpine, clomiphene, phenylbutazone, thiazide diuretics, antihistamines, anticholinergics, and phenothiazines; senile macular degeneration; serous retinopathy (central); and uveitis (posterior).

## Nursing considerations

• As necessary, teach the patient how to instill ophthalmic medication.

Alopecia—hair loss—occurs most commonly on the scalp. It usually develops gradually and may be diffuse or patchy. Scarring alopecia, or permanent hair loss, results from hair follicle destruction, which erases follicular openings and smooths the skin surface. Nonscarring alopecia, or temporary hair loss, results from damage that spares follicular openings, allowing regrowth.

Alopecia can result from drugs; radiotherapy; skin, connective tissue, endocrine, nutritional, and psychological disorders; neoplasms; infection; burns; and the effects of toxins.

## History

If the patient isn't receiving radiation or chemotherapy, ask when he first noticed the hair loss or thinning. Does it occur elsewhere on the body? Does it itch? Ask about recent weight change, anorexia, nausea, vomiting, and altered bowel habits; urinary changes; fatigue; irritability; stiffness; heat or cold intolerance; and exposure to insecticides. Ask the female patient about menstrual problems and pregnancies. Ask the male patient about impotence or decreased libido. Ask about hair care, a family history of alopecia, or nervous habits, such as twirling hair around a finger.

## Physical exam

Assess the extent and pattern of scalp hair loss. Inspect the underlying skin for follicular openings, erythema, loss of pigment, scaling, induration, broken hair shafts, and hair regrowth.

Examine remaining skin. Note lesions, jaundice, edema, hyperpigmentation, pallor, or duskiness. Examine nails for vertical or horizontal pitting, thickening, brittleness, or whitening. Observe for muscle weakness and ptosis. Palpate for lymphadenopathy, enlarged thyroid or salivary glands, and abdominal or chest masses. Take vital signs.

## Causes

*Arterial insufficiency.* Patchy alopecia occurs in this disorder, typically on the legs, feet, and toes, accompanied by atrophic skin and thickened nails.

*Fungal infections.* Tinea capitis (ringworm), the most common fungal infection, produces irregular balding areas, scaling, and erythematous lesions.

*Hodgkin's disease.* Permanent alopecia may occur if the lymphoma infiltrates the scalp, along with edema, pruritus, and hyperpigmentation.

*Hypothyroidism.* Facial, scalp, and genital hair thins and grows dull, coarse, and brittle. Loss of the outer third of the eyebrows is characteristic.

*Lupus erythematosus.* In both discoid and systemic lupus, hair tends to become brittle and may fall out in patches. Short, broken hairs commonly appear above the forehead.

*Protein deficiency.* Hair becomes brittle, fine, dry, and thin; occasionally, its pigment changes. Muscle wasting is characteristic.

*Seborrheic dermatitis.* Erupting in areas with many sebaceous glands and in skin folds, this disorder most commonly produces hair loss on the scalp. Alopecia begins at the vertex and frontal areas and may spread to other scalp areas.

*Secondary syphilis.* This infection produces temporary, patchy hair loss that gives the scalp and beard a "moth-eaten" appearance. It also produces loss of eyelashes and eyebrows.

*Other causes.* Alopecia areata; alopecia mucinosa; arsenic poisoning; burns; cutaneous T-cell lymphoma; dissecting cellulitis of the scalp; drugs, such as chemotherapeutic agents, oral contraceptives, colchicine, heparin, warfarin, vitamin A, trimethadione, indomethacin, methysergide, valproic acid, carbamazepine, gentamicin, allopurinol, lithium, beta-adrenergic blockers, and antithyroid agents; exfoliative dermatitis; folliculitis decalvans; hypopituitarism; lichen planus; myotonic dystrophy; progressive systemic sclerosis; radiotherapy; sarcoidosis; skin metastases; thallium poisoning; and thyrotoxicosis.

## Nursing considerations

• Encourage gentle hair care. Suggest a wig, cap, or scarf, if appropriate. Tell the patient to cover his head in cold weather to prevent heat loss.

# Vision loss

Vision loss—the inability to perceive visual stimuli—can be sudden or gradual and temporary or permanent. The deficit can range from a slight impairment of vision to total blindness.

## ▶ Emergency interventions
Inform the doctor immediately if sudden vision loss occurs. If the patient has *perforating* or *penetrating ocular trauma*, don't touch the eye. If you suspect *central artery occlusion*, perform light massage over his closed eyelid. Increase carbon dioxide blood levels, as ordered. If you suspect *acute closed-angle glaucoma*, help the doctor measure intraocular pressure (IOP) with a tonometer. Expect to administer timolol drops and I.V. acetazolamide.

## History
If vision loss is gradual, ask the patient if it affects one eye or both and all or only part of the visual field. Ask if he has experienced photosensitivity. Question him about the location, intensity, and duration of any eye pain. Obtain an ocular history and a family history of eye problems or systemic diseases that may lead to eye problems.

## Physical exam
Carefully inspect both eyes. Using a flashlight, examine the cornea and iris. Observe the size, shape, and color of the pupils, and evaluate the direct and consensual light reflex, accommodation, extraocular muscle function, and visual acuity.

## Causes
*Cataract.* Gradual blurring may precede vision loss. The pupil may turn milky white.

*Concussion.* Vision may be temporarily blurred, double, or lost. Other findings: headache and changes in level of consciousness and behavior.

*Glaucoma. Acute closed-angle glaucoma* may cause rapid blindness. Findings include rapid onset of unilateral inflammation and pain, nonreactive pupillary response, reduced acuity, photophobia, and halo vision. Usually bilateral, *chronic open-angle glaucoma* progresses slowly. It causes peripheral vision loss, aching eyes, halo vision, and reduced acuity.

*Ocular trauma.* Vision loss is sudden and may be unilateral or bilateral, total or partial, and permanent or temporary.

*Optic neuritis.* Unilateral vision loss is temporary but severe. The patient also develops pain around the eye.

*Retinal artery occlusion (central).* Unilateral vision loss occurs suddenly and may lead to permanent blindness. Direct pupillary response is sluggish, and consensual response is normal.

*Retinal detachment.* Painless vision loss may be gradual or sudden and total or partial.

*Retinal vein occlusion (central).* A unilateral decrease in visual acuity occurs with variable vision loss. IOP may be elevated.

*Senile macular degeneration.* Painless blurring or loss of central vision may occur. Visual acuity may worsen at night.

*Stevens-Johnson syndrome.* Marked vision loss may be accompanied by purulent conjunctivitis, eye pain, and difficulty opening the eyes.

*Temporal arteritis.* Findings include visual blurring or loss and unilateral headache.

*Vitreous hemorrhage.* Sudden unilateral vision loss may result from intraocular trauma, ocular tumors, or systemic disease.

*Other causes.* Amaurosis fugax; amblyopia; congenital rubella or syphilis; corneal dystrophies; diabetic retinopathy; drugs, such as chloroquine, phenylbutazone, digitalis, indomethacin, ethambutol, quinine sulfate, and methanol; endophthalmitis; herpes zoster; keratitis; Marfan's syndrome; optic nerve glioma; Paget's disease; pituitary tumor; retinitis pigmentosa; retinoblastoma; retrolental fibroplasia; trachoma; and uveitis.

## Nursing considerations
• Instruct the patient to wash his hands often, to avoid touching the unaffected eye with anything that has come in contact with the affected eye, and to avoid rubbing his eyes.

# Amenorrhea

The absence of menstrual flow, amenorrhea can be primary or secondary. In primary amenorrhea, menstruation fails to begin before the age of 18.

In secondary amenorrhea, it begins at an appropriate age but later ceases for 3 or more months in the absence of normal physiologic causes, such as pregnancy, lactation, or menopause.

Pathologic amenorrhea results from obstructed menstrual outflow or anovulation.

## History

Determine if the amenorrhea is primary or secondary. If it's primary, ask the patient at what age her mother first menstruated; age of menarche is fairly consistent in families. Assess the patient's physical, mental, and emotional development.

With secondary amenorrhea, determine the date, frequency, and duration of the patient's previous menstrual cycles. Ask about breast swelling or weight changes. Note long-term illnesses, use of oral contraceptives, exercise habits (especially running), stress, and eating habits.

## Physical exam

Study the patient's appearance. Does she have secondary sex characteristics? Signs of virilization? If you perform a pelvic examination, check for anatomic factors that could block flow.

## Causes

*Anorexia nervosa.* Amenorrhea may or may not occur. Findings include weight loss, compulsive behavior, blotchy or sallow complexion, constipation, reduced libido, dry skin, loss of scalp hair, skeletal muscle atrophy, and sleep disturbances.

*Corpus luteum cysts.* Amenorrhea commonly begins suddenly. Cysts also may produce acute abdominal pain and breast swelling.

*Hypothalamic tumor.* In addition to amenorrhea, a hypothalamic tumor can cause endocrine and visual field defects, gonadal underdevelopment or dysfunction, and short stature.

*Hypothyroidism.* Amenorrhea may occur. Early findings include fatigue, forgetfulness, cold intolerance, unexplained weight gain, and constipation. Later signs include bradycardia, decreased mental acuity, dry skin, hoarseness, periorbital edema, ptosis, dry hair, and brittle nails.

*Pituitary infarction.* Usually, postpartum lactation fails and menses don't resume. Other findings may include headaches, visual field defects, oculomotor palsies, altered level of consciousness.

*Pituitary tumor.* Amenorrhea may be the first sign of a pituitary tumor. Findings may include headache, visual disturbances, and acromegaly.

*Polycystic ovary syndrome.* Typically, menarche occurs at a normal age, followed by irregular menstrual cycles, oligomenorrhea, and secondary amenorrhea. Other findings may include obesity, hirsutism, a deepening voice, enlarged ovaries.

*Pseudoamenorrhea.* An anatomic anomaly obstructs menstrual flow, causing primary amenorrhea and possibly abdominal cramps.

*Thyrotoxicosis.* Thyroid hormone overproduction may result in amenorrhea. Findings include enlarged thyroid (goiter), nervousness, heat intolerance, sweating, tremors, palpitations, tachycardia, dyspnea, weakness, and weight loss.

*Other causes.* Adrenal tumor; adrenocortical hyperplasia; adrenocortical hypofunction; Asherman's syndrome; cervical stenosis; congenital absence of the ovaries or uterus; drugs, such as cyclophosphamide, busulfan, chlorambucil, phenothiazines, and oral contraceptives; Kallmann's syndrome; mosaicism; ovarian insensitivity to gonadotropins; pelvic inflammatory disease; pseudocyesis; radiation therapy; Sertoli-Leydig cell tumor; surgery; testicular feminization; Turner's syndrome; uterine hypoplasia; vaginal agenesis.

## Nursing considerations

• After diagnosis, answer the patient's questions about the type of treatment that will be provided and its expected outcome.

• Provide emotional support. Encourage the patient to discuss her fears. Refer her for psychological counseling, if necessary.

**A**

Violent behavior refers to the use of physical force to violate, injure, or abuse an object or person. Marked by sudden loss of self-control, violent behavior may also be self-directed. It may result from organic and psychiatric disorders or the effects of drugs.

## History

Determine if the patient has a history of violent behavior. Is he intoxicated or suffering symptoms of alcohol or drug withdrawal? Does he have a history of family violence, including corporal punishment and child or spouse abuse?

Watch for clues indicating that the patient is losing control and possibly becoming violent. Has he exhibited abrupt behavioral changes? Is he unable to sit still? Increased activity may indicate an attempt to discharge aggression. Does he suddenly cease activity (suggesting the calm before the storm)? Does he make verbal threats or angry gestures? Is he jumpy, extremely tense, or laughing? Increasing emotional intensity may herald loss of control.

## Physical exam

If your patient's violent behavior is a new development, suspect an organic disorder. Obtain a medical history. Watch for a sudden change in his level of consciousness. Disorientation, failure to recall recent events, or a display of tics, jerks, tremors, or asterixis all suggest an organic disorder.

## Causes

*Organic disorders.* Violent behavior may result from metabolic and neurologic dysfunction. Common causes include epilepsy, brain tumor, encephalitis, head injury, endocrine disorders, metabolic disorders (such as uremia and calcium imbalance), and severe physical trauma.

*Psychiatric disorders.* Violent behavior occurs as a protective mechanism in response to a perceived threat in psychotic disorders such as schizophrenia. A similar response may occur in personality disorders, such as antisocial or borderline personality.

*Other causes.* Alcohol abuse or withdrawal; barbiturate withdrawal; and drugs, such as amphetamines, hallucinogens, lidocaine, and procaine penicillin.

## Nursing considerations

• Violent behavior is most prevalent in certain hospital areas, including emergency rooms, critical care units, and crisis and acute psychiatric units. Natural disasters and accidents increase the potential for violent behavior.

• If your patient becomes violent or potentially violent, remain composed and make efforts to control the situation. First, protect yourself. Remain at a distance from the patient, call for assistance, and don't overreact. Make sure you have enough personnel for a show of force or, if necessary, for subduing him. Encourage the patient to move to a quiet location. Reassure him, explain what's happening, and tell him that he's safe. If he makes violent threats, take them seriously, and inform those at whom the threats are directed.

• If ordered, administer drugs to combat the patient's psychotic symptoms.

• Your own attitudes can affect your ability to care for a violent patient. If you feel fearful or judgmental, ask another staff member for help.

# Amnesia

A disturbance in or loss of memory, amnesia may be partial or complete, anterograde or retrograde. Anterograde amnesia is memory loss for events *after* onset of a trauma or disease; retrograde amnesia is memory loss for events *before* onset. Depending on the cause, amnesia may arise suddenly or slowly and may be temporary or permanent. It is common in patients with seizures, head trauma, and Alzheimer's disease.

## History

Because the patient may not be aware of his amnesia, gather information from his family or friends. Note the patient's appearance, behavior, mood, and train of thought. Ask when the amnesia first appeared and what types of things the patient can't remember. Does the amnesia encompass a recent or a remote time period?

Test the patient's recent memory with such questions as "How did you get here?" "What was the day before yesterday?" Test his intermediate memory by asking "Who was the president before this one?" Test remote memory by asking "How old are you?" "Where were you born?"

## Physical exam

Take the patient's vital signs. Assess his level of consciousness (LOC). Check his pupils: They should be equal in size and should constrict quickly when exposed to direct light. Test motor function by having the patient move his arms and legs through their range of motion. Evaluate sensory function with pinpricks on his skin.

## Causes

*Alzheimer's disease.* Amnesia progresses over months or years, producing severe and permanent memory loss. Other findings include agitation, inability to concentrate, poor personal hygiene, confusion, irritability, and emotional lability; later, aphasia, dementia, incontinence, muscle rigidity.

*Head trauma.* Depending on the trauma's severity, amnesia may last minutes, hours, or longer, and can cause permanent memory loss. Other findings may include altered respirations and LOC; headache; dizziness; confusion; blurred or double vision; motor and sensory disturbances.

*Hysteria.* Hysterical amnesia, a complete and long-lasting memory loss, begins and ends abruptly. It's typically accompanied by confusion.

*Seizure.* In temporal lobe seizures, amnesia occurs suddenly and can last seconds or minutes. The patient may recall an aura or nothing at all. An irritable focus on the brain's left side primarily causes verbal amnesia; on the right side, graphic and verbal amnesia. Other signs include decreased LOC during the seizure, confusion, motor and sensory disturbances, and blurred vision.

*Vertebrobasilar circulatory disorders.* Ischemia, infarction, embolus, or hemorrhage typically causes complete amnesia that begins abruptly, lasts several hours, and ends abruptly. Other findings include dizziness, decreased LOC, ataxia, blurred or double vision, vertigo, nausea, vomiting.

*Wernicke-Korsakoff syndrome.* Amnesia can become permanent without treatment. Findings include apathy, inability to concentrate or put events into sequence, confabulation to fill memory gaps.

*Other causes.* Cerebral hypoxia; drugs, such as general anesthetics, barbiturates, and some benzodiazepines; electroconvulsive therapy; herpes simplex encephalitis; temporal lobe surgery.

## Nursing considerations

- As ordered, prepare the patient for diagnostic tests, such as computed tomography scan, electroencephalography, or cerebral angiography.
- Provide reality orientation for the patient with retrograde amnesia. Encourage his family members to supply familiar photos, objects, or music.
- Adjust patient teaching, depending on the type of amnesia. Include his family in teaching sessions. Write down all instructions, including medication dosages and schedules.
- For the patient with severe amnesia, consider safety, elimination, and nutrition. If necessary, arrange for placement in an extended-care facility.

**A**

# Vesicular rash

A vesicular rash is a scattered or linear distribution of vesicles—sharply circumscribed lesions that are usually less than 0.5 cm in diameter and filled with clear, cloudy, or bloody fluid. Lesions larger than 0.5 cm in diameter are called bullae. A vesicular rash may be mild or severe and temporary or permanent.

## History
Ask when the patient's rash began, how it spread, and if it has appeared before. Did other skin lesions precede the vesicles? Obtain a drug history, including recent use of any topical medications. Also ask about associated signs and symptoms, allergies, recent infections, and insect bites. Ask if the patient has a family history of skin disorders.

## Physical exam
Examine the patient's skin and note the location, general distribution, color, shape, and size of the lesions. Check for crusts, scales, scars, macules, papules, or wheals. Palpate the vesicles or bullae to determine if they're flaccid or tense. Assess whether the outer layer of epidermis separates easily from the basal layer.

## Causes
*Burns.* Vesicles and bullae may appear with erythema, swelling, pain, and moistness.

*Dermatitis.* In *contact dermatitis*, small vesicles may erupt surrounded by redness and marked edema. Vesicles may ooze, scale, and cause severe pruritus. *Dermatitis herpetiformis* produces a chronic inflammatory eruption marked by vesicular, papular, bullous, pustular, or erythematous lesions. In *nummular dermatitis*, groups of pinpoint vesicles and papules appear on erythematous or pustular lesions that are nummular or annular.

*Dermatophytid.* Vesicular lesions appear on the hands. Extremely pruritic and tender, lesions may be accompanied by fever, anorexia, generalized adenopathy, and splenomegaly.

*Erythema multiforme.* Erythematous macules, papules and, occasionally, vesicles and bullae, erupt suddenly. A rash may occur symmetrically over the hands, arms, feet, legs, face, and neck. Vesiculobullous lesions commonly appear on the lips and buccal mucosa, then rupture and ulcerate, producing a thick, yellow or white exudate.

*Herpes simplex.* Vesicles have an erythematous base and may appear on the lips or genitalia singly or in groups. Vesicles are preceded by itching, tingling, burning, or pain; are 2 to 3 mm in diameter; and do not coalesce. Upon rupturing, they form a painful ulcer followed by a yellowish crust.

*Herpes zoster.* Fever and malaise precede a vesicular rash along a dermatome, deep pain, pruritus, and paresthesia or hyperesthesia, usually on the trunk and sometimes on the arms and legs.

*Insect bites.* Vesicles appear on red hivelike papules and may become hemorrhagic.

*Pompholyx.* Vesicular lesions are symmetrical and may become pustular. Pruritic lesions may appear on the palms or soles.

*Porphyria cutanea tarda.* Bullae usually affect areas exposed to sun, friction, trauma, or heat. Papulovesicular lesions may evolve into erosions or ulcers and scars. Chronic skin changes include hyperpigmentation or hypopigmentation, hypertrichosis, and sclerodermoid lesions.

*Scabies.* Small vesicles erupt on an erythematous base, possibly at the end of a curved, threadlike burrow 1 to 10 cm long. A swollen nodule or red papule holds the itch mite. Pustules and excoriations may occur. Lesions may form on the elbows, wrists, axillae, and waistline; the glans, shaft, and scrotum (men); or the nipples (women).

*Tinea pedis.* Vesicles and scaling occur between the toes and over the entire sole. Severe infection causes inflammation and pruritus.

*Other causes.* Pemphigus, toxic epidermal necrolysis.

## Nursing considerations
• If necessary, start an I.V. infusion to compensate for fluid and electrolyte losses that may occur during a large skin eruption.

The absence of sensitivity to pain, analgesia is a sign of central nervous system disease, commonly indicating the type and location of a spinal cord lesion. It occurs with loss of temperature sensation and possibly other sensory deficits, such as paresthesia, loss of proprioception and vibratory sense, and tactile anesthesia in disorders involving the peripheral nerves, spinal cord, and brain. When associated only with thermanesthesia, analgesia suggests an incomplete spinal cord lesion.

▶ **Emergency interventions**

If the patient complains of analgesia over a large body area, accompanied by paralysis, suspect spinal cord injury. Have another nurse notify the doctor immediately. Immobilize the patient's spine in proper alignment, using a cervical collar and a long backboard. If a collar or backboard isn't available, position the patient supine on a flat surface, placing sandbags around his head, neck, and torso. Use caution when moving him. Continuously monitor respiratory rate and rhythm, and observe for accessory muscle use; a complete lesion above T6 may cause muscle paralysis. Have an artificial airway and a manual resuscitation bag ready; be prepared to initiate emergency resuscitation.

**History**

Focus on the onset of analgesia and any recent trauma—a fall, sports injury, or automobile accident. Note any incidence of cancer in the patient or his family.

**Physical exam**

Once the patient's spine and respiratory status are stabilized, take his vital signs and assess his level of consciousness. Test pupillary, corneal, cough, and gag reflexes to rule out brain stem and cranial nerve involvement. If the patient is conscious, assess his speech and ability to swallow.

Observe his gait and posture, and assess his balance and coordination. Evaluate muscle tone and strength. Test for other sensory deficits over all dermatomes by applying light tactile stimulation with a tongue blade or cotton swab. If necessary, use a pin to check for pain sensitivity. Test temperature sensation over all dermatomes, using two test tubes—one filled with hot water, the other with cold water. In each arm and leg, test vibration sense (using a tuning fork), proprioception, and superficial and deep tendon reflexes. If the patient is paralyzed, palpate his muscles to determine whether paralysis is spastic or flaccid.

**Causes**

*Anterior cord syndrome.* Bilateral analgesia and thermanesthesia occur below the lesion, with flaccid paralysis and hypoactive deep tendon reflexes.

*Central cord syndrome.* Typically, analgesia and thermanesthesia occur bilaterally, extending over the arms, back, and shoulders. Early weakness in the hands progresses to weakness and muscle spasms in the arms and shoulder girdle.

With brain stem involvement, findings may include facial analgesia and thermanesthesia, vertigo, nystagmus, atrophy of the tongue, and dysarthria. The patient may also have dysphagia, urine retention, anhidrosis, decreased intestinal motility, and hyperkeratosis.

*Spinal cord hemisection.* Contralateral analgesia and thermanesthesia occur below the level of the lesion. Loss of proprioception, spastic paralysis, and hyperactive deep tendon reflexes develop ipsilaterally. The patient may experience urine retention with overflow incontinence.

*Other causes.* Local and topical anesthetics.

**Nursing considerations**

• Prepare the patient for spinal X-rays, and maintain spinal alignment and stability during transport to the laboratory.

• Provide meticulous skin care, massage, use of lamb's wool pads, and frequent repositioning.

• Guard against scalding by testing the patient's bathwater temperature before he bathes; advise him to test it at home using a thermometer or a body part with intact sensation.

**A**

Vertigo is an illusion of movement in which the patient feels that he's revolving in space (subjective vertigo) or that his surroundings are revolving around him (objective vertigo). He may complain of feeling pulled sideways, as if drawn by a magnet.

Vertigo usually begins abruptly and may be temporary or permanent, mild or severe. It worsens when the patient moves and commonly subsides when he lies down. In many cases, it's confused with dizziness — a sensation of imbalance and light-headedness that does not include a whirling sensation. However, unlike dizziness, vertigo is often accompanied by nausea, vomiting, nystagmus, and tinnitus or hearing loss. Although limb coordination is unaffected, vertiginous gait may occur.

## History

Ask the patient to describe the onset and duration of vertigo. Do he or his surroundings seem to be moving? How often do the attacks occur? Do they follow position changes, or are they unpredictable? During an attack, can the patient walk, does he lean to one side, or has he ever fallen? Ask if he experiences motion sickness and if he prefers one position during an attack. Obtain a recent drug history and note any evidence of alcohol abuse.

## Physical exam

Perform a neurologic assessment, focusing particularly on cranial nerve VIII function. Observe the patient's gait and posture for abnormalities.

## Causes

*Acoustic neuroma.* A mild, intermittent vertigo may occur after onset of unilateral sensorineural hearing loss. Other findings: tinnitus, postauricular or suboccipital pain and, possibly, facial paralysis.

*Brain stem ischemia.* This condition produces sudden, severe vertigo that becomes episodic and later persistent. Associated findings include ataxia, nausea, vomiting, increased blood pressure, tachycardia, nystagmus, and lateral deviation of the eyes toward the side of the lesion.

*Head trauma.* Persistent vertigo, occurring soon after the injury, accompanies spontaneous or positional nystagmus and, possibly, hearing loss. Associated findings include headache, nausea, vomiting, and decreased level of consciousness.

*Herpes zoster auricularis.* Sudden onset of vertigo may be accompanied by facial paralysis, hearing loss in the affected ear, and herpetic vesicular lesions in the auditory canal.

*Labyrinthitis.* Severe vertigo begins abruptly and may or may not recur. Other findings include nausea, vomiting, progressive sensorineural hearing loss, and nystagmus.

*Ménière's disease.* Vertigo begins abruptly and may last minutes, hours, or days. Unpredictable episodes of severe vertigo and unsteady gait may cause the patient to fall.

*Multiple sclerosis.* Episodic vertigo may occur early and become persistent. Other early findings include diplopia, visual blurring, and paresthesia.

*Posterior fossa tumor.* Positional vertigo lasts for a few seconds. The patient may have papilledema, headache, memory loss, nausea, vomiting, nystagmus, apneustic or ataxic respirations, and increased blood pressure.

*Vestibular neuritis.* Severe vertigo usually begins abruptly and lasts several days, without tinnitus or hearing loss. Other findings include nausea, vomiting, and nystagmus.

*Other causes.* Alcohol intoxication; caloric testing; middle ear surgery; toxic levels of certain drugs, such as salicylates, aminoglycosides, antibiotics, quinine, and oral contraceptives; and use of overly warm or cold eardrops or irrigating solutions.

## Nursing considerations

• Place the patient with vertigo in a comfortable position. Keep the side rails up if he's in bed, or help him to a chair if he's standing. Monitor his vital signs and level of consciousness. Darken the room and keep him calm. If ordered, administer drugs to control nausea and vomiting and to decrease labyrinthine irritability.

**V**

An abnormal deficiency of sweat in response to heat, anhidrosis can be generalized (complete) or localized (partial). Generalized anhidrosis can lead to life-threatening impairment of thermoregulation. Localized anhidrosis rarely interferes with thermoregulation. Anhidrosis results from neurologic and skin disorders and from congenital, atrophic, or traumatic changes to sweat glands.

## ▶ Emergency interventions

If you detect anhidrosis in a patient with hot, flushed skin, ask him if he's also experiencing nausea, dizziness, palpitations, and substernal tightness. If so, quickly take rectal temperature and other vital signs, and assess his level of consciousness (LOC). If rectal temperature above 102.2° F (39° C) occurs with tachycardia, tachypnea, altered blood pressure, and decreased LOC, suspect life-threatening anhidrotic asthenia (heatstroke). Have another nurse notify the doctor immediately, while you start rapid cooling measures, immersing the patient in ice or very cold water and giving I.V. fluid replacements. Frequently check vital signs and neurologic status until the patient's temperature drops below 102° F. Then place him in an air-conditioned room.

## History

If anhidrosis is localized or the patient reports local hyperhidrosis or fever, take a brief history. Ask him to characterize his sweating during heat spells or strenuous activity. Is it slight or profuse? Ask about exposure to heat, onset of anhidrosis or hyperhidrosis, neurologic and skin disorders, systemic diseases, and drug use.

## Physical exam

Inspect skin color, texture, and turgor. If you detect skin lesions, document their location, size, color, texture, and pattern.

## Causes

*Anhidrotic asthenia.* This life-threatening disorder causes acute, generalized anhidrosis. In early stages, patient's rectal temperature may exceed 102.2° F. Other findings include severe headache and muscle cramps, fatigue, nausea and vomiting, dizziness, palpitations, substernal tightness, and elevated blood pressure followed by hypotension.

*Cerebral lesions.* Cerebral cortex and brain stem lesions may cause anhidrotic palms and soles, along with various motor and sensory disturbances specific to the site of the lesions.

*Horner's syndrome.* A supraclavicular spinal cord lesion produces facial anhidrosis with hyperhidrosis. Other findings include ipsilateral pupillary constriction and ptosis.

*Miliaria profunda.* A severe condition can progress to anhidrotic asthenia. Typically, however, it produces localized anhidrosis with compensatory facial hyperhidrosis.

*Miliaria rubra (prickly heat).* A severe condition can progress to anhidrotic asthenia. Typically, though, it produces localized anhidrosis. Small, erythematous papules appear on the trunk and neck.

*Peripheral neuritis.* Anhidrosis over the legs commonly appears with compensatory hyperhidrosis over the head and neck. Other findings include glossy red skin; paresthesia, hyperesthesia, or anesthesia in the hands and feet; diminished or absent deep tendon reflexes; flaccid paralysis and muscle wasting; footdrop; and burning pain.

*Spinal cord lesions.* Anhidrosis may occur symmetrically below the lesion, with hyperhidrosis in adjacent areas. Other findings may include loss of motor and sensory function below the lesion and impaired cardiovascular and respiratory function.

*Other causes.* Anticholinergics, burns, miliaria crystallina, and Shy-Drager syndrome.

## Nursing considerations

● Advise the patient to remain in cool environments, to move slowly in warm weather, and to avoid strenuous exercise and hot foods.
● Warn him if any drugs he's receiving have anhidrotic effects.

A

# Venous hum

A venous hum is a functional or innocent murmur heard above the clavicles throughout the cardiac cycle. Loudest during diastole, it's low-pitched, rough, or noisy. The hum commonly accompanies a thrill or, possibly, a high-pitched whine. It's best heard by applying the bell of the stethoscope to the medial aspect of the right supraclavicular area, with the patient seated upright.

A venous hum is a common and normal finding in children and pregnant women. However, it also occurs in hyperdynamic states, such as anemia and thyrotoxicosis. The hum results from increased blood flow through the internal jugular veins, especially on the right side, which causes audible vibrations in the tissues.

Occasionally, this sign may be mistaken for an intracardiac murmur or a thyroid bruit. However, a venous hum disappears with jugular vein compression and waxes and wanes with head turning. In contrast, an intracardiac murmur and a thyroid bruit persist despite jugular compression and head turning.

## History
Determine if the patient has a history of anemia or thyroid disorders. If he does, ask what medication or other treatments he has received. If he doesn't have a history of these disorders, ask if he has experienced any associated symptoms, such as palpitations, dyspnea, nervousness, tremors, heat intolerance, weight loss, fatigue, weakness, or malaise.

## Physical exam
Take the patient's vital signs, noting especially tachycardia, hypertension, a bounding pulse, and widened pulse pressure. Auscultate the patient's heart for gallops or murmurs. Examine his skin and mucous membranes for pallor.

## Causes
*Anemia.* A venous hum is common with severe anemia (hemoglobin level below 7 g/dl). Other findings may include pale skin and mucous membranes, dyspnea, crackles, tachycardia, bounding pulse, atrial gallop, systolic bruits over both carotid arteries, bleeding tendencies, weakness, fatigue, and malaise.

*Thyrotoxicosis.* This disorder may cause a loud venous hum, audible whether the patient is sitting or supine. Auscultation may also reveal an atrial or ventricular gallop. Other findings commonly include tachycardia, palpitations, weight loss despite increased appetite, an enlarged thyroid, dyspnea, nervousness, tremors, diaphoresis, and heat intolerance. Exophthalmos may be present.

## Nursing considerations
• Prepare the patient for ordered diagnostic tests, which may include an electrocardiogram, a complete blood count, and thyroid hormone ($T_3$ and $T_4$) assays.

# Anorexia

A lack of appetite despite the need for food, anorexia is a common symptom of GI and endocrine disorders. It's characteristic of certain psychological disturbances and can result from anxiety, chronic pain, poor oral hygiene, increased blood temperature, and alterations in taste or smell. Short-term anorexia rarely jeopardizes the patient's health. Chronic anorexia, however, can lead to life-threatening malnutrition.

## History

Ask the patient about changes in his weight. Explore his dietary habits, what types of food he likes and dislikes and why. Ask about dental problems, difficulty swallowing, vomiting and diarrhea after meals, physical exercise, stomach or bowel disorders, drug and alcohol use. If there is no organic basis for anorexia, consider psychological factors.

## Physical exam

Take the patient's vital signs and weight. Check for signs of malnutrition. If the patient has any of these signs, consistently refuses food, and has lost 7% to 10% of his body weight within the last month, notify the doctor.

## Causes

*Alcoholism.* Chronic anorexia leading to malnutrition commonly accompanies this disorder. Other findings include signs of liver damage, paresthesia, tremors, increased blood pressure, bruising, GI bleeding, and abdominal pain.

*Anorexia nervosa.* Chronic anorexia begins insidiously and leads to life-threatening malnutrition. Findings include skeletal muscle atrophy, loss of fatty tissue, constipation, amenorrhea, blotchy or sallow skin, alopecia, and sleep disturbances.

*Appendicitis.* Anorexia closely follows the abrupt onset of epigastric pain, nausea, and vomiting. Other findings: abdominal rigidity, rebound tenderness, constipation, fever, tachycardia.

*Chronic renal failure.* Chronic anorexia is common and insidious. It's accompanied by nausea, vomiting, mouth ulcers, ammonia breath odor, GI bleeding, constipation or diarrhea, drowsiness, confusion, tremors, pallor, dry skin, pruritus, alopecia, purpuric lesions, and edema.

*Cirrhosis.* Anorexia occurs early. May be accompanied by weakness, nausea, vomiting, constipation or diarrhea, and dull abdominal pain.

*Crohn's disease.* Chronic anorexia causes marked weight loss and possibly diarrhea, abdominal pain, fever, abdominal mass, and weakness.

*Hepatitis.* In both viral and nonviral hepatitis, findings include fatigue, malaise, headache, arthralgia, myalgia, photophobia, cough, sore throat, rhinitis, nausea and vomiting, mild fever, hepatomegaly, and lymphadenopathy.

*Hypopituitarism.* Anorexia usually develops slowly. Findings include amenorrhea; decreased libido; lethargy; cold intolerance; dry skin; brittle hair; and decreased temperature, blood pressure, and pulse rate.

*Hypothyroidism.* Anorexia is common. Early findings include fatigue, forgetfulness, cold intolerance, unexplained weight gain, constipation.

*Ketoacidosis.* Anorexia usually arises gradually. It's accompanied by dry, flushed skin; fruity breath odor; polydipsia; hypotension; weak, rapid pulse; dry mouth; abdominal pain; and vomiting.

*Other causes.* Adrenocortical hypofunction; cancer; depressive syndrome; drugs, such as amphetamines, chemotherapeutic agents, and sympathomimetics; gastritis; pernicious anemia; radiation therapy; and total parenteral nutrition.

## Nursing considerations

• Provide high-calorie snacks or frequent, small meals. Encourage the patient's family to supply his favorite foods to help stimulate his appetite. Take a 24-hour diet history daily.
• If the patient exaggerates his food intake, ask the dietitian to maintain strict calorie and nutrient counts for the patient's meals. In severe malnutrition, provide supplemental nutritional support.
• Monitor the patient's vital signs and white blood cell count, and closely observe any wounds.

Common in women of childbearing age, vaginal discharge is mucoid, clear or white, nonbloody, and odorless. This discharge may occur normally. However, a marked increase in discharge or a change in discharge color, odor, or consistency may signal disease.

## History

Ask the patient to describe the onset, color, consistency, odor, and texture of her vaginal discharge. How does the discharge differ from her usual vaginal secretions? Is the onset related to her menstrual cycle? Also ask about associated genitourinary symptoms. Does she have spotting after coitus or douching? Ask about recent changes in her sexual habits and hygiene practices. Is she or could she be pregnant? Has she ever been treated for a vaginal infection? Ask about her current use of medications, especially antibiotics, oral estrogen, and contraceptives.

## Physical exam

Examine the external genitalia and note the character of the discharge. Observe vulvar and vaginal tissues for redness, edema, and excoriation. Palpate the inguinal lymph nodes to detect tenderness or enlargement, and palpate the abdomen for tenderness. As ordered, assist with a pelvic examination and obtain discharge specimens for testing.

## Causes

*Atrophic vaginitis.* A thin, scant, white vaginal discharge may be accompanied by pruritus, burning, tenderness, and bloody spotting after coitus or douching.

*Candidiasis.* A profuse, white, curdlike discharge with a yeasty, sweet odor may appear abruptly, commonly just before menses. Lightly attached to the labia and vaginal walls, exudate may be accompanied by vulvar redness and edema. A fine, red dermatitis may cover the inner thighs.

**Chlamydia** *infection.* A yellow, mucopurulent, odorless or acrid vaginal discharge may be accompanied by dysuria and dyspareunia.

*Endometritis.* A scant, serosanguineous discharge with a foul odor may occur. Other findings may include fever and back and abdominal pain.

**Gardnerella** *vaginitis.* This infection causes a thin, foul-smelling, green or grayish white discharge that adheres to the vaginal walls. Signs of vaginal irritation may also occur.

*Gonorrhea.* A yellow or green, foul-smelling discharge may be expressed from Bartholin's or Skene's ducts. Other findings include dysuria, urinary frequency and incontinence, and vaginal redness and swelling.

*Gynecologic cancer.* A chronic, watery, bloody or purulent, possibly foul-smelling discharge may be accompanied by abnormal vaginal bleeding and, later, weight loss and pelvic, back, and leg pain.

*Herpes simplex (genital).* A copious, mucoid discharge may occur, along with painful, indurated vesicles and ulcerations on the labia, vagina, cervix, anus, thighs, or mouth.

*Trichomoniasis.* This infection may cause a foul-smelling discharge that may be frothy, greenish yellow, and profuse, or thin, white, and scant. Other findings may include pruritus and a red, inflamed vagina with tiny petechiae.

*Other causes.* Antibiotics; chancroid; contraceptive creams and jellies; estrogen-containing drugs, including oral contraceptives; frequent douching; genital warts; irritants, such as feminine hygiene products, bubble baths, and colored or perfumed toilet papers; prolonged presence of a foreign body, such as a tampon or diaphragm, in the vagina; and radiation therapy.

## Nursing considerations

• Teach the patient to keep her perineum clean and dry. Also tell her to wear cotton-crotched underwear and pantyhose and to avoid wearing tight-fitting clothing and nylon underwear.
• Tell the patient with a vaginal infection to continue taking her prescribed medication. She should avoid intercourse until symptoms clear and should make sure her partner uses condoms until she completes her course of medication.

# Anosmia

The absence of the sense of smell, anosmia usually results from nasal congestion or obstruction, but it occasionally heralds a serious neural defect. Temporary anosmia can result from irritation, swelling, or obstruction of the nasal mucosa caused by heavy smoking, rhinitis, or sinusitis. Permanent anosmia usually indicates a lesion in the olfactory nerve pathway. Anosmia can also result from the use of cocaine or inhalation of acid fumes and may be reported by patients suffering from hysteria, depression, or schizophrenia.

## History

Ask about the onset and duration of anosmia and related symptoms — stuffy nose, nasal discharge or bleeding, postnasal drip, sneezing, dry or sore mouth and throat, loss of taste or appetite, tearing, facial or eye pain. Ask about nasal disease, allergies, head trauma, smoking, and the use of nose drops or sprays. Rule out cocaine use.

## Physical exam

Inspect and palpate nasal structures for obvious injury, inflammation, deformities, and septal deviation or perforation. Observe the nasal mucosa, and the size and color of the turbinates. Check for polyps. Note any nasal discharge. Palpate the sinus areas for tenderness and contour.

Assess for nasal obstruction by occluding one nostril at a time with your thumb as the patient breathes; listen for breath sounds and for sounds of moisture or mucus. Test olfactory nerve function by having the patient identify common odors.

## Causes

*Anterior cerebral artery occlusion.* Permanent anosmia may follow vascular damage involving the olfactory nerve. Other findings include contralateral weakness and numbness, confusion, and impaired motor and sensory functions.

*Head trauma.* Permanent anosmia may follow damage to the olfactory nerve. Other findings may include epistaxis, headache, nausea and vomiting, altered level of consciousness, blurred or double vision, raccoon's eyes, Battle's sign, and otorrhea.

*Lead poisoning.* Anosmia may be permanent or temporary, depending on the damage to the nasal mucosa. Other findings include abdominal pain, weakness, headache, nausea, vomiting, constipation, wristdrop or footdrop, lead line on the gums, metallic taste, seizures, and delirium.

*Lethal midline granuloma.* Permanent anosmia accompanies this slowly progressive disease. Examination reveals ulcerative granulation tissue in the nose, sinuses, and palate; often widespread crust formation and tissue necrosis; septal cartilage destruction; and possible purulent rhinorrhea, serous otitis media, and inflammation of the eyelids and lacrimal apparatus.

*Nasal or sinus neoplasms.* Anosmia may be permanent if the neoplasm destroys or displaces the olfactory nerve. Associated signs and symptoms may include unilateral or bilateral epistaxis, swelling and tenderness in the affected area, exophthalmos, diplopia, and decreased tearing.

*Pernicious anemia.* Anosmia is accompanied by weakness; sore, pale tongue; and numbness and tingling in the extremities.

*Other causes.* Diabetes mellitus; drugs, such as decongestants, reserpine, amphetamines, phenothiazines, and estrogen; polyps; radiation therapy; rhinitis; septal fracture; septal hematoma; sinusitis; and surgery.

## Nursing considerations

• If anosmia results from nasal congestion, administer local decongestants or antihistamines. Provide a vaporizer or humidifier to moisturize mucosa and encourage nasal discharge. Advise against excessive use of local decongestants, which can cause rebound nasal congestion.

• If anosmia doesn't result from nasal congestion, prepare the patient for ordered diagnostic tests, such as sinus transillumination, skull X-ray, or computed tomography scan.

# Vaginal bleeding, postmenopausal

Postmenopausal vaginal bleeding—bleeding that occurs 6 or more months after menopause— is an important indicator of gynecologic cancer. It may also result from infection, local pelvic disorders, estrogenic stimulation, and physiologic thinning and drying of the vaginal mucous membranes. Usually the patient develops brown or red spotting either spontaneously or after coitus or douching, but she may report an oozing of fresh blood or a bright red hemorrhage. Many women, especially those with a history of heavy menstrual flow, minimize the importance of this sign, seriously delaying diagnosis.

## History

Determine the patient's current age and her age at menopause. Ask when she first noticed the abnormal bleeding. Obtain a thorough obstetric and gynecologic history. When did she begin menstruating? Were her periods regular? If not, ask her to describe any menstrual irregularities. How old was she when she first had intercourse? How many sexual partners has she had? Has she had any children? Has she had fertility problems? If possible, obtain an obstetric and gynecologic history of the patient's mother, and ask about a family history of gynecologic cancer. Determine if the patient has any associated symptoms and if she's currently taking estrogen.

## Physical exam

Observe the external genitalia, noting the character of any vaginal discharge and the appearance of the labia, vaginal rugae, and clitoris. Carefully palpate the patient's breasts and lymph nodes for nodules or enlargement. As ordered, assist the doctor with pelvic and rectal examinations.

## Causes

*Atrophic vaginitis.* When bloody staining occurs, it usually follows coitus or douching. A white vaginal discharge may appear, accompanied by pruritus, dyspareunia, and a burning sensation in the vagina and labia. Other findings include sparse pubic hair, a pale vagina with decreased rugae and small hemorrhagic spots, clitoral atrophy, and shrinking of the labia minora.

*Cervical cancer.* The patient may develop vaginal spotting or heavier bleeding. Bleeding usually occurs after coitus or douching but may be spontaneous. Related findings include persistent vaginal discharge and postcoital pain. As cancer spreads, back and sciatic pain, leg swelling, anorexia, weight loss, and weakness may occur.

*Cervical or endometrial polyps.* Spotting (possibly as a mucopurulent pink discharge) may appear after coitus, douching, or straining at stool. Endometrial polyps may produce no symptoms.

*Endometrial cancer.* An early sign, bleeding may be brownish and scant or bright red and profuse. It commonly follows coitus or douching. Later on, bleeding becomes more severe and may be accompanied by pelvic, rectal, low back, and leg pain.

*Ovarian tumors (feminizing).* The patient may develop heavy bleeding unrelated to coitus or douching. Other findings include a palpable pelvic mass, increased cervical mucus, breast enlargement, and spider angiomas.

*Vaginal cancer.* A thin, watery vaginal discharge may precede spotting or bleeding. Bleeding may be spontaneous but usually follows coitus or douching. A firm, ulcerated vaginal lesion may be present. Dyspareunia, urinary frequency, bladder and pelvic pain, rectal bleeding, and vulvar lesions may develop later.

*Other causes.* Excessive or prolonged estrogen administration.

## Nursing considerations

• Prepare the patient for diagnostic tests, such as ultrasonography to outline a cervical or uterine tumor; endometrial biopsy and dilatation and fractional curettage to obtain tissue for histologic examination; testing for occult blood in the stool; and vaginal and cervical cultures.
• Discontinue estrogen administration, as ordered, until the condition is diagnosed.

V

Urine output of less than 75 ml daily, anuria indicates urinary tract obstruction or acute renal failure. Anuria rarely occurs and rarely goes undetected. But without immediate treatment, it can rapidly cause uremia and other complications.

## ▶ Emergency interventions

First, determine if urine is forming. If so, notify the doctor and prepare to catheterize the patient. An obstruction may hinder catheter insertion; urine return may be cloudy and foul-smelling. If you collect more than 75 ml of urine, suspect lower urinary tract obstruction; less than 75 ml, renal dysfunction or obstruction higher in the urinary tract.

## History

Ask about changes in the usual voiding pattern. Determine the amount of fluid normally ingested each day, the amount ingested in the last 24 to 48 hours, and the time and amount of his last urination. Review his history, noting kidney disease, urinary tract obstruction or infection, prostate enlargement, renal calculi, neurogenic bladder, or congenital abnormalities. Ask about abdominal, renal, or urinary tract surgery, and drug use.

## Physical exam

Take the patient's vital signs. Palpate the abdomen for asymmetry, distention, or bulging. Inspect the flank area for edema or erythema. Percuss and palpate the bladder. Palpate the kidneys anteriorly and posteriorly, and percuss them at the costovertebral angle. Auscultate over the renal arteries, listening for bruits.

## Causes

*Acute tubular necrosis.* Oliguria or anuria of longer than 2 weeks' duration is a common finding in this disorder. It precedes the onset of diuresis, which is accompanied by polyuria. Other findings may include signs of hyperkalemia, uremia, and congestive heart failure.

*Cortical necrosis (bilateral).* This disorder is marked by a sudden change from oliguria to anuria, with gross hematuria, flank pain, and fever.

*Glomerulonephritis (acute).* Anuria or oliguria occur. Other findings include mild fever, malaise, flank pain, hematuria, edema, elevated blood pressure, headache, nausea, vomiting, abdominal pain, and signs of pulmonary congestion.

*Papillary necrosis (acute).* Bilateral papillary necrosis produces anuria or oliguria, flank pain, costovertebral angle tenderness, renal colic, abdominal pain and rigidity, fever, vomiting, decreased bowel sounds, hematuria, and pyuria.

*Renal artery occlusion (bilateral).* This disorder produces anuria or severe oliguria, often accompanied by severe, continuous upper abdominal and flank pain; nausea and vomiting; decreased bowel sounds; and fever up to 102° F (38.9° C).

*Urinary tract obstruction.* Severe obstruction can produce acute and sometimes total anuria, alternating with or preceded by burning and pain on urination, overflow incontinence or dribbling, increased urinary frequency and nocturia, voiding of small amounts, or altered urine stream.

*Other causes.* Antibiotics, diagnostic tests, hemolytic-uremic syndrome, renal vein occlusion (bilateral), and vasculitis.

## Nursing considerations

• If catheterization fails to initiate urine flow, prepare the patient for diagnostic studies. If tests reveal an obstruction, prepare the patient as ordered for insertion of a nephrostomy or ureterostomy tube to drain the urine. If tests fail to reveal an obstruction, prepare the patient for further kidney function studies.

• Monitor and record the patient's vital signs, intake and output, and weight. Restrict his daily fluid allowance to 600-ml more than the previous day's total urine output. Restrict foods and juices high in potassium and sodium, and make sure the patient maintains a balanced diet. Provide low-sodium hard candy to help decrease his thirst.

Urticaria, also called hives, is a vascular skin reaction characterized by the eruption of pruritic wheals—smooth, slightly elevated patches with well-defined erythematous margins and pale centers. It's produced by the local release of histamine or other vasoactive substances during hypersensitivity reactions.

Acute urticaria evolves rapidly and usually has a detectable cause. It commonly results from hypersensitivity to certain drugs, foods, insect bites, inhalants, or contactants, or it may result from emotional stress. Although individual lesions usually subside in 12 to 24 hours, new crops of lesions may erupt continuously, thereby prolonging the attack.

Urticaria lasting longer than 6 weeks is classified as chronic. The lesions may recur for months or years, and the underlying cause is usually unknown. Occasionally, psychogenic urticaria is diagnosed.

Angioedema, or giant urticaria, is characterized by the acute eruption of wheals involving the mucous membranes and, occasionally, the arms, legs, or genitalia.

### ▶ Emergency interventions

If urticaria is acute, quickly assess the patient's respiratory status and take his vital signs. If you note signs of respiratory difficulty (such as air hunger, dyspnea, wheezing, or stridor) or impending anaphylactic shock (apprehension and uneasiness; warm, moist skin; or edema, especially facial), have a colleague call the doctor immediately. Start an I.V. infusion of dextrose 5% in water and, as appropriate, administer local epinephrine or apply ice to the affected site. Clear and maintain the airway, administer oxygen as needed, and institute cardiac monitoring. Have resuscitation equipment at hand, and be prepared to begin cardiopulmonary resuscitation or to assist with emergency intubation or tracheotomy if necessary.

### History

Ask the patient if urticaria follows any seasonal pattern. Do certain foods or drugs seem to aggravate it? Has he noticed any relationship to physical exertion? Is the patient routinely exposed to any chemicals on the job or at home? Obtain a detailed drug history, including prescription and over-the-counter drugs. Note any history of chronic or parasitic infections, skin disease, or GI disorders.

### Causes

*Anaphylaxis.* Diffuse urticaria and angioedema erupt rapidly, with wheals ranging from pinpoint to palm-sized or larger. Lesions are usually pruritic and stinging. Paresthesia commonly precedes eruption. Other findings include profound anxiety, weakness, diaphoresis, sneezing, shortness of breath, profuse rhinorrhea, nasal congestion, dysphagia, and warm, moist skin. Severe reactions may be life-threatening and are marked by signs of respiratory distress (caused by upper airway edema), cardiac arrhythmias, hypotension, and shock.

*Hereditary angioedema.* Nonpitting, nonpruritic edema may appear on an extremity or the face. Respiratory mucosal involvement can produce life-threatening acute laryngeal edema.

### Nursing considerations

• To help relieve the patient's discomfort, apply a bland skin emollient or one containing menthol and phenol, as ordered. Expect to give antihistamines, systemic corticosteroids or, if stress is a contributing factor, tranquilizers. Tepid baths and cool compresses may enhance vasoconstriction and decrease pruritus.

• Teach the patient to avoid the causative stimulus, if identified.

U

A subjective reaction to a real or imagined threat, anxiety is a nonspecific feeling of uneasiness or dread. It can be mild, moderate, or severe. Mild anxiety may cause slight physical or psychological discomfort; severe anxiety may be incapacitating or even life-threatening.

A normal response to real danger or stress, anxiety can also be caused by lack of sleep, poor diet, and excessive intake of caffeine or other stimulants. Excessive, unwarranted anxiety may indicate an underlying psychological problem.

## History
If the patient displays acute, severe anxiety, take his vital signs, determine his chief complaint, and try to calm him.

If the patient displays mild or moderate anxiety, ask about its duration and precipitating factors. Find out if his anxiety is exacerbated by stress, lack of sleep, or excessive caffeine intake and alleviated by rest, tranquilizers, or exercise.

Obtain a complete history, noting any drug use.

## Physical exam
Focus on complaints that may trigger or be aggravated by anxiety. If the patient's anxiety isn't accompanied by significant physical signs, suspect a psychological cause. Assess the patient's level of consciousness and observe his behavior. If appropriate, refer him for psychiatric evaluation.

## Causes
*Adult respiratory distress syndrome.* Acute anxiety occurs along with tachycardia, mental sluggishness and, in severe cases, hypotension.

*Anaphylactic shock.* Onset is usually signaled by acute anxiety accompanied by urticaria, angioedema, pruritus, and shortness of breath.

*Angina pectoris.* Acute anxiety may precede or follow an attack of angina pectoris, which produces sharp, crushing substernal or anterior chest pain often relieved by nitroglycerin or rest.

*Asthma.* In allergic asthma attacks, acute anxiety occurs with dyspnea, wheezing, productive cough, accessory muscle use, hyperresonant lung fields, diminished breath sounds, coarse crackles, cyanosis, tachycardia, and diaphoresis.

*Autonomic hyperreflexia (AHR).* The earliest sign of AHR may be acute anxiety accompanied by severe headache and dramatic hypertension.

*Congestive heart failure.* In this disorder, acute anxiety is commonly the first symptom of inadequate oxygenation. Other findings include restlessness, shortness of breath, tachypnea, decreased level of consciousness, and edema.

*Hyperventilation syndrome.* Produces acute anxiety, pallor, circumoral and peripheral paresthesia and, occasionally, carpopedal spasms.

*Myocardial infarction.* A life-threatening disorder, it commonly causes acute anxiety with crushing substernal pain.

*Postconcussion syndrome.* Chronic anxiety or attacks of acute anxiety may occur. Other findings include irritability, insomnia, and dizziness.

*Pulmonary edema.* The disorder causes acute anxiety with dyspnea, orthopnea, cough with frothy sputum, tachycardia, tachypnea, crackles, ventricular gallop, hypotension, and thready pulse.

*Pulmonary embolism.* Acute anxiety usually is accompanied by dyspnea, tachypnea, chest pain, tachycardia, blood-tinged sputum, and fever.

*Other causes.* Affective disorder; cardiogenic shock; chronic obstructive pulmonary disease; conversion disorder; drugs, especially sympathomimetics, central nervous system stimulants, and antidepressants; hyperthyroidism; hypochondriacal neurosis; hypoglycemia; obsessive-compulsive disorder; pheochromocytoma; phobic disorder; pneumonia; pneumothorax; posttraumatic stress disorder; rabies; and somatization disorder.

## Nursing considerations
• Provide a calm, quiet atmosphere and make the patient comfortable.
• Try anxiety-reducing measures, such as distraction, relaxation techniques, or biofeedback.

**A**

# Urine cloudiness

Normally clear, straw-colored, and slightly aromatic, urine may become cloudy, murky, or turbid when bacteria, mucus, fat, leukocytes, erythrocytes, or epithelial cells are present. In alkaline urine, cloudiness indicates the presence of phosphates. Although urine cloudiness is a characteristic sign of urinary tract infection (UTI), cloudiness can also result from prolonged storage of a urine specimen at room temperature.

## History
Ask the patient if he has experienced any symptoms of UTI, such as dysuria, urinary urgency or frequency, or pain in the flank, low back, or suprapubic area. Also ask if he's had recurrent UTIs or recent surgery or any other treatment involving the urinary tract.

## Physical exam
Obtain a urine specimen to check for pus or mucus. Using a reagent strip, test for blood and pH. Palpate the suprapubic area and flanks for tenderness.

If you note cloudy urine in a patient with an indwelling urinary catheter, especially if he has a concurrent fever, remove the catheter immediately. Insert a new catheter if the patient must have one in place.

## Causes
*Urinary tract infection.* Cloudy urine is common in this disorder. Other urinary changes include urgency, frequency, hematuria, dysuria, nocturia and, in males, urethral discharge. Urinary hesitancy, bladder spasms, costovertebral angle tenderness, and suprapubic, low back, or flank pain may occur. Additional findings include fever, chills, malaise, nausea, and vomiting.

*Vegetarian diet.* A high-alkali diet (one that contains excess quantities of vegetables, citrus fruits, and dairy products but lacks meats) may cloud urine.

*Other causes.* In men, contamination with spermatozoa or prostatic fluid after prostatectomy; in women, contamination with spermatozoa after intercourse.

## Nursing considerations
• As ordered, collect urine specimens for urinalysis and culture and sensitivity tests. Meticulous collection is vital for accurate laboratory data. If the patient is collecting the specimen, explain the importance of cleaning the meatal area thoroughly. The culture specimen should be caught midstream, in a sterile container; the urinalysis specimen, in a clean container, preferably at the first voiding of the day. Careful midstream, clean-catch collection is preferred to catheterization, which can reinfect the bladder with urethral bacteria.
• Increase the patient's fluid intake, and administer antibiotics and urinary anesthetics (such as phenazopyridine), as ordered.
• To monitor the effectiveness of therapy, continually check the appearance of the patient's urine.

**U**

Also called dysphasia, aphasia is impaired expression or comprehension of written or spoken words, reflecting a disease or injury of the brain's language centers. Depending on its severity, aphasia may impede communication slightly or make it impossible. It can be classified as expressive, receptive, anomic, or global aphasia. Anomic aphasia eventually resolves in more than 50% of patients, but global aphasia is irreversible.

## ▶ Emergency interventions

If the patient develops aphasia suddenly, have another nurse notify the doctor immediately. Assess the patient for signs of increased intracranial pressure (ICP) — pupillary changes, decreased level of consciousness (LOC), vomiting, seizures, bradycardia, widening pulse pressure, and irregular respirations. If you detect signs of increased ICP, administer mannitol I.V., as ordered, to decrease cerebral edema. Keep emergency resuscitation equipment available. If ordered, prepare the patient for surgery.

## History

Perform a thorough neurologic assessment, starting with a patient history obtained from his family or companion because of his impairment. Ask about headaches, hypertension, seizures, drug use, and the patient's ability to communicate and perform routine activities before aphasia began.

## Physical exam

Check for signs of neurologic deficit — ptosis or fluid leakage from the nose and ears. Take the patient's vital signs. Although his verbal responses may be unreliable, assess his LOC. Assess pupillary response, eye movements, and motor function, especially mouth and tongue movement and swallowing. To assess motor function, demonstrate and have the patient imitate responses, rather than provide verbal directions.

## Causes

*Alzheimer's disease.* Anomic aphasia may progress to receptive and global aphasia. Other findings include memory loss, poor judgment, restlessness, myoclonus, muscle rigidity, and incontinence.

*Brain tumor.* Anomic aphasia may be an early sign of this disorder. As the tumor enlarges, other aphasias may occur along with behavioral changes, memory loss, motor weakness, seizures, auditory hallucinations, and visual field deficits.

*Cerebrovascular accident.* The most common cause of aphasia, it may produce receptive, expressive, or global aphasia. Other findings include decreased LOC, right-sided hemiparesis, homonymous hemianopia, paresthesia, and loss of sensation.

*Head trauma.* Any type of aphasia may occur. It usually starts suddenly and may be transient or permanent, depending on the extent of brain damage. Other findings may include blurred or double vision, headache, pallor, diaphoresis, numbness and paresis, cerebrospinal fluid otorrhea or rhinorrhea, altered respirations, tachycardia, disorientation, and signs of increased ICP.

*Transient ischemic attack (TIA).* Aphasia of any type usually occurs suddenly and resolves within 24 hours of the TIA. Other findings include transient hemiparesis, hemianopia, and paresthesia (all usually right-sided), dizziness, and confusion.

*Other causes.* Brain abscess, drug abuse, and encephalitis.

## Nursing considerations

• If the patient is confused, reorient him by frequently telling him what has happened, where he is and why, and the date.
• Speak to the patient in simple phrases, in a normal tone of voice, using demonstrations to clarify your directions when appropriate.
• Make sure he has necessary aids, such as eyeglasses or dentures, to facilitate communication.
• Refer the patient to a speech pathologist early. Support from social services may be necessary later if the patient can't return to work.

# Urinary urgency

Urinary urgency refers to a sudden compelling urge to urinate. Frequent efforts to void may produce urine output of only a few milliliters.

Urgency accompanied by bladder pain is a classic symptom of urinary tract infection (UTI). As inflammation decreases bladder capacity, the accumulation of even small amounts of urine leads to discomfort.

Urgency without bladder pain may point to an upper motor neuron lesion that has disrupted bladder control.

## History
Ask the patient about the onset of urinary urgency and whether he has ever experienced it before. Ask about other urologic and neurologic symptoms. Examine his medical history for recurrent or chronic UTIs and for surgery or procedures involving the urinary tract.

## Physical exam
Obtain a clean-catch specimen for urinalysis. Note urine character, color, and odor, and use a reagent strip to test for pH, glucose, and blood. Then palpate the suprapubic area and both flanks for tenderness. If the patient's history or symptoms suggest neurologic dysfunction, perform a neurologic examination.

## Causes
*Bladder calculus.* Bladder irritation can lead to urinary urgency and frequency, dysuria, hematuria, and suprapubic pain from bladder spasms.

*Multiple sclerosis.* Urinary urgency may occur with or without the frequent UTIs that may accompany this disorder. Like other associated findings, urinary urgency may wax and wane. In many cases, visual and sensory impairments are the earliest findings. Other findings include urinary frequency, incontinence, constipation, muscle weakness, paralysis, spasticity, intention tremor, hyperreflexia, ataxic gait, dysphagia, dysarthria, impotence, and emotional lability.

*Reiter's syndrome.* Urgency accompanies other symptoms of acute urethritis 1 to 2 weeks after sexual contact. Arthritic and ocular symptoms and skin lesions usually develop within several weeks.

*Spinal cord lesion.* The patient may develop urinary urgency when voluntary control of sphincter function weakens in incomplete cord transection. Other findings may include urinary frequency, difficulty initiating and inhibiting a urine stream, and bladder distention and discomfort. Neuromuscular effects distal to the lesion may include weakness, paralysis, hyperreflexia, sensory disturbances, and impotence.

*Urethral stricture.* Bladder decompensation produces urinary urgency, frequency, and nocturia. Early signs include hesitancy, tenesmus, and reduced caliber and force of the urine stream. Eventually, overflow incontinence may occur.

*Urinary tract infection.* Urinary urgency is a common symptom of this disorder. Other characteristic urinary changes include frequency, hematuria, dysuria, nocturia, and cloudy urine. Urinary hesitancy may also occur. Associated findings may include bladder spasms; costovertebral angle tenderness; suprapubic, low back, or flank pain; urethral discharge in males; and fever, chills, malaise, nausea, and vomiting.

*Other causes.* Amyotrophic lateral sclerosis and radiation therapy.

## Nursing considerations
• Prepare the patient for the diagnostic workup, including a complete urinalysis, culture and sensitivity studies, and possibly neurologic tests.
• Unless contraindicated, increase the patient's fluid intake to dilute the urine and diminish the feeling of urgency. As ordered, administer antibiotics and urinary anesthetics (such as phenazopyridine).

U

The cessation of spontaneous respiration, apnea can be temporary and self-limiting. More often, however, it's a life-threatening emergency that requires immediate intervention to prevent death. Its most common causes include trauma, cardiac arrest, neurologic disease, aspiration of a foreign object, bronchospasm, and drug overdose.

## ▶ Emergency interventions

If you detect apnea, first establish and maintain a patent airway. Position the patient supine and open his airway using the head-tilt or chin-lift technique. (*Caution:* Use the jaw-thrust technique on a patient with an obvious or suspected head or neck injury.) Next, quickly look, listen, and feel for spontaneous respiration; if it's absent, begin artificial ventilation until it occurs or until mechanical ventilation begins.

Because apnea may result from cardiac arrest (or may cause it), assess the patient's carotid pulse immediately after you've established a patent airway. If the patient's an infant or a small child, assess the brachial pulse instead. If you can't palpate a pulse, begin cardiac compression.

## History

Ask the patient (or a witness, if the patient can't answer) about the onset of apnea and the events preceding it. Note any reports of headache, chest pain, muscle weakness, sore throat, or dyspnea and any history of respiratory, cardiac, or neurologic disease, allergies, or drug use.

## Physical exam

Inspect the head, face, neck, and trunk for soft-tissue injury, hemorrhage, or skeletal deformity. Look for any clues, such as oral and nasal secretions (reflecting fluid-filled airways and alveoli) or facial soot and singed nasal hair (suggesting thermal injury to the tracheobronchial tree).

Auscultate over all lung lobes for adventitious breath sounds. Percuss the lung fields for increased dullness or hyperresonance. Auscultate the heart for murmurs, pericardial friction rub, and arrhythmias. Check for cyanosis, pallor, jugular vein distention, and edema. If appropriate, perform a neurologic assessment, evaluating level of consciousness, orientation, and mental status and testing cranial nerve and motor function, sensation, and reflexes in all extremities.

## Causes

*Airway obstruction.* Occlusion or compression of the trachea, central airways, or smaller airways can cause sudden apnea by blocking airflow and producing acute respiratory failure.

*Alveolar gas diffusion impairment.* An occlusion at the alveolocapillary membrane level or an accumulation of fluid within the alveoli produces apnea, causing acute respiratory failure. Apnea may arise suddenly or gradually and may be preceded by crackles and labored respirations.

*Brain stem dysfunction.* Primary or secondary brain stem dysfunction can cause apnea by destroying the brain stem's ability to initiate respirations. Apnea may arise suddenly or gradually and may be preceded by decreased level of consciousness and motor and sensory deficits.

*Pulmonary capillary perfusion decrease.* Apnea can stem from obstructed pulmonary circulation, most commonly due to heart failure or lack of circulatory patency. Other findings include hypotension, tachycardia, and edema.

*Respiratory muscle failure.* Trauma or disease can disrupt the mechanics of respiration, causing sudden or gradual apnea. Associated findings may include diaphragmatic or intercostal muscle paralysis from injury, or respiratory weakness or paralysis from acute or degenerative disease.

*Other causes.* Drugs, such as central nervous system depressants, I.V. benzodiazepines, and neuromuscular blocking agents; and pleural pressure gradient disruption.

## Nursing considerations

• Monitor the apneic patient's cardiac and respiratory status to prevent further apneic episodes.

# Urinary incontinence

Urinary incontinence — the uncontrollable passage of urine — results from bladder abnormalities or neurologic disorders. It may be transient or permanent and may involve large volumes of urine or scant dribbling.

## History
Ask the patient when he first noticed the incontinence. Did it begin suddenly or gradually? Have him describe his urinary pattern. Does incontinence usually occur during the day or at night? Does he have any urinary control? If so, ask him the usual times and amounts voided. Determine his normal fluid intake. Ask about other urinary problems. Also ask if he has ever sought treatment for incontinence.

Obtain a medical history, especially noting urinary tract infection, prostate conditions, spinal injury or tumor, cerebrovascular accident, or surgery involving the bladder, prostate, or pelvic floor.

## Physical exam
Have the patient empty his bladder. Inspect the urethral meatus for obvious inflammation or anatomic defect. Have female patients bear down; note any urine leakage. Gently palpate the abdomen for bladder distention. Perform a complete neurologic assessment, noting motor and sensory function and obvious muscle atrophy.

## Causes
*Benign prostatic hyperplasia.* Overflow incontinence (a dribble resulting from urine retention) may occur. Other findings include reduced caliber and force of the urine stream, urinary hesitancy, and a feeling of incomplete voiding.

*Bladder calculus.* Besides overflow incontinence, findings may include an irritable bladder, urinary frequency and urgency, dysuria, hematuria, and suprapubic pain.

*Bladder cancer.* Obstruction by a tumor may produce overflow incontinence. The initial sign is usually gross, painless hematuria. Other findings include frequency, dysuria, nocturia, dribbling, and suprapubic pain after voiding.

*Cerebrovascular accident.* Urinary incontinence may be transient or permanent. Associated findings may include impaired mentation, emotional lability, behavioral changes, altered level of consciousness, and seizures.

*Diabetic neuropathy.* Overflow incontinence may accompany painless bladder distention. Related findings include episodic constipation or diarrhea, impotence and retrograde ejaculation, orthostatic hypotension, syncope, and dysphagia.

*Guillain-Barré syndrome.* Urinary incontinence may occur early in this disorder. Progressive, profound muscle weakness usually starts in the legs and extends to the arms and facial nerves.

*Multiple sclerosis.* Urinary incontinence, urgency, and frequency are common. Other findings include sensory impairment, constipation, muscle weakness, paralysis, and spasticity.

*Prostatic cancer.* Urinary incontinence usually appears in the advanced stages along with urinary frequency and hesitancy, nocturia, dysuria, bladder distention, perineal pain, and constipation.

*Prostatitis (chronic).* Besides urinary incontinence, findings may include urinary frequency and urgency, dysuria, hematuria, bladder distention, persistent urethral discharge, dull perineal pain, and decreased libido.

*Spinal cord injury.* Complete cord transection above the sacral level may lead to overflow incontinence. Other findings include paraplegia, sexual dysfunction, sensory loss, muscle atrophy, anhidrosis, and loss of reflexes distal to the injury.

*Other causes.* Prostatectomy, urethral stricture.

## Nursing considerations
- Implement a bladder retraining program.
- To prevent stress incontinence (intermittent leakage resulting from a sudden physical strain), teach exercises to strengthen the pelvic floor muscles.
- If incontinence has a neurologic basis, monitor for urine retention, which may require periodic catheterizations. If appropriate, teach the patient self-catheterization techniques.

U

# Apneustic respirations

Characterized by prolonged, gasping inspiration and brief, inefficient expiration, this irregular breathing pattern is an important localizing sign of severe brain stem damage.

Involuntary breathing is primarily regulated by groups of neurons, or respiratory centers, in the medulla oblongata and the pons. In the medulla, neurons react to impulses from the pons and other areas to regulate respiratory rate and depth. In the pons, two respiratory centers regulate respiratory rhythm by interacting with the medullary respiratory center to smooth the transition from inspiration to expiration and back.

The apneustic center in the pons stimulates inspiratory neurons in the medulla to precipitate inspiration. These inspiratory neurons, in turn, stimulate the pneumotaxic center in the pons to precipitate expiration. Destruction of neural pathways by pontine lesions disrupts regulation of respiratory rhythm, causing apneustic respirations.

▶ **Emergency interventions**

Your first priority for the patient with apneustic respirations is to ensure adequate ventilation. Have another nurse notify the doctor while you prepare to insert an artificial airway and administer oxygen until mechanical ventilation can begin. Next, thoroughly assess the patient's neurologic status, using the Glasgow Coma Scale.

**History**

Obtain a brief patient history from a family member or companion, if possible.

**Physical exam**

Assess the patient's respiratory pattern. Apneustic respirations must be differentiated from bradypnea and hyperpnea (disturbances in rate and depth, but not in rhythm), Cheyne-Stokes respirations (rhythmic alterations in rate and depth, followed by periods of apnea), and Biot's respirations (irregularly alternating periods of hyperpnea and apnea).

**Cause**

*Pontine lesions.* Apneustic respirations invariably result from extensive damage to the upper or lower pons due to infarction, hemorrhage, herniation, severe infection, tumor, or trauma. Typically, they're accompanied by profound stupor or coma; pinpoint midline pupils; ocular bobbing (a spontaneous downward jerk, followed by a slow drift up to midline); quadriplegia or, less commonly, hemiplegia with pupils pointing toward the affected side; a positive Babinski's reflex; negative oculocephalic reflexes (doll's eyes phenomenon); and, possibly, decerebrate rigidity if the lesion hasn't destroyed the lateral ventricular nucleus.

**Nursing considerations**

• Constantly monitor the patient's neurologic and respiratory status. Notify the doctor immediately of prolonged apneic periods or signs of neurologic deterioration.
• Monitor the patient's arterial blood gas levels.
• If appropriate, prepare him for neurologic tests, such as electroencephalography and computed tomography scan.

**A**

Urinary hesitancy — difficulty starting a urine stream — can result from a urinary tract infection, a partial lower urinary tract obstruction, a neuromuscular disorder, or use of certain drugs. Occurring at all ages and in both sexes, it's most common in older men with prostate enlargement. Hesitancy usually arises gradually, often going unnoticed until urine retention causes bladder distention and discomfort.

## History
Ask the patient when he first noticed hesitancy and if he's ever had the problem before. Ask about other urinary problems, especially reduced force or interruption of the urine stream. Ask the patient if he's ever been treated for a prostate problem or urinary tract infection or obstruction. Obtain a drug history.

## Physical exam
Inspect the patient's urethral meatus for inflammation, discharge, and any other abnormalities. Test sensation in the perineum. Obtain a clean-catch specimen for urinalysis. In a male patient, the doctor may palpate the prostate gland.

## Causes
*Benign prostatic hyperplasia.* Depending on the extent of prostate enlargement and the lobes affected, early findings may include urinary hesitancy, reduced caliber and force of the urine stream, a feeling of incomplete voiding and, occasionally, urine retention. As the obstruction increases, more frequent urination may be accompanied by nocturia, incontinence, bladder distention, and possibly hematuria.

*Prostatic cancer.* Urinary hesitancy may occur in advanced stages, accompanied by frequency, dribbling, nocturia, dysuria, bladder distention, perineal pain, and constipation. Palpation reveals a hard, irregularly shaped prostate. Pallor, weakness, and weight loss may also occur.

*Spinal cord lesion.* If a lesion below the micturition center destroys the sacral nerve roots, it causes urinary hesitancy, tenesmus, and constant dribbling from retention and overflow incontinence. Urinary frequency and urgency, dysuria, and nocturia may also occur. Other findings may include motor weakness or paralysis below the level of the lesion, paresthesia, fecal incontinence, and sexual dysfunction.

*Urethral stricture.* Partial obstruction of the lower urinary tract secondary to trauma or infection produces urinary hesitancy, tenesmus, and decreased force and caliber of the urine stream. Urinary frequency and urgency, nocturia, and eventually overflow incontinence may develop. Pyuria indicates accompanying infection.

*Urinary tract infection.* Besides hesitancy, characteristic urinary changes include frequency, possible hematuria, dysuria, nocturia, and cloudy urine. Associated findings may include bladder spasms; costovertebral angle tenderness; suprapubic, low back, or flank pain; and urethral discharge in males. Fever, chills, malaise, nausea, and vomiting may also occur.

*Other causes.* Anticholinergics and drugs with anticholinergic properties, such as tricyclic antidepressants and some nasal decongestant preparations and cold remedies; congenital urethral obstruction; epispadias; hypospadias; and neural tube defects.

## Nursing considerations
- Monitor the patient's voiding pattern, and frequently palpate for bladder distention.
- Apply local heat to the perineum or the abdomen to enhance muscle relaxation and aid urination.
- Also teach the patient to perform Valsalva's maneuver or Credé's maneuver.
- As ordered, prepare the patient for appropriate diagnostic tests, such as cystometrography or observation cystourethroscopy.

U

The inability to perform purposeful movements in the absence of weakness, sensory loss, poor coordination, or lack of comprehension or motivation, apraxia is an uncommon neurologic sign that usually indicates a lesion in the cerebral cortex.

Classified as *ideational (sensory), ideomotor,* or *ideokinetic,* depending on the stage at which voluntary movement is impaired, apraxia can also be classified by type of motor or skill impairment. For example, *facial* and *gait apraxia* involve specific motor groups. *Constructional apraxia* refers to the inability to copy simple drawings or patterns, *dressing apraxia* to the inability to dress oneself correctly, *callosal apraxia* to normal motor function on one side of the body and the inability to reproduce movements on the other side.

## ▶ Emergency interventions

Watch for signs of increased intracranial pressure (ICP), such as headache and vomiting. If you detect these, elevate the head of the bed 30 degrees, and monitor the patient for altered pupil size and reactivity, bradycardia, widened pulse pressure, and irregular respirations. Have emergency resuscitation equipment nearby, and be prepared to give mannitol I.V. to decrease cerebral edema.

If you detect seizures, stay with the patient and have another nurse notify the doctor immediately. Avoid restraining the patient. Help him to a lying position, loosen tight clothing, and place a pillow or another soft object beneath his head.

If the patient's teeth are clenched, don't force anything into his mouth. If his mouth is open, protect the tongue by placing a soft object, such as a washcloth, between his teeth. Turn the patient's head to provide an open airway.

## History

Ask about previous neurologic disease. If the patient fails to report such disease, notify the doctor and begin a neurologic assessment.

Ask about previous cerebrovascular disease, atherosclerosis, neoplastic disease, infection, or hepatic disease. Assess the apraxia to help determine its type.

Ask the patient if he has recently experienced headache or dizziness.

## Physical exam

First, take the patient's vital signs and assess his level of consciousness. Be alert for any evidence of aphasia or dysarthria. Then test motor function, looking for weakness and tremors. Next, test sensory function. Check deep tendon reflexes, and test for visual field deficits.

## Causes

*Alzheimer's disease.* This disorder may cause gradual and irreversible ideomotor apraxia. It can also cause amnesia, anomia, decreased attention span, apathy, aphasia, restlessness, agitation, paranoid delusions, incontinence, social withdrawal, ataxia, and tremors.

*Brain tumor.* Progressive apraxia may be preceded by decreased mental acuity, headache, dizziness, and seizures. It may occur with or directly after early signs of increased ICP, such as pupillary changes.

*Cerebrovascular accident (CVA).* Apraxia commonly begins suddenly; it may resolve spontaneously or may persist. Other findings may include confusion, stupor or coma, hemiplegia, visual field deficits, aphasia, agnosia, dysarthria, and urinary incontinence.

*Other causes.* Brain abscess, hemodialysis, and hepatic encephalopathy.

## Nursing considerations

• Prepare the patient for diagnostic studies.
• Because weakness, sensory deficits, confusion, and seizures may accompany apraxia, take measures to ensure the patient's safety.
• Encourage the patient to participate in normal activities. Demonstrate tasks in simple steps, giving him enough time to imitate them. Have family members help in rehabilitation.

Urinary frequency is an increased incidence of the urge to void. Usually caused by decreased bladder capacity, frequency is a cardinal sign of urinary tract infection. Other causes include urologic disorders, neurologic dysfunction, or pressure on the bladder from a nearby tumor or organ enlargement.

## History

Ask the patient how many times a day he voids compared with his previous pattern of voiding. Ask about the onset and duration of frequency and about associated urinary or neurologic symptoms. Also inquire about past urologic and neurologic disorders and about recent urologic procedures. Ask a male patient about a history of prostate enlargement. Ask a female patient of childbearing age whether she is or could be pregnant.

## Physical exam

Obtain a clean-catch midstream specimen for urinalysis and culture and sensitivity tests. Palpate the patient's suprapubic area, abdomen, and flanks, noting any tenderness. Examine his urethral meatus for redness, discharge, or swelling. Perform a neurologic examination if the patient's history warrants it.

## Causes

*Benign prostatic hyperplasia.* Urinary frequency may be accompanied by nocturia, incontinence, and hematuria. Other findings include reduced caliber and force of the urine stream, urinary hesitancy, tenesmus, a feeling of incomplete voiding, and bladder distention.

*Bladder calculus.* The patient may develop urinary frequency and urgency, dysuria, hematuria, suprapubic pain, and overflow incontinence.

*Bladder cancer.* Urinary frequency, dribbling, and nocturia may develop. Other findings may include intermittent hematuria and suprapubic pain.

*Multiple sclerosis.* Urinary frequency, urgency, and incontinence are common. Other findings include visual problems, sensory impairment, constipation, muscle weakness, paralysis, spasticity, hyperreflexia, intention tremor, ataxic gait, dysarthria, impotence, and emotional lability.

*Prostatic cancer.* Urinary frequency may be accompanied by hesitancy, dribbling, nocturia, dysuria, bladder distention, perineal pain, and constipation.

*Prostatitis. Acute prostatitis* causes urinary frequency along with urgency, dysuria, nocturia, and purulent urethral discharge. Other findings include fever, chills, low back pain, myalgia, arthralgia, and perineal fullness. *Chronic prostatitis* produces similar findings to a lesser degree. Other effects may include painful ejaculation, persistent urethral discharge, and sexual dysfunction.

*Rectal tumor.* Findings include urinary frequency, changes in bowel habits, blood or mucus in the stool, and a feeling of incomplete evacuation.

*Reproductive tract tumor.* In female patients, urinary frequency may accompany abdominal distention, menstrual disturbances, vaginal bleeding, weight loss, pelvic pain, and fatigue.

*Spinal cord lesion.* Urinary frequency results from weakened voluntary sphincter control. Other findings include urgency, hesitancy, bladder distention, weakness, paralysis, sensory disturbances, hyperreflexia, and impotence.

*Urethral stricture.* Urinary frequency is accompanied by urgency and nocturia. Other findings include hesitancy, tenesmus, and reduced caliber and force of the urine stream.

*Urinary tract infection.* This common cause of urinary frequency may also produce dysuria, hematuria, cloudy urine, and, in males, urethral discharge. The patient may report fever, chills, nausea and vomiting, bladder spasms, or a feeling of warmth during urination.

*Other causes.* Anxiety neurosis, pregnancy, radiation therapy, and Reiter's syndrome.

## Nursing considerations

• If the patient's mobility is impaired, keep a bedpan or commode near his bed.

Usually the result of musculoskeletal disorders, arm pain can also be caused by neurovascular or cardiovascular disorders. Its location, onset, and character provide clues to its cause. The pain may affect the entire arm or only the upper arm or forearm. It may arise suddenly or gradually and be constant or intermittent, sharp or dull, burning or numbing, shooting or penetrating.

## History

If the pain began after an injury, ask the patient or his companion to recount the incident. Ask the patient to describe the pain and when it began, and to point out related painful areas. Ask if the pain worsens in the morning or evening, if it affects his job or restricts his movements, and if anything relieves it. Ask about other illnesses, a family history of gout or arthritis, and drug therapy. Ask him about edema and if the pain has worsened in the last 24 hours. Also ask what activities he has been performing.

## Physical exam

Assess for injuries requiring immediate treatment. If you've ruled out severe injuries, check pulses, capillary refill time, sensation, and movement distal to the affected area. Inspect the arm for deformity, assess the level of pain, and immobilize the arm.

Observe the way the patient walks, sits, and holds his arm. Compare the affected arm with the opposite arm for symmetry, movement, muscle atrophy, strength, and reflexes. Palpate it for swelling, nodules, and tender areas.

If the patient reports numbness or tingling, check his sensation to vibration and pinprick. Compare bilateral hand grasps and shoulder strength.

If the patient has a cast, splint, or restrictive dressing, check circulation, sensation, and mobility distal to the dressing.

## Causes

*Angina.* This disorder may cause inner arm pain as well as chest and jaw pain. Typically, the pain follows exertion and persists for a few minutes. Accompanied by dyspnea, diaphoresis, and apprehension, the pain is relieved by rest or vasodilators.

*Cervical nerve root compression.* Compression of the cervical nerves supplying the upper arm produces chronic arm and neck pain.

*Compartment syndrome.* Severe pain with passive muscle stretching is the cardinal sign. Ominous signs include paralysis and absent pulse.

*Fractures.* In fractures of the cervical vertebrae, humerus, scapula, clavicle, radius, or ulna, pain can occur at the injury site and radiate throughout the arm. Pain at a fresh fracture site is intense and worsens with movement.

*Myocardial infarction.* In this life-threatening disorder, the patient may complain of left arm pain and characteristic deep, crushing chest pain. He may display weakness, pallor, nausea, vomiting, diaphoresis, altered blood pressure, tachycardia, dyspnea, and feelings of impending doom.

*Neoplasm of the arm.* This disorder produces continuous, deep, and penetrating arm pain that worsens at night. Skin breakdown, impaired circulation, and paresthesia may occur.

*Osteomyelitis.* Typical signs include a sudden onset of localized arm pain and fever, accompanied by local tenderness, painful and restricted movement and, later, swelling.

*Other causes.* Biceps rupture, cellulitis, muscle contusion, and muscle strain.

## Nursing considerations

● If you suspect a fracture, apply a sling or a splint and monitor for worsening pain, numbness, or decreased circulation distal to the injury site.

● Monitor vital signs. Be alert for tachycardia, hypotension, and diaphoresis. Withhold food, fluids, and analgesics until the doctor evaluates potential fractures. Elevate the patient's arm and apply ice. Clean abrasions and lacerations, and apply dry, sterile dressings if necessary.

● Prepare the patient for diagnostic tests.

**A**

An excretion from the urinary meatus, urethral discharge may be purulent, mucoid, or thin; sanguineous or clear; and scant or profuse. It usually develops suddenly, most commonly in men with a prostate infection.

## History

Ask the patient when he first noticed the discharge, and have him describe its color, consistency, and quantity. Does he have any pain on urination? Any difficulty initiating a urine stream? Ask about other associated symptoms, such as fever, chills, and perineal fullness. Explore his history for any incidence of prostate problems, sexually transmitted disease, or urinary tract infection. Ask if he's had recent sexual contact or a new sexual partner.

## Physical exam

Inspect the patient's urethral meatus for inflammation and swelling. Using proper technique, obtain a culture specimen. Then obtain a urine specimen for urinalysis and possibly a three-glass urine specimen. In a male patient, the doctor may palpate the prostate gland.

## Causes

*Prostatitis. Acute prostatitis* produces purulent urethral discharge. Other findings include sudden fever, chills, myalgia, perineal fullness, low back pain, and arthralgia. Urination becomes increasingly frequent and urgent, and the urine may appear cloudy. Dysuria, nocturia, and some degree of urinary obstruction may also occur. When palpated rectally, the prostate is markedly tender, indurated, swollen, firm, and warm. Although it commonly produces no symptoms, *chronic prostatitis* may produce a persistent urethral discharge that's thin, milky or clear, and sometimes sticky. The discharge appears at the meatus after a long interval between voidings, commonly in the morning. Other findings include a dull aching in the prostate or rectum, sexual dysfunction, and urinary disturbances, such as frequency, urgency, and dysuria.

*Reiter's syndrome.* Urethral discharge and other signs of acute urethritis occur 1 to 2 weeks after sexual contact. Arthritic and ocular symptoms and skin lesions usually develop within several weeks.

*Urethral neoplasm.* The patient may develop a painless urethral discharge that's initially opaque and gray. Later, the discharge becomes yellowish and blood-tinged.

*Urethritis.* This inflammatory disorder commonly produces a scant or profuse urethral discharge. The discharge may be thin and clear, mucoid, or thick and purulent. Other effects include urinary hesitancy, urgency, and frequency; dysuria; and itching and burning around the meatus.

## Nursing considerations

• Advise the patient with acute prostatitis to discontinue sexual activity until acute symptoms subside. However, encourage the patient with chronic prostatitis to regularly engage in sexual activity. To help this patient relieve symptoms, suggest that he take hot sitz baths several times daily, increase his fluid intake, void frequently, and avoid caffeine, tea, and alcohol. Monitor him for urine retention.

• Carefully evaluate a child with urethral discharge for evidence of sexual and physical abuse.

**U**

Also called liver flap or flapping tremor, asterixis is a coarse, bilateral tremor characterized by rapid, nonrhythmic extensions and flexions. It's most commonly observed in the wrists and fingers but also appears in the ankles, the corners of the mouth, the eyelids, and the tongue and usually signals the onset of coma in end-stage hepatic, renal, or pulmonary disease.

## History
Assess neurologic status and vital signs, comparing them with the patient's baseline and reporting acute changes to the doctor immediately. Continue to monitor neurologic status, vital signs, and urine output. Watch for signs of respiratory insufficiency. Be prepared to assist with endotracheal intubation and ventilatory support.

If the patient has hepatic disease, assess for early signs of hemorrhage, including restlessness, tachypnea, and cool, moist, pale skin. Hypotension, oliguria, hematemesis, and melena are late signs of hemorrhage. If any of these signs develops, notify the doctor immediately. Prepare to insert a large-bore I.V. line for fluid and blood replacement. Position the patient flat in bed with legs elevated 20 degrees. Begin or continue giving oxygen.

If the patient has renal disease, review the therapy he's received. If it's dialysis, ask about the frequency of treatments. Ask a family member if the patient's level of consciousness (LOC) is significantly decreased. Assess for hyperkalemia and metabolic acidosis. If you detect tachycardia, nausea, diarrhea, abdominal cramps, muscle weakness, hyperreflexia, or Kussmaul's respirations, notify the doctor immediately. Prepare to administer sodium bicarbonate, calcium gluconate, dextrose, insulin, or sodium polystyrene sulfonate (Kayexalate), as ordered.

If the patient has pulmonary disease, assess for labored respirations, tachypnea, accessory muscle use, and cyanosis. If you detect any of these signs, notify the doctor immediately. Prepare to assist with ventilatory support via nasal cannula, mask, or intubation and mechanical ventilation.

## Physical exam
To elicit asterixis, have the patient extend his arms, dorsiflex his wrists, and spread his fingers. Briefly observe for asterixis. If the patient has a decreased LOC but can follow verbal commands, ask him to squeeze two of your fingers. Rapid clutching and unclutching indicate asterixis. Or elevate the patient's leg off the bed and dorsiflex the foot. Observe for asterixis in the ankle. If the patient can close his eyes and mouth tightly, observe for irregular tremulous movements of the eyelids and corners of the mouth. If he can stick out his tongue, observe for continuous quivering.

## Causes
*Hepatic encephalopathy.* This life-threatening disorder initially causes slight personality changes and a slight tremor, which progresses to asterixis—the hallmark of hepatic encephalopathy.

*Severe respiratory insufficiency.* Characterized by life-threatening respiratory acidosis, this disorder produces headache, restlessness, confusion, apprehension, and decreased reflexes.

*Uremic syndrome.* This life-threatening disorder initially causes lethargy, somnolence, confusion, disorientation, behavior changes, and irritability. Asterixis is accompanied by stupor, paresthesia, muscle twitching, fasciculation, and footdrop.

## Nursing considerations
• Elevate the head of the bed to relieve dyspnea and orthopnea. Administer oil baths, avoiding soap, to relieve itching from jaundice and uremia.
• Provide enteral or parenteral nutrition if the patient is intubated or has a decreased LOC. Monitor serum and urine glucose levels to evaluate parenteral nutrition.
• Reposition the patient every 2 hours to prevent skin breakdown. Observe strict hand-washing and aseptic technique when changing dressings and caring for invasive lines.

# Uremic frost

Uremic frost—a fine white powder, believed to be urate crystals, that covers the skin—is a characteristic sign of end-stage renal failure. Urea compounds and other waste substances that can't be excreted by the kidneys in urine are excreted in sweat and remain as powdery deposits on the skin when the sweat evaporates. The frost usually appears on the face, neck, axillae, groin, and genitalia.

Because of advances in managing renal failure, uremic frost is now relatively rare. However, it does occur in patients with chronic renal failure who, because of advanced age or the severity of accompanying illnesses, do not undergo dialysis.

## Physical exam

Uremic frost usually appears well after a diagnosis of chronic renal failure has been established. As a result, your assessment will be limited to inspecting the skin to determine the extent of uremic frost.

## Cause

*End-stage chronic renal failure.* Uremic frost heralds the preterminal stage of chronic renal failure. The patient may also have pruritus, hypertension, lassitude, fatigue, irritability, and decreased level of consciousness. Additional findings may include muscle cramps, gross myoclonus, peripheral neuropathies, and seizures. Anorexia, nausea and vomiting, constipation or diarrhea, and oliguria or anuria may occur along with GI bleeding, petechiae, and ecchymoses. Integumentary effects may include mouth and gum ulceration, skin pigment changes and excoriation, and brown arcs under nail margins. Acidosis results in Kussmaul's respirations. The patient may also have ammonia breath odor (uremic fetor).

## Nursing considerations

• Because this patient is prone to seizures from uremic encephalopathy, take seizure precautions. Monitor his vital signs frequently, pad the bed's side rails, and keep an artificial airway and suction equipment at hand.
• Because the patient is prone to respiratory or cardiac arrest from metabolic acidosis or hyperkalemia, constantly monitor his respiratory and cardiac status. As necessary, administer supplemental oxygen and be prepared to assist with intubation and mechanical ventilation. Establish an I.V. line to administer fluids and medication. Also begin cardiac monitoring, and be prepared to initiate cardiopulmonary resuscitation, if indicated.
• Enhance patient comfort by providing regular position changes to prevent skin breakdown and by bathing the patient often with tepid water and minimal soap to remove the frost. Trim his fingernails to prevent scratching.
• Because the appearance of uremic frost invariably signals impending death, prepare the patient and his family for this eventuality, and provide emotional support. Death from uremia is typically peaceful, following a deep coma.

Ataxia refers to incoordination and irregularity of voluntary, purposeful movements. *Cerebellar ataxia* results from disease of the cerebellum and its pathways to and from the cerebral cortex, brain stem, and spinal cord. It causes gait, trunk, limb, and possibly speech disorders. *Sensory ataxia* results from impaired position sense caused by interruption of afferent nerve fibers in the peripheral nerves, posterior roots, posterior columns of the spinal cord, or medial lemnisci, or by a lesion in both parietal lobes. Gait disorders result.

## ▶ Emergency interventions

Assess the ataxic patient for signs of increased intracranial pressure and impending herniation. Assess his level of consciousness (LOC). Watch for pupillary abnormalities, motor weakness or paralysis, neck stiffness or pain, and vomiting. Check vital signs. Elevate the head of the bed. Have emergency resuscitation equipment ready.

## History

Ask about previous cerebrovascular accident, multiple sclerosis, diabetes, central nervous system infection, neoplastic disease, and a family history of ataxia. Ask about alcohol abuse or exposure to industrial toxins such as mercury. Determine if the ataxia arose suddenly or gradually. If necessary, perform the Romberg test to distinguish between cerebellar and sensory ataxia. In gait ataxia, ask the patient if he tends to fall to one side or if falling occurs more often at night.

## Causes

*Cerebellar abscess.* Limb ataxia on the side opposite the lesion, gait ataxia, and truncal ataxia are common. Typically, the initial symptom is headache behind the ear or in the occipital region.

*Cerebellar hemorrhage.* In this life-threatening disorder, ataxia usually occurs acutely but is transient. It affects the trunk, gait, or limbs.

*Cerebrovascular accident.* Along with ataxia, this life-threatening disorder may cause motor weakness, altered LOC, sensory loss, vertigo, nausea, vomiting, ocular motor palsy, and dysphagia.

*Friedreich's ataxia.* The spinal cord and cerebellum are affected, causing gait ataxia, followed by truncal, limb, and speech ataxia. Other features include pes cavus, kyphoscoliosis, cranial nerve palsy, and motor and sensory deficits.

*Metastatic carcinoma.* Carcinoma that metastasizes to the cerebellum may cause gait ataxia, along with headache, dizziness, nystagmus, and decreased LOC.

*Multiple sclerosis.* Nystagmus and cerebellar ataxia commonly occur, but they aren't always accompanied by limb weakness and spasticity.

*Olivopontocerebellar atrophy.* This disorder produces gait ataxia and, later, limb and speech ataxia. It's accompanied by choreiform movements, dysphagia, and loss of sphincter tone.

*Posterior fossa tumor.* Gait, truncal, or limb ataxia is an early sign of this tumor. It's accompanied by vomiting, headache, papilledema, vertigo, ocular motor palsy, decreased LOC, and motor and sensory changes.

*Wernicke's disease.* Gait ataxia occurs and, rarely, intention tremor or speech ataxia. Other findings include nystagmus, diplopia, ocular palsies, confusion, tachycardia, exertional dyspnea, and postural hypotension.

*Other causes.* Behçet's disease; cranial trauma; diabetic neuropathy; diphtheria; drugs, such as anticonvulsants, anticholinergics, tricyclic antidepressants, and aminoglutethimide; encephalomyelitis; Guillain-Barré syndrome; hepatocerebral degeneration; hyperthermia; hypothyroidism; pellagra; poisoning; polyarteritis nodosa; polyneuropathy; porphyria; spinocerebellar ataxia; syringomyelia; tabes dorsalis.

## Nursing considerations

• As ordered, prepare the patient for diagnostic studies. Promote rehabilitation goals and help ensure the patient's safety. Provide a cane or walker for extra support. Ask the patient's family to check his home for hazards.

Also called gunbarrel vision or tubular vision, tunnel vision refers to a severe constriction of the visual field that leaves only a small central area of sight. The patient may describe a sensation of looking through a tunnel or gun barrel. Verifying tunnel vision requires a comprehensive visual field examination performed by an ophthalmologist or optometrist.

Tunnel vision may be unilateral or bilateral and usually develops gradually. It results from chronic open-angle glaucoma, advanced retinal degeneration, and laser photocoagulation therapy. Be aware that tunnel vision is also a common complaint of malingerers.

## History

Ask the patient when he first noticed a loss of peripheral vision. Then have him describe the progression of vision loss. Next, ask him to describe in detail exactly what and how far he can see peripherally. Explore the patient's personal and family history for ocular problems. Have any family members experienced progressive blindness beginning at an early age?

## Physical exam

To rule out malingering, observe the patient as he walks. A patient with severely limited peripheral vision may frequently bump into objects (and may even have bruises), whereas a malingerer will manage to avoid them.

## Causes

*Chronic open-angle glaucoma.* Bilateral tunnel vision occurs late and slowly progresses to complete blindness. Other late findings include mild eye pain, halo vision, and reduced visual acuity (especially at night) that cannot be corrected with glasses.

*Retinal pigmentary degeneration.* This group of hereditary disorders, which includes retinitis pigmentosa, produces an annular scotoma that progresses concentrically, causing tunnel vision. Eventually, the patient becomes completely blind, usually by age 50. The earliest symptom—impaired night vision—usually appears in the first or second decade of life. Ophthalmoscopic examination may reveal narrowed retinal blood vessels and a pale optic disk.

*Other causes.* Tunnel vision can result from laser photocoagulation therapy, which aims to correct retinal detachment.

## Nursing considerations

- If your assessment findings suggest tunnel vision, refer the patient to an ophthalmologist or optometrist for further evaluation.
- To protect the patient with tunnel vision from injury, be sure to remove all potentially dangerous objects and orient him to his surroundings.
- If tunnel vision is permanent, teach the patient to move his eyes from side to side when he walks to avoid bumping into objects.
- Since any visual impairment is frightening, provide emotional support and clearly explain diagnostic procedures, such as tonometry, perimeter examination, and visual field testing.

# Athetosis

An extrapyramidal sign, athetosis is characterized by slow, continuous, and twisting involuntary movements. Typically, these movements involve the face, neck, and distal extremities, such as the forearm, wrist, and hand. Facial grimaces, jaw and tongue movements, and occasional phonation are associated with neck movements.

Athetosis worsens during stress and voluntary activity and may subside during relaxation and even disappear during sleep. Commonly a lifelong affliction, athetosis is sometimes difficult to distinguish from chorea. But typically, athetoid movements are slower than choreiform movements.

This sign usually begins during childhood, resulting from hypoxia at birth, kernicterus, or genetic disorders. In adults, athetosis most commonly results from vascular or neoplastic lesions, degenerative disease, or drug toxicity.

## History

Take a prenatal and postnatal history, covering maternal and child health, labor and delivery, and possible trauma. Obtain a family health history; genetic disorders can cause athetosis. Ask about current drug therapy.

Ask about the decline in the patient's functional abilities: When was he last able to roll over, sit up, or carry out daily activities? Find out what problems — uncontrollable movements, mental deterioration, or speech impediment — prompted him to seek medical help. Ask about the effects of rest, stress, and routine activity on symptoms.

## Physical exam

Test the patient's muscle strength and tone, range of motion, fine muscle movements, and ability to perform rapidly alternating movements. Observe limb muscles during voluntary movements for the rhythm and duration of contraction and relaxation.

## Causes

*Brain tumor.* If this disorder affects the basal ganglia, contralateral choreoathetosis and dystonia result. Other signs vary markedly with the type of tumor and its degree of invasion.

*Calcification of the basal ganglia.* This unilateral or bilateral disorder is characterized by choreoathetosis and rigidity. Usually, it arises in adolescence or early adult life.

*Cerebral infarction.* In this disorder, contralateral athetosis is accompanied by altered level of consciousness. The patient may also display contralateral paralysis of the face or limbs.

*Hepatic encephalopathy.* Episodic or persistent choreoathetosis occurs in the chronic stage of this encephalopathy. It's accompanied by cerebellar ataxia, myoclonus of the face and limbs, asterixis, dysarthria, and dementia.

*Huntington's disease.* In this hereditary degenerative disease, athetosis and chorea develop in early or middle adult life. Other findings include dystonia, dysarthria, facial apraxia, rigidity, depression, and mental deterioration.

*Wilson's disease.* In this inherited metabolic disorder, choreoathetoid movements initially involve the fingers and hands and then spread to the arms, head, trunk, and legs. Other findings include Kayser-Fleischer rings, arm and hand tremors, facial and muscular rigidity, dysarthria, dysphagia, drooling, and progressive dementia.

*Other causes.* Drugs, such as levodopa and phenytoin, phenothiazines and other antipsychotics; and Pick's disease.

## Nursing considerations

• As ordered, prepare the patient for diagnostic tests, such as urine and blood studies, lumbar puncture, electroencephalography, and computed tomography scan.

• Supply the patient with assistive devices, such as a long-handled shoehorn, to help him carry out fine motor tasks. When appropriate, assist in rehabilitation. Encourage swimming, stretching, and balance and gait exercises to help maintain coordination, slow deterioration, and minimize antisocial behavior.

# Tremors

The most common involuntary muscle movement, tremors are regular rhythmic oscillations that result from alternate contraction and relaxation of opposing muscle groups. *Resting tremors* occur when an extremity is at rest and subside with movement. *Intention tremors* occur with movement and subside with rest. *Postural (or action) tremors* appear when an extremity or the trunk is actively held in a particular posture or position. *Essential tremors* are slow postural tremors.

## History

Ask the patient about the tremor's onset (sudden or gradual) and about its duration, progression, and any aggravating or alleviating factors. Does the tremor interfere with his normal activities? Does the patient have other symptoms?

Explore the patient's personal and family medical history for neurologic, endocrine, or metabolic disorders. Obtain a complete drug history, noting the use of phenothiazines. Ask about alcohol use.

## Physical exam

Assess the patient's overall appearance and demeanor, noting mental status. Test range of motion and strength in all major muscle groups while observing involuntary movements. Check deep tendon reflexes, and observe the patient's gait.

## Causes

*Alcohol withdrawal syndrome.* Resting and intention tremors may accompany diaphoresis, tachycardia, elevated blood pressure, restlessness, anxiety, irritability, and insomnia. Severe withdrawal may produce delirium tremens.

*Cerebellar tumor.* An early sign, intention tremor may occur with ataxia, nystagmus, incoordination, and muscle weakness and atrophy.

*Hypoglycemia (acute).* A rapid, fine intention tremor may be accompanied by confusion, weakness, tachycardia, diaphoresis, and cold, clammy skin. Patient complaints may include mild generalized headache, profound hunger, nervousness, and blurred or double vision.

*Manganese toxicity.* Besides a resting tremor, findings may include chorea, propulsive gait, cogwheel rigidity, personality changes, amnesia, and masklike facies.

*Multiple sclerosis.* An intention tremor may be accompanied by nystagmus, muscle weakness, paralysis, spasticity, hyperreflexia, ataxic gait, dysphagia, and dysarthria.

*Parkinson's disease.* An insidious resting tremor begins in the fingers ("pill-rolling" tremor) and may eventually affect the foot, eyelids, jaw, lips, and tongue. Leg involvement produces flexion-extension foot movement. Lightly closing the eyelids causes them to flutter. The jaw may move up and down, and the lips may purse. Other findings include cogwheel or lead-pipe rigidity, bradykinesia, monotone voice, masklike facies, and drooling.

*Porphyria.* A resting tremor with rigidity may be accompanied by chorea and athetosis.

*Thalamic syndrome.* Central midbrain syndromes produce contralateral ataxic tremors and other abnormal movements, along with Weber's syndrome, paralysis of vertical gaze, and stupor or coma.

*Thyrotoxicosis.* A rapid, fine intention tremor of the hands and tongue may occur along with clonus, hyperreflexia, and Babinski's reflex.

*Wernicke's disease.* An intention tremor is an early sign. Other characteristics include ocular abnormalities, ataxia, and apathy.

*Wilson's disease.* Slow "wing-flapping" tremors in the arms and pill-rolling tremors in the hands appear early. Rusty brown rings of pigment may develop around the corneas.

*Other causes.* Alkalosis; benign familial essential tremor; drugs, such as amphetamines, antipsychotics, lithium, metoclopramide, metyrosine, sympathomimetics, and phenytoin; general paresis; hypercapnia; and kwashiorkor.

## Nursing considerations

• Assist the patient with activities of daily living and take precautions against injury, as necessary.

An aura is a sensory or motor phenomenon that marks the initial stage of a seizure or the approach of a classic migraine headache. It may be classified as cognitive, affective, psychosensory, or psychomotor.

The aura associated with classic migraine headache results from cranial vasoconstriction. Diagnostically important, it helps distinguish classic migraine from other types of headache.

Typically, the aura develops over 10 to 30 minutes and varies in intensity and duration. If the patient recognizes the aura as a warning sign, he may be able to prevent the headache by taking appropriate drugs.

## History

When an aura rapidly progresses to the ictal phase of a seizure, quickly evaluate the seizure and be alert for life-threatening complications, such as apnea.

When an aura heralds a classic migraine, make the patient as comfortable as possible. Place him in a dark, quiet room and administer drugs to prevent headache, as ordered.

Later, obtain a thorough history of the patient's headaches. Ask him to describe any sensory or motor phenomena that precede each headache. Find out how long each headache typically lasts. Does anything make it worse, such as bright lights, noise, or caffeine? Does anything make it better? Ask the patient about drugs for pain relief.

## Causes

*Classic migraine headache.* This disorder is preceded by a vague premonition and then, usually, a visual aura involving flashes of light. The aura develops over 10 to 30 minutes and may intensify until it completely obscures the patient's vision.

A classic migraine may also cause numbness or tingling of the lips, face, or hands; slight confusion; and dizziness before the characteristic unilateral, throbbing headache appears. This headache slowly intensifies and, when it peaks, may cause photophobia, nausea, and vomiting.

*Seizure disorder.* When associated with a seizure, an aura stems from an irritable focus in the brain that spreads throughout the cortex. Although an aura was once considered a sign of impending seizure, it's now considered an actual stage of the seizure.

Typically, it occurs seconds to minutes before the ictal phase. Its intensity, duration, and type depend on the origin of the irritable focus. For example, an aura of bitter taste may accompany a frontal lobe lesion.

Unfortunately, an aura is difficult to describe because the postictal phase of a seizure temporarily alters the patient's level of consciousness, impairing his memory of the event.

## Nursing considerations

• Advise the patient to keep a diary of factors that precipitate migraine headaches, as well as associated symptoms to evaluate the effectiveness of drug therapy and recommended life-style changes. Measures to reduce stress may play a role.

# Tracheal tugging

Also known as Oliver's or Porter's sign, tracheal tugging refers to a visible recession of the larynx and trachea that occurs in synchrony with cardiac systole. It commonly results from an aneurysm or a tumor near the aortic arch.

Best observed with the patient's neck hyperextended, the tugging movement reflects abnormal transmission of aortic pulsations caused by compression and distortion of the heart, esophagus, great vessels, airways, and nerves. It may signal dangerous compression or obstruction of major airways.

▶ **Emergency interventions**
Upon observing tracheal tugging, assess the patient for signs of respiratory distress, such as tachypnea, stridor, accessory muscle use, cyanosis, and agitation. If the patient's in distress, have a colleague call the doctor immediately while you check airway patency. Administer oxygen and prepare to intubate the patient, if necessary. As ordered, insert an I.V. line for fluid and drug access, and institute cardiac monitoring.

## History
Ask about associated symptoms, especially pain, and about any history of cardiovascular disease, cancer, chest surgery, or trauma.

## Physical exam
Examine the neck and chest for abnormalities. Palpate the neck for masses, enlarged lymph nodes, abnormal arterial pulsations, and tracheal deviation. Percuss and auscultate the lung fields for abnormal sounds, and auscultate the heart for murmurs.

## Causes
*Aortic arch aneurysm.* A large aneurysm can distort and compress surrounding tissues and structures, producing tracheal tugging. Severe pain may occur in the substernal area, sometimes radiating to the back or side of the chest. A sudden increase in pain may herald impending rupture. Assessment may reveal a visible pulsatile mass in the first or second intercostal space or suprasternal notch, a diastolic murmur of aortic regurgitation, and an aortic systolic murmur and thrill. Other findings may include dyspnea; stridor; hoarseness; dysphagia; brassy cough; hemoptysis; distended jugular veins; edema of the face, neck, or arm; and atelectasis of the left lung.

*Hodgkin's disease.* Development of a tumor adjacent to the aortic arch can cause tracheal tugging. Initial findings include usually painless cervical lymphadenopathy, sustained or remittent fever, fatigue, malaise, pruritus, night sweats, and weight loss. Swollen lymph nodes may become tender and painful. Later findings include dyspnea and stridor; dry cough; dysphagia; distended neck veins; edema of the face, neck, or arm; hepatosplenomegaly; hyperpigmentation, jaundice, or pallor; and neuralgia.

*Non-Hodgkin's lymphoma.* Tracheal tugging may reflect anterior mediastinal lymphadenopathy or tumor development next to the aortic arch. Other findings include painless peripheral lymphadenopathy, fever, fatigue, malaise, night sweats, and weight loss.

*Thymoma.* Tracheal tugging may occur if a tumor develops in the anterior mediastinum. Other findings include cough, chest pain, dysphagia, dyspnea, hoarseness, a palpable neck mass, distended neck veins, and edema of the face, neck, or upper arm.

## Nursing considerations
• Prepare the patient for diagnostic procedures, which may include chest X-ray, computed tomography scan, lymphangiography, aortography, bone marrow biopsy, liver biopsy, echocardiography, and a complete blood count.
• Place the patient in semi-Fowler's position to ease respiration.
• Administer cough suppressants and pain medications, as ordered, keeping alert for signs of respiratory depression.

**T**

Also called plantar reflex, Babinski's reflex is dorsiflexion of the great toe with extension and fanning of the other toes — an abnormal reflex elicited by firmly stroking the sole of the foot. In some patients, this reflex can be triggered by noxious stimuli, such as pain, noise, or even bumping of the bed. It indicates corticospinal damage and helps differentiate neurologic and metabolic coma. Babinski's reflex may occur unilaterally or bilaterally and may be temporary or permanent.

## Physical exam
After eliciting a positive Babinski's reflex, assess the patient for other neurologic signs. Evaluate muscle strength in each extremity by having the patient push or pull against your resistance. Passively flex and extend the extremity to assess muscle tone. Check coordination by asking the patient to perform a repetitive activity. Test deep tendon reflexes in the elbow, antecubital area, wrist, knee, and ankle with a reflex hammer. Then assess pain sensation and proprioception in the feet. As you move the patient's toes up and down, ask him to identify the direction without looking at his feet. Notify the doctor immediately of any changes in his neurologic status.

## Causes
*Brain tumor.* Unilateral or bilateral Babinski's reflex may occur, accompanied by hyperactive deep tendon reflexes, spasticity, seizures, cranial nerve dysfunction, hemiparesis or hemiplegia, decreased pain sensation, unsteady gait, incoordination, headache, emotional lability, and decreased level of consciousness.

*Cerebrovascular accident (CVA).* If the CVA involves the cerebrum, it produces unilateral Babinski's reflex, hemiplegia or hemiparesis, unilateral hyperactive deep tendon reflexes, hemianopia, and aphasia. If it involves the brain stem, it produces bilateral Babinski's reflex, bilateral weakness or paralysis, bilateral hyperactive deep tendon reflexes, cranial nerve dysfunction, incoordination, and unsteady gait.

*Hepatic encephalopathy.* Babinski's reflex occurs late in this disorder when the patient slips into a coma. It's accompanied by hyperactive reflexes and fetor hepaticus.

*Meningitis.* Bilateral Babinski's reflex commonly occurs, preceded by fever, chills, and malaise and accompanied by nausea and vomiting.

*Multiple sclerosis (MS).* In most patients with this demyelinating disorder, Babinski's reflex occurs bilaterally. It follows initial signs and symptoms of MS, most commonly paresthesia, nystagmus, and blurred or double vision.

*Rabies.* Bilateral Babinski's reflex appears in the excitation phase of rabies. This phase occurs 2 to 10 days after the onset of prodromal symptoms, such as fever, malaise, and irritability.

*Spinal cord injury.* In acute injury, spinal shock temporarily erases all reflexes. As shock resolves, Babinski's reflex occurs. Rather than signaling the return of neurologic function, it confirms corticospinal damage.

*Spinal cord tumor.* Bilateral Babinski's reflex occurs with variable loss of pain and temperature sensation, proprioception, and motor function.

*Spinal paralytic poliomyelitis.* Babinski's reflex occurs 5 to 7 days after the onset of fever in this disorder. It's accompanied by progressive weakness, paresthesia, muscle tenderness, spasticity, irritability, and atrophy.

*Other causes.* Amyotrophic lateral sclerosis, familial spastic paralysis, Friedreich's ataxia, head trauma, pernicious anemia, spinal tuberculosis, and syringomyelia.

## Nursing considerations
• Babinski's reflex usually causes incoordination, weakness, and spasticity, increasing the patient's risk of injury. To prevent injury, assist the patient with activities, especially ambulation. Keep his environment tidy.
• Prepare the patient for diagnostic tests, as necessary.

# Tracheal deviation

If the patient's trachea deviates from its normal position, it commonly signals an underlying condition that can compromise pulmonary function and lead to respiratory distress. Normally, the trachea is located at the midline of the neck—except at the bifurcation, where it shifts slightly to the right.

## ▶ Emergency interventions
If the patient exhibits signs of respiratory distress, notify the doctor. If possible, place the patient in semi-Fowler's position to aid respiratory excursion and improve oxygenation. Give supplemental oxygen, and prepare to intubate the patient, if necessary. Insert an I.V. line for fluid and drug administration, and prepare to assist with chest tube insertion, as ordered.

## History
Ask about a history of respiratory or cardiac disorders, trauma, or infection. If the patient smokes, determine how much. Ask about associated symptoms, especially breathing difficulty, pain, and cough.

## Physical exam
Palpate for subcutaneous crepitation in the neck and chest—a sign of tension pneumothorax.

## Causes
*Hiatal hernia.* Tracheal deviation may result from intrusion of abdominal viscera into the pleural space. Other findings may include respiratory distress, pyrosis, regurgitation or vomiting, and chest or abdominal pain.

*Mediastinal tumor.* When large, this tumor can press against the trachea and nearby structures, causing deviation. Other late-stage findings may include dysphagia, stridor, dyspnea, brassy cough, hoarseness, and stertorous respirations with suprasternal retraction.

*Pleural effusion.* A large pleural effusion may lead to tracheal deviation. Other findings may include dry cough, dyspnea, pleuritic pain, pleural friction rub, tachypnea, decreased chest motion, decreased or absent breath sounds, egophony, flatness on percussion, decreased tactile fremitus, fever, and weight loss.

*Pulmonary fibrosis.* Tracheal deviation may result from asymmetrical fibrosis. Other findings may include dyspnea, cough, clubbing, and fever.

*Pulmonary tuberculosis.* Deviation may occur with a large cavitation. Other findings may include asymmetrical chest excursion, dullness on percussion, increased tactile fremitus, amphoric breath sounds, and inspiratory crackles.

*Tension pneumothorax.* Tracheal deviation is a hallmark sign of this life-threatening condition.

The patient experiences a sudden onset of respiratory distress with sharp chest pain, dry cough, severe dyspnea, tachycardia, wheezing, cyanosis, accessory muscle use, nasal flaring, air hunger, and asymmetrical chest movement. Restless and anxious, the patient may also have subcutaneous crepitation in the neck and upper chest, decreased vocal fremitus, decreased or absent breath sounds on the affected side, distended neck veins, and hypotension.

*Thoracic aortic aneurysm.* The trachea usually deviates to the right. Associated findings may include stridor; dyspnea; wheezing; brassy cough; hoarseness; dysphagia; edema of the face, neck, or arm; distended chest wall and neck veins; and substernal, neck, shoulder, or lower back pain, possibly with paresthesia or neuralgia.

*Other causes.* Atelectasis, kyphoscoliosis, and retrosternal thyroid.

## Nursing considerations
- Because of the high risk of respiratory distress, monitor the patient's respiratory and cardiac status constantly, and have emergency equipment readily available.
- Prepare the patient for diagnostic tests, such as chest X-ray, ECG, and arterial blood gas analysis.
- In elderly patients, tracheal deviation to the right may occur normally.

**T**

# Back pain

Back pain may be acute or chronic, constant or intermittent. It may remain localized in the back or radiate along the spine or down one or both legs. Intrinsic back pain results from muscle spasm, nerve root irritation, fracture, or a combination of these mechanisms. It occurs most commonly in the lower back or lumbosacral area and may also be referred from the abdomen, possibly signaling life-threatening perforated ulcer, acute pancreatitis, or dissecting abdominal aortic aneurysm.

▶ **Emergency interventions**
If the patient reports acute, severe back pain, take his vital signs and have another nurse notify the doctor immediately. If the patient describes deep lumbar pain unaffected by activity, palpate for a pulsating epigastric mass. If present, suspect dissecting abdominal aortic aneurysm. Start an I.V. line and administer oxygen. If the patient describes severe epigastric pain that radiates through the abdomen to the back, assess for absent bowel sounds and abdominal rigidity. If these signs are present, suspect a perforated ulcer or acute pancreatitis. Start an I.V. line, administer oxygen, and insert a nasogastric tube, as ordered.

**History**
When stabilized, ask the patient when and how the pain began. Ask him to describe the pain. Does it radiate to the buttocks or legs? Or does it seem to originate in the abdomen and radiate to the back? Also ask him what makes the pain better or worse. Ask about past injuries and illnesses, diet, and alcohol intake. Obtain a drug history.

**Physical exam**
Observe skin color, especially in the legs, and palpate skin temperature. Palpate leg pulses, and ask the patient about numbness and tingling in the legs. Palpate the back for tenderness. Then evaluate and compare reflexes.

**Causes**
*Abdominal aortic aneurysm (dissecting).* A pulsating abdominal mass may be palpated in the epigastrium; after rupture, it no longer pulsates. Other signs include absent femoral and pedal pulses, and lower blood pressure in the legs than in the arms.
*Endometriosis.* Deep sacral pain and severe, cramping pain occur in the lower abdomen. The pain worsens just before or during menstruation.
*Intervertebral disk rupture.* Gradual or sudden low back pain develops with or without leg pain. It's exacerbated by activity, coughing, and sneezing, and is eased by rest.
*Pancreatitis (acute).* This life-threatening disorder produces continuous upper abdominal pain that may radiate to both flanks and to the back.

Early findings include abdominal tenderness, nausea, vomiting, and fever.
*Prostatic carcinoma.* Chronic, aching back pain may be the only symptom, but cloudy urine or hematuria may also occur.
*Spondylolisthesis.* This major structural disorder may produce no symptoms or may cause low back pain with or without nerve root involvement. Other findings include paresthesia, buttocks pain, and pain radiating down the leg.
*Transverse process fracture.* This fracture causes severe localized back pain with muscle spasm.
*Vertebral compression fracture.* Initially, this fracture may be painless. Several weeks later, it causes back pain aggravated by weight bearing.
*Other causes.* Acute pyelonephritis; ankylosing spondylitis; appendicitis; cholecystitis; chordoma; lumbosacral sprain; metastatic tumors, including myeloma; perforated ulcer; Reiter's syndrome; renal calculi; spinal neoplasm; spinal stenosis; and vertebral osteomyelitis and osteoporosis.

**Nursing considerations**
• Withhold analgesics until the doctor makes a tentative diagnosis. Place a pillow under the patient's knees. Encourage relaxation techniques.
• Instruct the patient not to wear a corset or lumbosacral support in bed. Teach him about other ordered pain relief measures.

# Tinnitus

Tinnitus literally means ringing in the ears, although the term encompasses various abnormal sounds. The patient may describe tinnitus as the sound of escaping air, running water, or the inside of a seashell. It may also be described as a sizzling, buzzing, humming, roaring, or musical sound.

## History
Ask the patient about the onset, pattern, pitch, location, and intensity of tinnitus. Is it accompanied by other symptoms, such as vertigo, headache, or hearing loss? Next, take a health history, including a complete drug history.

## Physical exam
Using an otoscope, inspect the patient's ears and examine the tympanic membrane. To check for hearing loss, perform the Weber and Rinne tuning fork tests. Auscultate for bruits in the neck; then compress the jugular or carotid artery to see if this affects tinnitus. Finally, examine the nasopharynx for masses that might cause eustachian tube dysfunction and tinnitus.

## Causes
*Acoustic neuroma.* Tinnitus occurs before unilateral sensorineural hearing loss and vertigo.

  *Anemia.* Severe anemia may produce mild, reversible tinnitus accompanied by such symptoms as dim vision, syncope, and irritability.

  *Atherosclerosis of the carotid artery.* Tinnitus is constant but can be stopped by applying pressure over the carotid artery. The patient feels confused, weak, and unsteady when he rises in the morning or stands up quickly.

  *Cervical spondylosis.* Usually, a stiff neck and pain aggravated by activity produce tinnitus. Other findings may include brief vertigo, nystagmus, hearing loss, and pain that radiates down the arms.

  *Chronic exposure to noise.* Tinnitus and bilateral hearing loss may be permanent.

  *Ear canal obstruction.* Tinnitus may occur with conductive hearing loss, itching, and a feeling of fullness or pain in the ear.

  *Eustachian tube patency.* Audible breath sounds, loud and distorted voice sounds, and a sense of fullness in the ear may accompany tinnitus.

  *Glomus jugulare or tympanicum tumor.* Usually, vibratory tinnitus is the first symptom. Other features include a reddish blue mass behind the tympanic membrane and progressive conductive hearing loss.

  *Hypertension.* Bilateral, high-pitched tinnitus may occur in severe hypertension.

  *Intracranial arteriovenous malformation.* A large malformation may cause pulsating tinnitus accompanied by a bruit over the mastoid process.

  *Labyrinthitis (suppurative).* Tinnitus may be accompanied by severe attacks of vertigo, unilateral or bilateral sensorineural hearing loss, nystagmus, dizziness, nausea, and vomiting.

  *Ménière's disease.* Attacks of low-pitched tinnitus may be accompanied by vertigo and fluctuating sensorineural hearing loss. Usually unilateral, these attacks last from 10 minutes to several hours. Severe nausea, vomiting, diaphoresis, and nystagmus may also occur.

  *Ossicle dislocation.* Tinnitus may be accompanied by sensorineural hearing loss and bleeding from the middle ear.

  *Otosclerosis.* The patient may describe ringing, roaring, or whistling tinnitus. Other findings include progressive hearing loss and vertigo.

  *Tympanic membrane perforation.* Tinnitus is usually the chief complaint in a small perforation. Other findings include hearing loss, pain, vertigo, and a feeling of fullness in the ear.

  *Other causes.* Acute otitis externa; drugs, including quinine, alcohol, indomethacin, aminoglycoside antibiotics, and vancomycin; otitis media; palatal myoclonus; and salicylate overdose.

## Nursing considerations
• Administer vasodilators, tranquilizers, and anticonvulsants, as ordered.
• Encourage use of biofeedback, a hearing aid, or tinnitus maskers, as ordered.

**T**

# Barrel chest

In barrel chest, the normal elliptical configuration of the chest is replaced by a rounded one in which the anteroposterior diameter enlarges to approximate the transverse diameter. The diaphragm is depressed and the sternum pushed forward with the ribs attached in a horizontal — not angular — fashion. As a result, the chest appears continuously in the inspiratory position.

Typically a late sign of chronic obstructive pulmonary disease (COPD), barrel chest results from augmented lung volumes caused by chronic airflow obstruction. It may go unnoticed by the patient because of its gradual development. In elderly people, senile kyphosis of the thoracic spine may be mistaken for barrel chest. But unlike barrel chest, senile kyphosis lacks signs of pulmonary disease.

### History
Begin by asking about a history of pulmonary disease. Note chronic exposure to environmental irritants, such as asbestos. Also ask about the patient's smoking habits. Then explore other symptoms of pulmonary disease. Does the patient have a cough? Is it productive or nonproductive? If it's productive, have him describe sputum color and consistency. Does the patient experience shortness of breath? Is it related to activity? Although dyspnea is common in COPD, many patients fail to associate it with the disease. Instead, they'll blame "old age" or "getting out of shape" for causing dyspnea.

### Physical exam
Auscultate for abnormal breath sounds, such as crackles and wheezes. Then percuss the chest; hyperresonant sounds indicate trapped air, whereas dull or flat sounds indicate mucus buildup. Be alert for accessory muscle use, intercostal retractions, and tachypnea, which may signal respiratory distress. If these signs develop, notify the doctor immediately.

Finally, assess the patient's general appearance. Look for central cyanosis in the cheeks, the nose, and the mucosa inside the lips. Look for peripheral cyanosis in the nail beds. If cyanosis develops, notify the doctor immediately. Also note fingernail clubbing, a late sign of COPD.

### Causes
*Asthma.* Typically, barrel chest develops only in chronic asthma. An acute asthmatic attack causes severe dyspnea, wheezing, and productive cough. It can also cause prolonged expiratory time, accessory muscle use, tachycardia, tachypnea, perspiration, and flushing.

*Chronic bronchitis.* A late sign in chronic bronchitis, barrel chest is characteristically preceded by productive cough and exertional dyspnea. This form of COPD may also cause cyanosis, tachypnea, wheezing, prolonged expiratory time, and accessory muscle use.

*Emphysema.* In this form of COPD, barrel chest is also a late sign. Typically, the disorder begins insidiously, with dyspnea the predominant symptom. Eventually, emphysema may also cause chronic cough, anorexia, weight loss, malaise, accessory muscle use, pursed-lip breathing, tachypnea, peripheral cyanosis, and fingernail clubbing.

### Nursing considerations
• Advise the patient to avoid bronchial irritants — especially smoking — which may exacerbate COPD. Have him notify the doctor of purulent sputum production, which may indicate upper respiratory infection.
• Instruct him to space his activities to help minimize exertional dyspnea.
• To ease breathing, have the patient sit and lean forward, resting his hands on his knees to support the upper torso (tripod position). This position allows maximum diaphragmatic excursion, facilitating chest expansion.

# Tics

A tic is an involuntary, repetitive movement of a specific group of muscles—usually those of the face, neck, shoulders, trunk, and hands. Typically, this sign occurs suddenly and intermittently. It may involve a single isolated movement, such as lip smacking, grimacing, blinking, sniffing, tongue thrusting, throat clearing, hitching up one shoulder, or protruding the chin. Or it may involve a complex set of movements. Mild tics, such as twitching of an eyelid, are especially common.

Usually, tics are psychogenic and may be aggravated by stress or anxiety. Psychogenic tics commonly begin between the ages of 5 and 10 as voluntary, coordinated, and purposeful actions that the child feels compelled to perform to decrease anxiety. Unless the tics are severe, the child may be unaware of them. The tics may subside as the child matures, or they may persist into adulthood. Tics are also associated with one rare affliction—Gilles de la Tourette's syndrome.

To distinguish tics from minor seizures, remember that tics aren't associated with transient loss of consciousness or amnesia.

## History
Ask the parents how long the child has had the tic. Can they identify any precipitating factors? Ask about stress in the child's life, such as difficult school work.

## Physical exam
Carefully observe the tic. Is it a purposeful or involuntary movement? Note whether it's localized or generalized, and describe it in detail.

## Causes
*Gilles de la Tourette's syndrome.* The patient develops a tic that involves the face or neck. Usually, this sign first appears between the ages of 2 and 15. Eventually, the tic spreads to the muscles of the shoulders, arms, trunk, and legs. It may be accompanied by violent movement and outbursts of obscenities (coprolalia). The patient snorts, barks, and grunts and may emit explosive sounds, such as hissing, when he speaks. He may involuntarily repeat another person's words (echolalia) or movements (echopraxia). Occasionally, Tourette's syndrome subsides spontaneously or undergoes a prolonged remission; however, the syndrome may persist throughout life.

*Psychogenic factors.* Tics commonly develop when a child experiences overwhelming anxiety, usually associated with normal maturation. When his ego can no longer balance conflicting influences from his desires, his conscience, and the environment, symptoms can develop.

## Nursing considerations
• As ordered, administer tranquilizers to relieve the source of anxiety causing the tic.
• When treating a patient with Gilles de la Tourette's syndrome, expect to administer haloperidol or pimozide to control tics and reduce anxiety.
• Provide support to the patient who is undergoing psychotherapy to learn to cope with anxiety.
• Help the patient to identify and eliminate any avoidable stress and to learn positive new ways to deal with anxiety.

# Battle's sign

Ecchymosis over the mastoid process of the temporal bone, Battle's sign is often the only outward sign of basilar skull fracture, which can go undetected by skull X-rays. If left untreated, this type of fracture can be fatal because of associated injury to the nearby cranial nerves and brain stem as well as to blood vessels and the meninges. Therefore, Battle's sign must be reported to the doctor immediately.

Appearing behind one or both ears, Battle's sign is easily overlooked or hidden by the patient's hair. During emergency care of the trauma victim, it may be overshadowed by imminently life-threatening or more apparent injuries.

Force exerted on the head great enough to fracture the base of the skull causes Battle's sign by damaging supporting tissues of the mastoid area. It may also result from seepage of blood from the fracture site to the mastoid. Battle's sign usually develops 24 to 36 hours after the fracture and may persist for several days to weeks.

## History
Ask about recent traumatic injury to the head. Did the patient sustain a severe blow to the head? Was he involved in a motor vehicle accident? Note level of consciousness as the patient responds. Does he respond quickly or slowly? Are his answers appropriate, or does he appear confused?

## Physical exam
Check vital signs; be alert for widening pulse pressure and bradycardia, signs of increased intracranial pressure. Assess cranial nerve function, focusing on nerves III, IV, VI, VII, and VIII. Evaluate pupillary size and response to light as well as motor and verbal responses. Relate this data to the Glasgow Coma Scale. Note cerebrospinal fluid (CSF) leakage from the nose or ears.

Ask about postnasal drip, which may reflect CSF drainage down the throat. Also look for the halo sign—blood encircled by a yellowish ring—on bed linens or dressings. To confirm that drainage is CSF, test it with a glucose reagent strip; CSF is positive for glucose, whereas mucus is not. Follow up the neurologic examination with a complete physical examination to detect other injuries associated with basilar skull fracture.

## Cause
*Basilar skull fracture.* Battle's sign may be the only outward sign of this fracture. Or it may be accompanied by periorbital ecchymosis (raccoon eyes), conjunctival hemorrhage, nystagmus, ocular deviation, epistaxis, anosmia, a bulging tympanic membrane (from CSF or blood accumulation), visible fracture lines on the external auditory canal, tinnitus, hearing difficulty, facial paralysis, and vertigo.

## Nursing considerations
- Expect the patient with basilar skull fracture to be on bed rest for several days to weeks. Keep him flat to decrease pressure on dural tears and minimize CSF leakage. Monitor his neurologic status closely.
- Avoid nasogastric intubation and nasopharyngeal suction, which may cause cerebral infection. Also caution the patient against blowing his nose, which may worsen a dural tear.
- The doctor may order skull X-rays and a computed tomography scan to help confirm basilar skull fracture and to evaluate the severity of head injury. Typically, basilar skull fracture and any associated dural tears heal spontaneously within several days to weeks. However, if the patient has a large dural tear, a craniotomy may be necessary to repair the tear with a graft patch.

B

Subnormal temperature, or hypothermia, refers to a core body temperature under 98.6° F (37° C). If the patient's body temperature falls between 82° and 92° F (27.8° and 33.3° C), this indicates *moderate hypothermia*. If the patient's body temperature falls between 62° and 81° F (16.7° and 27.2° C), this indicates *deep hypothermia*. *Profound hypothermia*, a temperature between 39° and 61° F (3.9° and 16.1° C), usually leads to death.

During deep or profound hypothermia, the thermoregulatory center in the hypothalamus becomes depressed. This disrupts the brain's ability to regulate body temperature. Metabolic processes and nerve conduction become progressively slower, resulting in coma and, eventually, respiratory and circulatory failure.

## ▶ Emergency interventions

You may use active or passive measures to rewarm the patient. Active external rewarming may consist of immersing the patient in warm water or applying electric blankets or heating pads. For the patient with a temperature below 85° F (29.4° C), or for one who is comatose, be prepared to assist with peritoneal dialysis, hemodialysis, intragastric lavage with warm fluids, or inhalation warming.

Passive rewarming techniques require you to remove the patient from the cold environment and wrap him in something warm and dry, such as a blanket. If the patient is extremely hypothermic, you may speed up the rewarming process by removing his clothing and wrapping him in the blanket with another person.

## History

Find out if the patient has recently been exposed to cold temperatures or immersed in cold water. If so, for how long was he exposed? Does the patient have adequate heat in his home? Is he homeless? Find out if he has recently received a blood transfusion or undergone surgery. Explore the patient's medical history for thyroid, adrenal, liver, or cerebrovascular disease and for diabetes mellitus. Has he ingested any substances that could induce hypothermia, such as alcohol or barbiturates?

## Physical exam

Observe the patient's skin color, and check capillary refill time. Note the rate and depth of breathing and any abnormal respiratory pattern. Does the patient have difficulty breathing? Inspect his oral mucosa for signs of cyanosis, and assess for abdominal distention. Check peripheral pulses. If fractures have been ruled out, slowly move the patient's arms and legs through a small range of motion to detect any muscle stiffness. Auscultate the lungs and abdomen for hyperresonance and dullness. Percuss the deep tendon reflexes and note any abnormalities. Check all lung fields for adventitious or diminished breath sounds. Then assess the patient's bowel sounds.

## Causes

*Prolonged exposure to extremely low temperatures.* Deep or profound hypothermia may be accompanied by lethargy or coma, depressed respiratory rate and depth, bradycardia, and muscle stiffness.

*Other causes.* Advanced cirrhosis, alcohol or barbiturate ingestion, cerebrovascular accident, diabetes mellitus, hypoadrenalism, hypopituitarism, hypothyroidism, surgical procedures requiring cooling of the body, and transfusion of chilled blood products.

## Nursing considerations

• Note that temperatures do not have to be extremely low to induce hypothermia in elderly or debilitated patients.

A late and ominous sign of neurologic deterioration, Biot's respirations are characterized by breaths of equal volume interrupted by irregular periods of apnea—the cessation of spontaneous respiration. A rare breathing pattern, Biot's respirations may appear abruptly and reflect increased pressure on the medulla coinciding with brain stem herniation.

Biot's respirations are a sign of increased intracranial pressure (ICP) and may occur with spinal meningitis and other conditions involving the central nervous system, such as skull fractures; epidural, subdural, and intercerebral hematomas; and brain tumors.

## ▶ Emergency interventions

Because Biot's respirations signal life-threatening neurologic deterioration, you must notify the doctor immediately when you recognize them.

But first be sure that you've observed the patient's breathing pattern for several minutes to avoid confusing Biot's respirations with Cheyne-Stokes respirations, which are sometimes mistaken for each other. Remember that, whether deep or shallow, the volume of each breath in Biot's respirations is equal. Conversely, Cheyne-Stokes respirations wax and wane, with breaths fluctuating from shallow to deep to shallow.

Prepare to assist the doctor with intubation and mechanical ventilation. Then you should take the patient's vital signs, especially noting increased systolic pressure.

## Cause

*Brain stem herniation.* Biot's respirations are characteristic in this neurologic emergency. Associated signs include pupillary changes, such as inequality and unresponsiveness to light; decorticate or decerebrate posture; bradycardia; and increased systolic pressure.

## Nursing considerations

• Monitor vital signs frequently. Elevate the head of the patient's bed 30 degrees to help reduce ICP.
• Perform neurologic assessment frequently, using the Glasgow Coma Scale. The Glasgow Coma Scale, which grades level of consciousness in relation to eye-opening and motor and verbal responses, is a useful tool for evaluating the severity of a head injury and predicting its outcome.

A Glasgow Coma Scale score of 14 to 15 indicates a minor head injury. A score of 9 to 13 indicates a moderate head injury. A score of less than 8 indicates a severe head injury.
• If ordered, prepare the patient for emergency surgery to relieve pressure on the brain stem caused by a hematoma or space-occupying lesion.
• If necessary, prepare the patient for a computed tomography scan, which may be ordered to confirm the cause of brain stem herniation.
• Because Biot's respirations typically reflect a grave prognosis, give the patient's family emotional support.

**B**

Also known as epiphora, increased tearing refers to an abnormal overflow of tears.

## History

Begin by asking when tearing began. Is it constant or intermittent? Minimal or excessive? Is tearing accompanied by pain? Ask about recent eye trauma, ocular and systemic disorders, and current medications. Ask if the patient reads extensively or works with small objects.

## Physical exam

After taking vital signs, examine both eyes (unless the history suggests a perforating or penetrating injury). Carefully inspect the external structures. Do the eyelashes contain debris?

Examine the eyelids for lesions and edema. Ask the patient to look straight ahead at a fixed object while you check for ptosis. Are the lid margins turned inward or outward? Examine the eyeballs. Do they appear sunken or bulging? Examine the conjunctiva for redness and abnormal drainage. Also note the color of the sclera. Examine the cornea and iris for scars, irregularities, and foreign bodies. Evaluate extraocular muscle function, and test the patient's visual acuity.

## Causes

*Conjunctival foreign bodies and abrasions.* Besides increased tearing, the patient may have localized conjunctival injection, severe eye pain, and photophobia.

*Conjunctivitis.* Increased tearing is accompanied by conjunctival injection and itching. *Allergic conjunctivitis* causes ropy or stringy discharge. *Bacterial conjunctivitis* causes copious, purulent discharge; burning; and a foreign-body sensation. *Viral conjunctivitis* causes a foreign-body sensation, slight exudate, and lid edema.

*Corneal abrasion.* Increased tearing may be accompanied by severe corneal pain that's aggravated by blinking.

*Corneal foreign body.* Besides increased tearing, the patient may have blurred vision, a foreign-body sensation, photophobia, eye pain, miosis, and conjunctival injection.

*Corneal ulcers.* Increased tearing is accompanied by severe photophobia, eye pain that's aggravated by blinking, blurred vision, conjunctival injection, and a white, opaque cornea.

*Dacryocystitis.* This disorder produces increased tearing and purulent discharge. Other findings include pain and tenderness around the tear sac with marked eyelid edema and redness near the lacrimal punctum.

*Episcleritis.* Besides increased tearing, findings include photophobia and eye pain and tenderness.

*Herpes zoster.* Increased tearing results from infection of the trigeminal nerve. It's accompanied by severe unilateral facial and eye pain and the eruption of vesicles.

*Psoriasis vulgaris.* When lesions affect the eyelids and extend into the conjunctiva, they may cause irritation with increased tearing and a foreign-body sensation.

*Raeder's paratrigeminal syndrome.* The patient may have increased tearing, ptosis, abnormal pupillary response, ipsilateral headache, and anhidrosis of the face and neck. Periodic symptomatic attacks last for 5 minutes or longer.

*Thyrotoxicosis.* Increased tearing may occur in both eyes. Other ocular effects may include ptosis, lid edema, photophobia, a foreign-body sensation, conjunctival injection, chemosis, and diplopia.

*Trachoma.* Increased tearing is accompanied by visible conjunctival follicles, red and edematous eyelids, pain, photophobia, and exudation.

*Other causes.* Blepharophimosis, eyelid contractions, punctum displacement, scleritis, and use of miotics.

## Nursing considerations

- Obtain a tear specimen for culture, as ordered.
- Prepare the patient for Schirmer's test and for irrigation of the lacrimal drainage system, as ordered. Instruct him not to touch the unaffected eye.

T

# Bladder distention

When an unusually large amount of urine accumulates in the bladder, the organ may distend beyond its normal limits. Distention can result from mechanical or anatomic obstructions, neuromuscular disorders, and drugs. Relatively common in all ages and both sexes, it occurs most frequently in older men who have prostate disorders.

Typically, bladder distention occurs gradually and remains asymptomatic until stretching of the bladder produces discomfort. Acute distention produces perineal fullness, pressure, and pain. If severe distention isn't corrected promptly, the risk of rupture increases.

▶ **Emergency interventions**
If the patient has severe distention, insert an indwelling urinary catheter, as ordered, to help relieve discomfort and prevent bladder rupture.

## History
Review the patient's voiding patterns. Find out the time and amount of his last voiding and the amount of fluid consumed since then. Ask if the patient has difficulty initiating urination, if urination occurs with urgency or without warning, and if it causes pain or irritation. Ask about the force and continuity of the patient's urine stream and if he feels that his bladder is empty after voiding.

Ask about urinary tract obstruction or infections; venereal disease; neurologic, intestinal, or pelvic surgery; lower abdominal or urinary tract trauma; and systemic or neurologic disorders. Note his drug history.

## Physical exam
Take the patient's vital signs, and percuss and palpate the bladder. Inspect the urethral meatus and measure its diameter. Describe the appearance and amount of any discharge. Test for perineal sensation and anal sphincter tone, and in the male patient, examine the prostate.

## Causes
*Benign prostatic hyperplasia.* Bladder distention gradually develops as the prostate enlarges. Other findings include urinary hesitancy, straining, and frequency; reduced force of the urine stream; nocturia; and postvoiding dribbling.

*Multiple sclerosis.* Urine retention results from interruption of upper motor neuron control of the bladder. Other findings include optic neuritis, paresthesia, impaired position and vibratory senses, diplopia, nystagmus, dizziness, abnormal reflexes, dysarthria, muscle weakness, emotional lability, Lhermitte's sign, and ataxia.

*Prostatitis.* In *acute prostatitis,* bladder distention occurs rapidly, along with perineal discomfort and fullness. In *chronic prostatitis,* bladder distention usually occurs gradually, along with perineal discomfort and fullness.

*Spinal neoplasms.* Neurogenic bladder results, followed by distention. Findings include a sense of pelvic fullness, back pain, constipation, tender vertebral processes, sensory deficits, and muscle weakness, flaccidity, and atrophy.

*Urethral stricture.* This disorder results in urine retention and bladder distention with chronic urethral discharge (most common symptom), urinary frequency and urgency, dysuria, decreased force and diameter of the urine stream, and pyuria.

*Other causes.* Bladder calculi; bladder neoplasms; catheterization; diabetes mellitus; drugs, such as parasympatholytics, ganglionic blockers, sedatives, anesthetics, and opiates; prostatic neoplasms; urethral calculi.

## Nursing considerations
• Monitor the patient's vital signs and the extent of bladder distention. Encourage him to change positions to alleviate discomfort. Give analgesics if ordered.
• If the patient doesn't require immediate urethral catheterization, suggest that he assume the normal voiding position. Teach him to perform Valsalva's maneuver, or gently perform Credé's maneuver.
• Prepare the patient for diagnostic tests or surgery, if necessary.

**B**

# Taste abnormalities

Types of taste abnormalities include *ageusia,* complete loss of taste; *hypogeusia,* partial loss of taste; and *dysgeusia,* distorted sense of taste. In *cacogeusia,* food may taste unpleasant or revolting.

Concentrated over the tongue's surface, taste buds can differentiate among sweet, salty, sour, and bitter stimuli. Taste and olfactory receptors work together to perceive more complex flavors. Taste abnormalities may result from any factor that interrupts transmission of taste stimuli to the brain. Such factors may include trauma, infection, vitamin or mineral deficiency, neurologic or oral disorders, mouth dryness, and drug use. Aging and smoking may interfere with taste as well.

## History
Note the patient's age, and ask when his taste abnormality began. Does the patient have a history of oral or other disorders? Has he recently had the flu? Any head trauma? Does he smoke? Is he receiving radiation treatments? Have the patient list drugs he's currently taking.

## Physical exam
To evaluate taste, gently withdraw the patient's tongue slightly with a gauze sponge. Then use a moistened applicator to place a few crystals of salt or sugar on one side of the tongue. Wipe the tongue clean, and ask the patient to identify the taste sensation. Repeat the test on the other side of the tongue. To test bitter taste sensation, apply a tiny amount of quinine to the base of the tongue. To test sour taste sensation, place electrodes on the surface of either side of the tongue, and use low-voltage direct current.

Evaluate sense of smell. Pinch off one nostril, and ask the patient to close his eyes and sniff through the open nostril to identify nonirritating odors, such as coffee, lime, and wintergreen. Repeat the test on the opposite nostril.

## Causes
*Basilar skull fracture.* Impaired taste may result if fracture affects the cranial nerves. Usually, the patient cannot taste aromatic flavors, although he can still identify sweet, salty, sour, and bitter stimuli. Other findings include anosmia, epistaxis, rhinorrhea, otorrhea, Battle's sign, raccoon's eyes, headache, nausea and vomiting, hearing and vision loss, and decreased level of consciousness.

*Bell's palsy.* Taste loss usually involves the anterior two-thirds of the tongue. Hemifacial muscle weakness or paralysis also occurs. Other signs include drooling, tearing, diminished or absent corneal reflex, and difficulty blinking the affected eye.

*Influenza.* After this viral infection, the patient may have hypogeusia, dysgeusia, or both. An impaired sense of smell is common.

*Oral cancer.* Oral tumors involving the tongue, especially the posterior portion and the lateral borders, may destroy or damage taste buds. The patient may also experience halitosis and difficulty chewing and speaking.

*Sjögren's syndrome.* Extreme mouth dryness may impair taste. Ocular dryness may cause burning and pain around the eyes and under the lids. Later, the patient develops photosensitivity, impaired vision, and eye fatigue and redness. Other findings may include mouth soreness; difficulty chewing, swallowing, and talking; a dry cough; hoarseness; epistaxis; dry, scaly skin; decreased sweating; abdominal distress; and polyuria.

*Viral hepatitis (acute).* Hypogeusia commonly precedes jaundice by 1 to 2 weeks. Other preicteric findings include altered sense of smell, anorexia, nausea, vomiting, fatigue, headache, photophobia, sore throat, cough, and muscle and joint aches.

*Other causes.* Common cold; Déjérine-Roussy syndrome and other thalamic syndromes; drugs, such as penicillamine, captopril, griseofulvin, lithium, rifampin, antithyroid preparations, procarbazine, vincristine, and vinblastine; irradiation of the head or neck; and vitamin $B_{12}$ or zinc deficiency.

## Nursing considerations
• Modify the patient's diet to enable him to distinguish and enjoy as many tastes as possible.

Also called hypotension, decreased blood pressure refers to inadequate blood pressure to perfuse or oxygenate the body's tissues.

Because normal blood pressure varies, every blood pressure reading must be compared against the patient's baseline. A reading under 90/60 mm Hg, or a drop of 30 mm Hg from the baseline, is considered decreased blood pressure.

## ▶ Emergency interventions

If the patient's systolic blood pressure is less than 80 mm Hg, or 30 mm Hg below his baseline, suspect shock. To confirm it, assess for a decreased level of consciousness. Check apical pulse for tachycardia and respirations for tachypnea; inspect for cool, clammy skin. Have another nurse notify the doctor immediately. Start an I.V. line and administer oxygen. Monitor the patient's intake and output. Keep his spinal column immobile.

## History

Ask the patient about weakness, blurred vision, chest pain, difficulty breathing, and dizziness. If these episodes occur when he stands, take his blood pressure with him lying down, sitting, then standing; compare readings. A drop in systolic or diastolic pressure of 10 to 20 mm Hg caused by position changes suggests postural hypotension.

## Physical exam

Inspect the skin for pallor, diaphoresis, and clamminess. Palpate peripheral pulses. Note paradoxical pulse. Auscultate for heart rate, rhythm, and sounds. Auscultate the lungs for abnormal breath sounds. Check respiratory rate and rhythm. Check for signs of hemorrhage, palpable masses, bruising, tenderness, abdominal rigidity, and bowel sounds.

## Causes

*Anaphylactic shock.* A dramatic fall in blood pressure and narrowed pulse pressure follow exposure to an allergen. Findings include anxiety, restlessness, itching, and pounding headache.

*Cardiac tamponade.* An accentuated fall in systolic pressure during inspiration, known as pulsus paradoxus, is characteristic in cardiac tamponade. Other findings include cyanosis, tachycardia, dyspnea, and Kussmaul's respirations.

*Cardiogenic shock.* Accompanying systolic pressure less than 80 mm Hg, or 30 mm Hg less than baseline, are narrowed pulse pressure, diminished Korotkoff sounds, peripheral cyanosis, and pale, cool, clammy skin.

*Diagnostic tests.* These include the gastric acid stimulation test using histamine, and X-ray studies using contrast media.

*Drugs.* Calcium channel blockers, diuretics, vasodilators, antihypertensives, anesthetics, narcotics, monoamine oxidase inhibitors, antianxiety agents, tranquilizers, and I.V. antiarrhythmics can cause low blood pressure.

*Hypovolemic shock.* Accompanying systolic pressure less than 80 mm Hg, or 30 mm Hg less than baseline, are diminished Korotkoff sounds, narrowed pulse pressure, and rapid, weak, or irregular pulse.

*Neurogenic shock.* Blood pressure decreases and bradycardia results. The patient's skin remains warm and dry.

*Septic shock.* Initial signs include fever, chills, and rash. Low blood pressure, tachycardia, and tachypnea may also develop. Later, decreased blood pressure accompanies narrowed pulse pressure.

*Other causes.* Acute adrenal insufficiency, alcohol toxicity, cardiac arrhythmias or contusion, congestive heart failure, diabetic ketoacidosis, hyperosmolar nonketotic syndrome, hypoxemia, myocardial infarction, pulmonary embolism, vasovagal syncope.

## Nursing considerations

• Check the patient's vital signs frequently. If blood pressure is extremely low, assist with insertion of an arterial catheter, or use a Doppler flowmeter, to allow close monitoring of pressures.

• Prepare the patient for diagnostic tests.

**B**

# Tachypnea

A common sign of cardiopulmonary disorders, tachypnea refers to an abnormally fast respiratory rate — 20 breaths or more per minute.

## ▶ Emergency interventions

If tachypnea is accompanied by cyanosis, chest pain, dyspnea, tachycardia, and hypotension, have a colleague notify the doctor at once. If the patient has paradoxical chest movement, splint his chest with your hands or with sandbags. Administer supplemental oxygen. Insert an I.V. line and begin cardiac monitoring. Prepare to assist with intubation and mechanical ventilation.

## History

Find out when the tachypnea began. Did it follow activity? Has it happened before? Ask about related findings, such as diaphoresis and recent weight loss. Is the patient anxious? Note whether he takes pain medication and if it's effective.

## Physical exam

Take vital signs and observe the patient. Does he seem restless? Auscultate for abnormal heart and lung sounds, and assess for jugular vein distention.

## Causes

*Adult respiratory distress syndrome.* Tachypnea and apprehension occur, perhaps with accessory muscle use, grunting expirations, suprasternal and intercostal retractions, crackles, and rhonchi.

*Anaphylactic shock.* Tachypnea develops quickly. Other findings include anxiety, pounding headache, skin flushing, and intense pruritus.

*Aspiration of a foreign body.* In *partial obstruction,* a dry, paroxysmal cough and rapid, shallow respirations develop abruptly. *Complete obstruction* may rapidly cause asphyxia and death.

*Asthma.* Attacks usually begin with mild wheezing and a dry cough that progresses to mucus expectoration. Tachypnea is common.

*Cardiac tamponade.* Tachypnea may accompany tachycardia, dyspnea, and pulsus paradoxus. Other findings include muffled heart sounds, pericardial friction rub, chest pain, and hypotension.

*Cardiogenic shock.* Besides tachypnea, the patient commonly has cold, pale, clammy, cyanotic skin; hypotension; tachycardia; narrowed pulse pressure; a ventricular gallop; oliguria; decreased level of consciousness; and neck vein distention.

*Emphysema.* Tachypnea is accompanied by dyspnea on exertion.

*Flail chest.* Tachypnea usually appears early. Other findings include paradoxical chest wall movement, rib bruises, localized chest pain, hypotension, and diminished breath sounds.

*Hypovolemic shock.* The patient has cool, pale skin; restlessness; thirst; and mild tachycardia.

*Mesothelioma (malignant).* Tachypnea and dyspnea occur on mild exertion. Other findings include shoulder and chest pain.

*Neurogenic shock.* Tachypnea commonly occurs with apprehension, bradycardia or tachycardia, oliguria, fluctuating body temperature, decreased level of consciousness, and warm, dry skin.

*Pneumonia (bacterial).* Tachypnea is preceded by a painful, hacking, dry cough that rapidly becomes productive.

*Pneumothorax.* Tachypnea may accompany severe, sharp, unilateral chest pain.

*Pulmonary edema.* Tachypnea may accompany dyspnea on exertion, paroxysmal nocturnal dyspnea and, later, orthopnea.

*Pulmonary embolism (acute).* Tachypnea occurs suddenly along with dyspnea and chest pain.

*Septic shock.* Tachypnea may accompany sudden fever and chills.

*Other causes.* Alcohol withdrawal syndrome, arrhythmias, bronchiectasis, chronic bronchitis, head trauma, hyperosmolar nonketotic syndrome, interstitial fibrosis, lung abscess, primary pulmonary hypertension, salicylate overdose, and tumors.

## Nursing considerations

• Calm the patient and administer low-flow oxygen, if needed.

**T**

# Blood pressure, increased

Also called hypertension, elevated blood pressure is an intermittent or sustained increase in blood pressure exceeding 140/86 mm Hg. It may develop suddenly or gradually. A sudden, severe rise in blood pressure (exceeding 200/120 mm Hg) indicates life-threatening hypertensive crisis.

Unfortunately, elevated blood pressure may simply reflect an inaccurate measurement. Each reading must be compared with the patient's baseline.

▶ **Emergency interventions**
If blood pressure exceeds 200/120 mm Hg, notify the doctor and maintain airway patency. Institute seizure precautions and prepare to give I.V. antihypertensive drugs and diuretics. Insert an indwelling catheter to monitor urine output.

## History
If the patient isn't in hypertensive crisis, ask about a family history of increased blood pressure, pheochromocytoma, and polycystic kidney disease. Obtain a drug history, including over-the-counter drugs. If the patient is already taking antihypertensive drugs, evaluate compliance.

## Physical exam
Using a funduscope, check for intraocular hemorrhage, exudate, and papilledema. Check for carotid bruits and neck vein distention. Assess skin color, temperature, and turgor. Palpate peripheral pulses. Auscultate for heart rate, rhythm, and sounds. Auscultate the lungs for abnormal breath sounds. Check respiratory rate and rhythm.

Take blood pressures with the patient supine, then sitting and standing. Normally, systolic pressure falls and diastolic pressure rises on standing. In postural hypotension, both pressures fall.

Palpate the abdomen for tenderness, masses, or liver enlargement. Auscultate for abdominal bruits. Palpate the liver and kidneys.

## Causes
*Aortic aneurysm (dissecting).* Initially, this life-threatening disorder causes a sudden rise in systolic pressure, but no change in diastolic pressure. In an *abdominal aneurysm,* there may be persistent abdominal and back pain, weakness, sweating, tachycardia, dyspnea, a pulsating abdominal mass, restlessness, confusion, and cool, clammy skin. In a *thoracic aneurysm,* there may be a ripping or tearing sensation in the chest.

*Drugs.* Central nervous system stimulants, sympathomimetics, corticosteroids, oral contraceptives, monoamine oxidase inhibitors, and cocaine can increase blood pressure.

*Hypertension. Essential hypertension* develops insidiously, marked by a gradual rise in blood pressure. The patient may be asymptomatic or report suboccipital headache, light-headedness, tinnitus, and fatigue. In *malignant hypertension,* diastolic pressure abruptly rises above 120 mm Hg, and systolic pressure may exceed 200 mm Hg.

*Pheochromocytoma.* Paroxysmal or sustained hypertension is characteristic, possibly accompanied by postural hypotension. Other findings: anxiety, diaphoresis, palpitations, and tremors.

*Polycystic kidney disease.* Elevated blood pressure is typically preceded by flank pain. Other signs include enlarged kidneys; enlarged, tender liver; and intermittent gross hematuria.

*Renovascular stenosis.* Systolic and diastolic pressures rise abruptly. Characteristic findings: bruits over the upper abdomen or in the costovertebral angles, hematuria, and acute flank pain.

*Other causes.* Aldosteronism, anemia, atherosclerosis, Cushing's syndrome, eclampsia, increased intracranial pressure, MI, pyelonephritis, thyrotoxicosis, and some treatments.

## Nursing considerations
• Stress the need for follow-up diagnostic tests.
• If the patient has essential hypertension, explain the need for long-term blood pressure control. Encourage weight loss, if necessary, and restricted sodium intake. Suggest an exercise program.
• Teach the patient how to monitor his blood pressure and when to notify his doctor.

**B**

Tachycardia is a heart rate greater than 100 beats/minute. The patient may complain of palpitations or of his heart "racing." This sign may result from emotional or physical stress or the use of stimulants, such as caffeine. It may also indicate a life-threatening disorder.

## ▶ Emergency interventions

After detecting tachycardia, assess for signs of reduced cardiac output. Have a colleague notify the doctor while you administer oxygen, begin cardiac monitoring, insert an I.V. line, and gather emergency resuscitation equipment.

## History

Ask if the patient has had palpitations before. If so, how were they treated? Is he dizzy, short of breath, weak, fatigued, or complaining of chest pain? Ask about a history of trauma, diabetes, drug use, and cardiac, pulmonary, or thyroid disorders.

## Physical exam

Inspect the patient's skin for pallor or cyanosis. Assess pulses, noting peripheral edema. Auscultate the heart and lungs.

## Causes

*Adult respiratory distress syndrome.* Besides tachycardia, findings may include crackles, dyspnea, tachypnea, and grunting respirations.

*Anaphylactic shock.* Tachycardia and hypotension develop quickly. Other findings include anxiety, severe pruritus, and a pounding headache.

*Aortic insufficiency.* Tachycardia is accompanied by a "water-hammer" bounding pulse and a large, diffuse apical heave. Auscultation may reveal an atrial or ventricular gallop.

*Aortic stenosis.* Findings include tachycardia; a weak, thready pulse; and atrial or ventricular gallop.

*Cardiac tamponade.* Tachycardia commonly occurs with pulsus paradoxus and tachypnea.

*Cardiogenic shock.* Tachycardia may accompany a weak, thready pulse; narrowing pulse pressure; hypotension; tachypnea; and cold, clammy skin.

*Chronic obstructive pulmonary disease.* Besides tachycardia, findings include a cough, tachypnea, dyspnea, pursed-lip breathing, accessory muscle use, cyanosis, crackles, and wheezing.

*Congestive heart failure.* Ventricular gallop, dyspnea, and orthopnea may occur.

*Diabetic ketoacidosis.* Tachycardia and a thready pulse may be accompanied by abnormally rapid, deep breathing; fruity breath odor; orthostatic hypotension; and abdominal pain.

*Hypertensive crisis.* Tachycardia and tachypnea are accompanied by increased blood pressure.

*Hypovolemic shock.* Tachypnea, restlessness, thirst, and pale, cool skin may occur.

*Hypoxemia.* Tachycardia may accompany tachypnea, dyspnea, and cyanosis. Confusion, syncope, and incoordination may also occur.

*Orthostatic hypotension.* Tachycardia accompanies dizziness, syncope, pallor, blurred vision, diaphoresis, and nausea.

*Pneumothorax.* Findings include tachycardia, dyspnea, chest pain, tachypnea, cyanosis, a dry cough, and absent or decreased breath sounds.

*Pulmonary embolism.* Tachycardia may follow sudden dyspnea and anginal or pleuritic chest pain. Other findings include tachypnea, restlessness, and a cough with blood-tinged sputum.

*Septic shock.* Findings may include tachycardia, chills, sudden fever, and warm, dry skin.

*Other causes.* Adrenocortical insufficiency; alcohol intoxication or withdrawal; anemia; cardiac arrhythmias; cardiac catheterization; cardiac contusion; cardiac surgery; drugs, such as sympathomimetics, phenothiazines, anticholinergics, thyroid drugs, vasodilators, nitrates, and alpha-adrenergic blockers; electrophysiologic studies; febrile illness; hyperosmolar nonketotic syndrome; hypoglycemia; hyponatremia; myocardial infarction; neurogenic shock; pacemaker malfunction; pheochromocytoma; and thyrotoxicosis.

## Nursing considerations

• Continue to monitor the patient closely.

If no bowel sounds can be heard while listening through a stethoscope for at least 5 minutes over each abdominal quadrant, a patient is considered to have absent bowel sounds, a condition also known as silent abdomen.

Bowel sounds cease when mechanical or vascular obstruction or neurogenic inhibition halts peristalsis. Mechanical obstruction—from adhesions, hernia, or tumor—causes dehydration. Vascular obstruction cuts off circulation to the intestinal walls, causing ischemia, necrosis, and shock.

Abrupt cessation of bowel sounds, when accompanied by abdominal pain, rigidity, and distention, signals a life-threatening crisis requiring immediate intervention. Absent bowel sounds following a period of hyperactivity are equally ominous.

## ▶ Emergency interventions

If you fail to detect bowel sounds and the patient reports sudden, severe abdominal pain and cramping or exhibits severe abdominal distention, call the doctor immediately. Prepare to assist with insertion of a nasogastric or intestinal tube to suction lumen contents and decompress the bowel. Administer I.V. fluids and electrolytes, as ordered, to offset any dehydration and imbalances caused by the dysfunctioning bowel. Because the patient may require surgery, withhold oral intake, as ordered. Take the patient's vital signs, and be alert for signs of shock. Measure abdominal girth as a baseline for gauging subsequent changes.

## History

Ask first about abdominal pain: When did it begin? Has it gotten worse? Where do you feel it? Also ask about a sensation of bloating and flatulence. Ask if the patient has had diarrhea, pencil-thin stools, or no bowel movements at all.

Ask about abdominal tumors, hernias, adhesions from past surgery, and recent accidents that may have caused vascular clots. Check for a history of acute pancreatitis, diverticulitis, or gynecologic infection. Ask about previous toxic conditions, spinal cord injury, and surgical history.

## Physical exam

Inspect the abdominal contour. Check for localized or generalized distention. Percuss and palpate the abdomen gently. Listen for dullness over fluid-filled areas and tympany over pockets of gas. Palpate for abdominal rigidity and guarding.

## Causes

*Complete mechanical intestinal obstruction.* Absent bowel sounds follow a period of hyperactive bowel sounds in this potentially life-threatening disorder. This silence accompanies acute, colicky abdominal pain in the quadrant of obstruction. Other findings include abdominal distention and bloating, constipation, and nausea and vomiting.

*Mesenteric artery occlusion.* In this life-threatening disorder, bowel sounds disappear after a brief period of hyperactive sounds. Sudden, severe midepigastric or periumbilical pain occurs next, followed by abdominal distention.

*Paralytic (adynamic) ileus.* The cardinal sign of this potentially life-threatening disorder is absent bowel sounds. Other findings include abdominal distention, discomfort, and constipation or passage of flatus and small, liquid stools.

*Other causes.* Abdominal surgery.

## Nursing considerations

- After you've inserted a nasogastric or an intestinal tube, elevate the head of the patient's bed at least 30 degrees, and turn the patient as ordered to facilitate passage of the tube through the GI tract. Don't tape an intestinal tube to the patient's face. Ensure tube patency by checking for drainage and for properly functioning suction devices, and irrigate as ordered. Monitor GI drainage losses.
- Give I.V. fluids and electrolytes, as ordered, and send a serum specimen to the laboratory for analysis at least once a day.
- Give drugs, as ordered, to control pain and stimulate peristalsis.

**B**

# Syncope

A common neurologic sign, syncope is transient loss of consciousness associated with impaired cerebral oxygenation. It usually occurs abruptly and lasts for seconds to minutes. In many cases, the patient lies motionless with his skeletal muscles relaxed but sphincter muscles controlled. Depth of unconsciousness varies; some patients can hear voices or see blurred outlines, whereas others are unaware of their surroundings.

Signs include striking pallor; a slow, weak pulse; hypotension; and almost imperceptible breathing. If loss of consciousness lasts for 15 to 20 seconds, the patient may develop convulsive, tonic-clonic movements.

Syncope may also follow vigorous coughing (tussive syncope) and emotional stress, injury, shock, or pain (vasovagal syncope). Hysterical syncope may also follow emotional stress but isn't accompanied by other vasodepressor effects.

## ▶ Emergency interventions

If you witness syncope, place the patient in a supine position, elevate his legs, and loosen any tight clothing. Ensure a patent airway and take vital signs. If you detect tachycardia, bradycardia, or an irregular pulse, have a colleague notify the doctor. Place the patient on a cardiac monitor to detect arrhythmias; if they occur, give oxygen and insert an I.V. line for drug administration. Be prepared to begin cardiopulmonary resuscitation and to assist with cardioversion, defibrillation, or insertion of a temporary pacemaker, as needed.

## History

Discuss episodes of syncope with the patient. Did he feel weak, light-headed, nauseous, or sweaty before fainting? Did he get up quickly from a chair or from lying down? During syncope, did he have muscle spasms or incontinence? How long was he unconscious? Upon awakening, was he alert or confused? Did he have a headache? Has he experienced syncope before? How often does it occur?

## Physical exam

Take the patient's vital signs and assess for injuries he may have incurred during his fall.

## Causes

*Aortic arch syndrome.* Syncope may be accompanied by weak or abruptly absent carotid pulses and unequal or absent radial pulses. Other findings include night sweats, pallor, nausea, anorexia, weight loss, arthralgia, Raynaud's phenomenon, chest pain, and hypotension in the arms.

*Aortic stenosis.* Syncope is accompanied by exertional dyspnea and anginal chest pain. Auscultation may reveal atrial and ventricular gallops as well as a harsh, crescendo-decrescendo systolic ejection murmur that's loudest at the right sternal border of the second intercostal space.

*Cardiac arrhythmias.* Syncope may follow palpitations, pallor, confusion, diaphoresis, dyspnea, and hypotension. In Adams-Stokes syndrome, syncope may occur several times daily.

*Carotid sinus hypersensitivity.* Triggered by compression of the carotid sinus, syncope lasts several minutes and is followed by mental clarity.

*Hypoxemia.* Findings include syncope, restlessness, confusion, tachycardia, and incoordination.

*Orthostatic hypotension.* Rising quickly from a recumbent position may produce syncope. It follows a drop of 10 to 20 mm Hg or more in systolic or diastolic blood pressure, tachycardia, pallor, dizziness, blurred vision, nausea, and diaphoresis.

*Transient ischemic attack.* Findings include syncope, decreased level of consciousness, vision changes, aphasia, dysarthria, unilateral numbness, and hemiparesis or hemiplegia.

*Other causes.* Drugs, such as quinidine, prazosin, griseofulvin, levodopa, and indomethacin; and vagal or glossopharyngeal neuralgia.

## Nursing considerations

• Monitor the patient's vital signs closely.
• Advise the patient to pace activities, to rise slowly, to avoid prolonged standing, and to sit or lie down if he feels faint.

Sometimes audible without a stethoscope, hyperactive bowel sounds reflect increased intestinal motility (peristalsis). They're commonly characterized as rapid, rushing, gurgling waves of sound and may stem from life-threatening bowel obstruction or GI hemorrhage. Hyperactive bowel sounds may also stem from GI infection, inflammatory bowel disease, food allergies, and stress.

## ▶ Emergency interventions

After detecting hyperactive bowel sounds, quickly check vital signs and ask the patient about associated symptoms, such as abdominal pain, vomiting, and diarrhea. If the patient reports cramping abdominal pain or vomiting, continue to auscultate for bowel sounds and have another nurse notify the doctor. If bowel sounds stop abruptly, suspect complete bowel obstruction and prepare to assist with GI suction and decompression, as ordered, and to give I.V. fluids and electrolytes. If ordered, prepare the patient for surgery.

Record the frequency, amount, color, and consistency of stools. If you detect excessive watery diarrhea or bleeding, prepare to administer antidiarrheal drugs, I.V. fluids and electrolytes, or blood transfusions, as ordered.

## History

Obtain a detailed medical and surgical history.

Ask the patient about hernia and abdominal surgery, a history of inflammatory bowel disease, and recent eruptions of gastroenteritis among family members, friends, or co-workers. If the patient has traveled recently, even within the United States, was he aware of any endemic illnesses?

Ask about stress, food allergies, and recent ingestion of unusual foods or fluids. Check for fever, which suggests infection.

## Physical exam

Having already auscultated, now gently inspect, percuss, and palpate the abdomen.

## Causes

*Crohn's disease.* Hyperactive bowel sounds usually arise insidiously. Other findings include diarrhea, cramping abdominal pain, anorexia, low-grade fever, abdominal distention and tenderness, and a fixed mass in the right lower quadrant.

*Food hypersensitivity.* Hyperactive bowel sounds follow ingestion of allergenic foods. Other findings may include diarrhea, nausea, and vomiting.

*Gastroenteritis.* Hyperactive bowel sounds follow sudden nausea and vomiting and accompany "explosive" diarrhea. Abdominal cramping is common.

*Gastrointestinal hemorrhage.* Hyperactive bowel sounds provide the most immediate indication of persistent bleeding. Other findings may include abdominal distention and pain, bloody diarrhea, and rectal passage of bright red blood clots and jellylike material.

*Mechanical intestinal obstruction.* Hyperactive bowel sounds occur simultaneously with cramping abdominal pain every few minutes in this potentially life-threatening disorder. In small-bowel obstruction, nausea and vomiting occur earlier and with greater severity than in large-bowel obstruction. In complete bowel obstruction, hyperactive sounds are also accompanied by abdominal distention and constipation.

*Ulcerative colitis (acute).* Hyperactive bowel sounds arise abruptly in this disorder. They're accompanied by bloody diarrhea, anorexia, abdominal pain, nausea, vomiting, fever, and tenesmus. Weight loss may occur.

## Nursing considerations

• If ordered, prepare the patient for diagnostic tests.
• Explain prescribed dietary changes to the patient. Stress commonly precipitates bowel hyperactivity, so teach him relaxation techniques.
• Encourage rest. Restrict the patient's physical activity, as ordered.

A loud, harsh, musical respiratory sound, stridor may begin as low-pitched "croaking" and progress to high-pitched "crowing." It results from obstruction in the trachea or larynx. Usually heard during inspiration, stridor may occur during expiration in severe upper airway obstruction.

## ▶ Emergency interventions

Upon hearing stridor, quickly check the patient's vital signs and assess for signs of partial airway obstruction — choking or gagging, tachypnea, dyspnea, shallow respirations, intercostal retractions, nasal flaring, tachycardia, cyanosis, and diaphoresis. (Abrupt cessation of stridor signals complete obstruction. Be alert for inspiratory chest movement, absent breath sounds, inability to talk, lethargy, and loss of consciousness.) If you suspect airway obstruction, have a colleague notify the doctor immediately while you perform back blows or abdominal thrusts. Administer oxygen by nasal cannula or face mask, or prepare for intubation or emergency tracheotomy and mechanical ventilation. Have equipment ready to suction any aspirated vomitus or blood. Connect the patient to a cardiac monitor and position him upright.

## History

Find out when the stridor began. Has the patient had it before? Does he have an upper respiratory infection? If so, how long has he had it? Ask about past allergies, tumors, and respiratory and vascular disorders. Note recent exposure to smoke or noxious fumes or gases. Next, explore associated signs and symptoms, such as pain or cough.

## Physical exam

Examine the patient's mouth for excessive secretions, foreign matter, inflammation, and swelling. Assess his neck for swelling, masses, subcutaneous crepitation, or scars. Observe the patient's chest for delayed, decreased, or asymmetrical chest expansion. Auscultate for wheezes, rhonchi, crackles, rubs, and other abnormal breath sounds. Percuss for dullness, tympany, or flatness. Note any burns or signs of trauma.

## Causes

*Airway trauma.* Sudden onset of stridor may be accompanied by dysphonia, dysphagia, hemoptysis, cyanosis, accessory muscle use, intercostal retractions, nasal flaring, tachypnea, progressive dyspnea, shallow respirations, and subcutaneous crepitation (in the neck or upper chest).

*Anaphylaxis.* Stridor results from upper airway edema. Other findings include nasal flaring, wheezing, accessory muscle use, intercostal retractions, and dyspnea.

*Aspiration of a foreign body.* Stridor occurs suddenly and may be accompanied by dry, paroxysmal coughing, gagging or choking, tachycardia, wheezing, intercostal retractions, diminished breath sounds, cyanosis, and shallow respirations.

*Inhalation injury.* Laryngeal edema and bronchospasm may result in stridor. Other findings include singed nasal hairs, orofacial burns, sooty sputum, and signs of respiratory distress.

*Laryngeal tumor.* A late sign, stridor may be accompanied by dysphagia, dyspnea, enlarged cervical nodes, and pain radiating to the ear.

*Mediastinal tumor.* Stridor results from the tumor compressing the trachea and bronchi. Other findings include hoarseness, brassy cough, tracheal shift or tug, stertorous respirations, and suprasternal retractions on inspiration.

*Retrosternal thyroid.* Stridor may be accompanied by dysphagia, cough, hoarseness, tracheal deviation, and signs of thyrotoxicosis.

*Thoracic aortic aneurysm.* If an aneurysm compresses the trachea, it may cause stridor along with dyspnea, wheezing, and a brassy cough.

*Other causes.* Acute laryngitis, bronchoscopy or laryngoscopy, hypocalcemia, neck surgery, and prolonged intubation.

## Nursing considerations

• Closely monitor the patient's vital signs. Prepare him for diagnostic tests, as ordered.

**S**

Bowel sounds diminished in regularity, tone, or loudness are termed hypoactive. These sounds don't herald an emergency; in fact, they're considered normal during sleep. But they may portend the absence of bowel sounds, which can indicate a life-threatening disorder.

Hypoactive bowel sounds are caused by decreased peristalsis, which can result from a developing bowel obstruction. Such obstruction may be mechanical, vascular, or neurogenic.

## History

After detecting hypoactive bowel sounds, assess for related symptoms. Ask the patient about the location, onset, duration, frequency, and severity of any pain. Cramping or colicky abdominal pain usually indicates a mechanical bowel obstruction; diffuse abdominal pain usually indicates intestinal distention in paralytic ileus.

Ask about recent vomiting, changes in bowel habits, constipation, and gas. Does the patient have a history of abdominal tumor or hernia, pancreatitis, bowel inflammation, gynecologic infection, toxic conditions such as uremia, severe pain, or trauma? Has he recently had radiation therapy or abdominal surgery, or ingested drugs?

## Physical exam

Inspect the abdomen for distention, surgical incisions, and obvious masses. Gently percuss and palpate the abdomen for masses, gas, fluid, tenderness, and rigidity. Measure abdominal girth to detect any subsequent increase in distention. Check for poor skin turgor, hypotension, narrowed pulse pressure, and other signs of dehydration and electrolyte imbalance.

## Causes

***Mechanical intestinal obstruction.*** Bowel sounds may become hypoactive after a period of hyperactivity. The patient may have acute, colicky abdominal pain in the quadrant of obstruction; nausea and vomiting; constipation; and abdominal distention and bloating.

***Mesenteric artery occlusion.*** After a brief period of hyperactivity, bowel sounds become hypoactive and then quickly disappear, signifying a life-threatening crisis. Other findings include fever, sudden and severe midepigastric or periumbilical pain followed by abdominal distention and possible bruits, vomiting, constipation, and signs of shock.

***Paralytic (adynamic) ileus.*** Bowel sounds are hypoactive and may disappear. Other findings include abdominal distention, generalized discomfort, and constipation or passage of flatus and small, liquid stools.

***Other causes.*** Drugs, such as opiates, anticholinergics, phenothiazines, vinca alkaloids, and general or spinal anesthetics; radiation therapy; and surgery.

## Nursing considerations

• Frequently assess the patient for signs of shock. Monitor vital signs and auscultate for bowel sounds every 2 to 4 hours. Immediately report sudden absence of bowel sounds, particularly when accompanied by severe pain, abdominal rigidity, guarding, and fever. Then prepare for emergency interventions.
• If the patient requires GI suction and decompression, restrict his oral intake and assist with tube insertion, as ordered. Then elevate the head of the bed at least 30 degrees, and turn the patient, as ordered, to facilitate passage of the tube through the GI tract. Don't tape an intestinal tube to the patient's face. Make sure the tube is patent and the suction devices are working properly. Irrigate the tube, as ordered, and monitor drainage.
• Continue to give I.V. fluids and electrolytes, as ordered, and send a serum specimen to the laboratory for analysis at least once a day.
• Provide comfort measures, as needed.
• If unexpelled flatus makes the patient uncomfortable, insert a rectal tube and leave it in place for 1 to 2 hours. During that time, turn the patient from side to side to help move gas through the intestines and out the tube.

**B**

Commonly associated with jaundice, clay-colored stools usually result from hepatic, gallbladder, or pancreatic disorders. Normally, bile pigments give the stool its characteristic brown color. However, hepatocellular degeneration or biliary obstruction may interfere with the formation or release of these pigments into the intestine, resulting in pale, putty-colored stools.

## History

Note when the patient first noticed clay-colored stools. Ask about associated signs and symptoms, such as abdominal pain, nausea and vomiting, fatigue, anorexia, weight loss, and dark urine. Does the patient have trouble digesting fatty foods or heavy meals? Does he bruise easily?

Review the patient's medical history for gallbladder, hepatic, or pancreatic disorders. Has he ever had biliary surgery? Has he recently undergone barium studies? (After barium studies, the patient has light-colored stools for several days; these may be mistaken for clay-colored stools.) Note a history of alcoholism or exposure to other hepatotoxins.

## Physical exam

After assessing the patient's general appearance, take his vital signs and check his skin and eyes for jaundice. Then examine the abdomen; inspect for distention and auscultate for hypoactive bowel sounds. Percuss and palpate for masses and rebound tenderness. Finally, obtain urine and stool specimens for laboratory analysis.

## Causes

*Bile duct cancer.* Clay-colored stools may be accompanied by jaundice, pruritus, and weight loss. Upper abdominal pain and bleeding tendencies may also occur.

*Biliary cirrhosis.* Clay-colored stools may accompany unexplained pruritus that worsens at bedtime, weakness, fatigue, weight loss, and vague abdominal pain. Signs and symptoms may be present for years.

*Cholangitis (sclerosing).* Clay-colored stools may be accompanied by chronic or intermittent jaundice, pruritus, and right upper abdominal pain.

*Cholelithiasis.* Stones in the biliary tract may cause clay-colored stools, especially when they obstruct the common bile duct. However, if the obstruction is intermittent, stools may alternate between normal and clay color. Associated findings may include dyspepsia and — in sudden, severe obstruction — biliary colic. Right upper quadrant pain intensifies over several hours and may radiate to the epigastrium or shoulder blades.

*Hepatic carcinoma.* Before clay-colored stools occur, the patient usually experiences weight loss, weakness, and anorexia. Later, he may develop jaundice, right upper quadrant pain, hepatomegaly, ascites, dependent edema, and fever.

*Pancreatic cancer.* Common bile duct obstruction may cause clay-colored stools. Associated findings include hepatomegaly, abdominal or back pain, jaundice, pruritus, nausea, vomiting, anorexia, weight loss, fatigue, weakness, and fever.

*Viral hepatitis.* Clay-colored stools signal the start of the icteric phase and are usually followed by jaundice within 1 to 5 days. Associated findings include mild weight loss, dark urine, anorexia, and tender hepatomegaly. During the icteric phase, the patient may become irritable and develop right upper quadrant pain, splenomegaly, enlarged cervical lymph nodes, and severe pruritus.

*Other causes.* Acute pancreatitis, biliary surgery.

## Nursing considerations

• Prepare the patient for diagnostic tests, such as liver enzyme and serum bilirubin measurements and stool analysis.

Bradycardia refers to a heart rate of fewer than 60 beats/minute. It occurs normally in young adults, trained athletes, and elderly people, and during sleep. It's also a normal response to vagal stimulation caused by coughing, vomiting, or straining during defecation. In response to these causes, the heart rate rarely drops below 40 beats/minute. When it results from pathologic causes, the heart rate may be as slow as 1 beat/minute.

By itself, bradycardia is a nonspecific sign. However, in conjunction with such symptoms as chest pain, dizziness, and shortness of breath, it can signal a life-threatening disorder.

## History
If the patient has no untoward signs, take a brief history. Ask if the patient or a family member has a history of slow pulse rate. Ask about any underlying metabolic disorders, such as hypothyroidism, which can precipitate bradycardia. Ask what medications the patient takes and if he's complying with the schedule and dosage.

## Physical exam
After detecting bradycardia, check for related signs of life-threatening disorders.

## Causes
*Cardiac arrhythmia.* Depending on the arrhythmia and the patient's tolerance of it, bradycardia may be transient or sustained, benign or life-threatening. Related findings may include hypotension, palpitations, dizziness, weakness, and fatigue.

*Cardiomyopathy.* This potentially life-threatening disorder causes transient or sustained bradycardia. Other findings may include dizziness, syncope, edema, fatigue, jugular vein distention, orthopnea, dyspnea, and peripheral cyanosis.

*Cervical spinal injury.* Bradycardia may be transient or sustained, depending on the severity of injury. Its onset coincides with sympathetic denervation. Other findings may include hypotension, decreased body temperature, slowed peristalsis, leg paralysis, and partial arm and respiratory muscle paralysis.

*Hypothermia.* Bradycardia usually appears when core temperature drops below 89.6° F (32° C). It's accompanied by shivering, peripheral cyanosis, muscle rigidity, bradypnea, and confusion leading to stupor.

*Hypothyroidism.* This disorder causes severe bradycardia along with fatigue, constipation, unexplained weight gain, and sensitivity to cold. Related signs include cool, dry, thick skin; sparse, dry hair; facial swelling; periorbital edema; thick, brittle nails; and confusion leading to stupor.

*Increased intracranial pressure.* Bradycardia is a late sign of this condition, along with rapid respirations, elevated systolic pressure, decreased diastolic pressure, and widened pulse pressure. Other findings include persistent headache, projectile vomiting, decreased level of consciousness, and fixed, unequal, possibly dilated pupils.

*Myocardial infarction (MI).* Mild or severe bradycardia occurs in about 65% of patients with an inferior MI. Other findings include an aching, burning, or viselike pressure in the chest, shoulder, arm, back, or epigastric area; nausea and vomiting; cool, clammy, and either pale or cyanotic skin; anxiety; and dyspnea.

*Other causes.* Diagnostic tests; drugs, such as beta-adrenergic and calcium channel blockers, cardiac glycosides, topical miotics, I.V. nitroglycerin, protamine sulfate, quinidine, and sympatholytics; and invasive treatments.

## Nursing considerations
• Continue to monitor vital signs frequently. Be especially alert for changes in cardiac rhythm, respiratory rate, and level of consciousness.
• Prepare the patient for diagnostic tests, which can include a complete blood count; cardiac enzyme, serum electrolyte, blood glucose, and thyroid function tests; arterial blood gas and blood urea nitrogen levels; and a 12-lead ECG. If appropriate, prepare the patient for 24-hour Holter monitoring.

**B**

# Stertorous respirations

Characterized by a harsh rattling or snoring sound, stertorous respirations usually result from the vibration of relaxed oropharyngeal structures during sleep or coma, causing partial airway obstruction. Less often, these respirations result from retained mucus in the upper airway.

## ▶ Emergency interventions

Check the patient's mouth and throat for edema, redness, and masses. If edema is marked, quickly take vital signs and notify the doctor immediately. Observe for signs and symptoms of respiratory distress, such as dyspnea, tachypnea, use of accessory muscles, intercostal muscle retractions, and cyanosis. Elevate the head of the bed 30 degrees to help ease breathing and reduce the edema. Administer supplemental oxygen by nasal cannula or face mask, and prepare to assist with intubation or tracheotomy and mechanical ventilation. Insert an I.V. line for fluid and drug access, and begin cardiac monitoring.

## History

When possible, question the patient's sleep partner about his snoring habits. Is she frequently awakened by the patient's snoring? Has she observed him talking or walking in his sleep? Ask about characteristic signs of sleep deprivation, such as personality changes or decreased mental acuity.

## Physical exam

If you detect stertorous respirations while the patient is sleeping, observe his breathing pattern for 3 to 4 minutes. Do noisy respirations cease when he turns on his side and recur when he assumes a supine position? Watch carefully for periods of apnea and note their length.

## Causes

*Airway obstruction.* Stertorous respirations accompanied by wheezing, dyspnea, and tachypnea may indicate partial airway obstruction. Later, intercostal retractions and nasal flaring may occur. If the obstruction becomes complete, the patient abruptly loses his ability to talk and displays diaphoresis, tachycardia, and inspiratory chest movement with absent breath sounds. Severe hypoxemia rapidly ensues, resulting in cyanosis, loss of consciousness, and cardiopulmonary collapse.

*Obstructive sleep apnea.* Spells of loud and disruptive snoring usually alternate with periods of sleep apnea, which usually end with loud, gasping sounds. Alternating tachycardia and bradycardia may occur. The patient may also experience somnambulism or talking during sleep. He may awaken in the morning with a generalized headache, feeling tired and unrefreshed, and may complain of excessive daytime sleepiness. Other findings include hypertension and ankle edema.

*Other causes.* Endotracheal surgery, intubation, or suction.

## Nursing considerations

• This sign occurs in about 10% of normal individuals, especially middle-aged, obese men. It may be aggravated by the the use of alcohol or sedatives before bed, which increases oropharyngeal flaccidity, and by sleeping in the supine position, which allows the tongue to slip back into the airway.
• In patients with airway obstruction, continue to monitor respiratory status carefully. As ordered, administer corticosteroids or antibiotics and cool, humidified oxygen to reduce palatal or uvular inflammation and edema.

**S**

# Bradypnea

A pattern of regular respirations with a rate of fewer than 12 breaths/minute, bradypnea commonly precedes life-threatening apnea or respiratory arrest. It results from neurologic and metabolic disorders and drug overdose, which depress the brain's respiratory control centers.

## ▶ Emergency interventions

Depending on the degree of central nervous system (CNS) depression, the patient with severe bradypnea may require constant stimulation to breathe. If the patient seems excessively sleepy, try to arouse him by shaking him and instructing him to breathe. Have another nurse immediately notify the doctor, and take the patient's vital signs.

Place him on an apnea monitor. Keep emergency airway equipment available and be prepared to assist with intubation and mechanical ventilation if spontaneous respirations cease. To prevent aspiration, position the patient on his side and clear his airway with suction or finger sweeps, if necessary.

## History

Obtain a brief history from the patient, if possible, or whoever accompanied him to the hospital. Ask about possible drug overdose, and try to determine which drugs the patient has taken, how much, when, and by what route. Check the patient's arms for needle marks, indicating possible drug abuse. You may need to administer I.V. naloxone, a narcotic antagonist.

If you rule out drug overdose, ask about chronic illnesses, such as diabetes and renal failure. Check for medical identification jewelry or a wallet card that identifies an underlying condition. Also ask whether the patient has a history of head trauma, brain tumor, neurologic infection, or stroke.

## Physical exam

Assess his neurologic status, checking pupil size and reactions, and evaluating his level of consciousness (LOC) and ability to move extremities.

## Causes

*Diabetic ketoacidosis.* Bradypnea occurs late in severe, uncontrolled diabetes. Other findings include decreased LOC, fatigue, weakness, fruity breath odor, and oliguria.

*Drugs.* An overdose of narcotic analgesics or, less commonly, sedatives, barbiturates, phenothiazines, and CNS depressants can cause bradypnea.

*Hepatic failure.* Occurring in end-stage hepatic failure, bradypnea may be accompanied by coma, hyperactive reflexes, a positive Babinski's sign, fetor hepaticus, and other signs.

*Increased intracranial pressure.* A late sign of this serious condition, bradypnea is preceded by decreased LOC, deteriorated motor function, and fixed, dilated pupils. The triad of bradypnea, bradycardia, and hypertension is a classic sign of late medullary strangulation.

*Renal failure.* Occurring in end-stage renal failure, bradypnea may be accompanied by seizures, decreased LOC, GI bleeding, hypotension or hypertension, uremic frost, and diverse other signs.

*Respiratory failure.* Bradypnea occurs in end-stage respiratory failure. Its accompanying signs include cyanosis, diminished breath sounds, tachycardia, mildly increased blood pressure, and decreased LOC.

## Nursing considerations

• The patient with bradypnea may develop apnea, so check his respiratory status frequently. Be prepared to give ventilatory support, if necessary.

• Don't leave the patient unattended. Keep his bed in the lowest position and raise the side rails. As ordered, obtain blood for arterial blood gas and electrolyte studies, and ready the patient for chest and skull X-rays and computed tomography scan.

• Administer drugs and oxygen, as ordered. Avoid giving CNS-depressant drugs because these exacerbate bradypnea. Similarly, give oxygen judiciously to a patient with chronic carbon dioxide retention, which may occur in chronic obstructive pulmonary disease.

# Splenomegaly

Because splenomegaly, or enlargement of the spleen, commonly occurs in many disorders (and in 5% of normal adults), it isn't a diagnostic sign by itself. Usually, though, splenomegaly points to infection, trauma, or hepatic, autoimmune, neoplastic, or hematologic disorders.

## ▶ Emergency interventions

If you detect left upper quadrant pain and signs of shock, such as tachycardia and tachypnea, suspect splenic rupture. Have a colleague notify the doctor immediately. Insert an I.V. line for emergency fluid and blood replacement and administer oxygen. Catheterize the patient to evaluate urine output, and begin cardiac monitoring. Prepare for surgery, if ordered.

## History

Ask the patient if he frequently has colds, sore throats, or other infections. Does he bruise easily? Ask about tiredness, left upper quadrant pain, abdominal fullness, and early satiety.

## Physical exam

If splenomegaly is *not* related to trauma, you may palpate lightly under the left costal margin. Also examine the patient's skin for pallor and ecchymoses. Palpate his axillae, groin, and neck for lymphadenopathy.

## Causes

*Cirrhosis.* Marked splenomegaly may occur in advanced stages along with jaundice, hepatomegaly, leg edema, hematemesis, and ascites. Signs of hepatic encephalopathy are common.

*Felty's syndrome.* Splenomegaly may be accompanied by joint pain and deformity, sensory or motor loss, rheumatoid nodules, palmar erythema, lymphadenopathy, and leg ulcers.

*Histoplasmosis.* Splenomegaly and hepatomegaly may accompany lymphadenopathy, jaundice, fever, anorexia, emaciation, and anemia.

*Hypersplenism (primary).* Splenomegaly may accompany signs of pancytopenia. If the patient has anemia, findings may include weakness, fatigue, malaise, and pallor.

*Infectious mononucleosis.* Splenomegaly is usually accompanied by sore throat, cervical lymphadenopathy, and fluctuating temperature with an evening peak of 101° to 102° F (38.3° to 38.9° C). Hepatomegaly, jaundice, and a maculopapular rash may also occur.

*Infective endocarditis (subacute).* The patient may develop an enlarged, nontender spleen along with a suddenly changing murmur or a new murmur accompanied by fever. Other findings include anorexia, pallor, weakness, night sweats, fatigue, tachycardia, weight loss, arthralgia, and petechiae.

*Leukemia (acute or chronic).* Moderate to severe splenomegaly occurs early and may be accompanied by pain, hepatomegaly, fatigue, fever, lymphadenopathy, gum swelling, bleeding tendencies, weight loss, and abdominal, bone, and joint pain.

*Lymphoma.* Splenomegaly is a late sign. Other findings include hepatomegaly, painless lymphadenopathy, scaly dermatitis with pruritus, fever, fatigue, and weight loss.

*Malaria.* Usually, splenomegaly is preceded by the malarial paroxysm of chills followed by high fever and diaphoresis.

*Pancreatic cancer.* Moderate to severe splenomegaly may occur if tumor growth compresses the splenic vein. Other findings include abdominal or back pain, anorexia, nausea and vomiting, weight loss, GI bleeding, jaundice, pruritus, skin lesions, weakness, and fatigue.

*Polycythemia vera.* A late sign, splenomegaly may lead to easy satiety, abdominal fullness, and left upper quadrant or pleuritic chest pain.

*Splenic rupture.* Splenomegaly may result from massive hemorrhage.

*Other causes.* Amyloidosis, brucellosis, hepatitis, sarcoidosis, thrombotic thrombocytopenic purpura.

## Nursing considerations

• Prepare the patient for diagnostic studies, such as radionuclide and computed tomography scans.

**S**

Breast dimpling—the puckering or retraction of skin on the breast—results from abnormal attachment of the skin to underlying tissue. It suggests an inflammatory or malignant mass beneath the skin surface and most often represents a late sign of breast cancer. Dimpling most commonly affects women over age 40 but occasionally occurs in men.

Because breast dimpling occurs over a mass or an induration, the patient usually discovers other signs before the dimpling. But a thorough breast examination may reveal dimpling and alert the patient and nurse to a breast problem.

## History
Obtain a medical, reproductive, and family history, noting high-risk factors for breast cancer. How old was the patient when she began menstruation? How old was she at menopause? Has her mother or a sister had breast cancer? Has she herself had a previous neoplasm, especially cancer in the other breast? Ask about her dietary habits.

Ask about changes in the shape of her breast and cyclical pain or tenderness. If she's lactating, has she recently experienced high fever, chills, malaise, muscle aches, fatigue, or other flulike symptoms? Can she remember sustaining any traumatic injury to the breast?

## Physical exam
Carefully inspect the dimpled area. Is it swollen, red, warm, or bruised? Have the patient tense her pectoral muscles by pressing her hips with both hands or raising her hands over her head. Does puckering increase? Gently pull the skin upward toward the clavicle. Is dimpling exaggerated?

Look for nipple retraction. Do both nipples point in the same direction? Are they flattened or inverted? If the patient reports nipple discharge, describe it. Observe the contour of both breasts.

Examine both breasts with your patient supine, then sitting, then leaning forward. Does the skin move freely over both breasts? If you palpate a lump, describe its size, location, consistency, mobility, and delineation. Gently mold the skin around the lump. Is dimpling exaggerated? Examine breast and axillary lymph nodes for enlargement.

## Causes
*Breast abscess.* Breast dimpling sometimes accompanies chronic breast abscess. Other findings include a firm, irregular, nontender lump and nipple retraction.

*Breast cancer.* Breast dimpling is an important but *late* sign of cancer. A neoplasm that causes dimpling is usually close to the skin and at least 1 cm in diameter, irregularly shaped, and fixed to underlying tissue. Bloody nipple discharge in the presence of a lump is a classic sign of breast cancer.

*Fat necrosis.* Breast dimpling from fat necrosis follows inflammation and trauma to fatty tissue of the breast. Findings include a hard, poorly delineated lump and nipple retraction.

*Mastitis.* Breast dimpling may signal bacterial mastitis, commonly resulting from duct obstruction and milk stasis during lactation. It's usually accompanied by erythema, swelling, induration, pain, and tenderness.

## Nursing considerations
• Provide a clear explanation of diagnostic tests that may be ordered, such as mammography, thermography, ultrasound, cytology of nipple discharge, and biopsy.

• Discuss breast self-examination, and provide follow-up teaching when the patient expresses a readiness to learn. Advise the lactating mother with mastitis to pump her breasts to prevent further milk stasis, to discard the milk, and to substitute formula until the breast infection responds adequately to antibiotics.

• Remember that any breast problem can arouse fears of mutilation, loss of sexuality, and death. Allow the patient to express her feelings.

# Spider angioma

A spider angioma (also called arterial spider, spider nevus, stellate angioma, or vascular spider) is a fiery red vascular lesion with an elevated central body, branching spiderlike legs, and a surrounding flush. A form of telangiectasia, this characteristic lesion ranges from a few millimeters to several centimeters in diameter and may appear alone or with other angiomas. On palpation, they may be slightly warmer than the surrounding skin and may have a pulsating central body.

Most commonly, angiomas appear on the face and neck. Angiomas on the shoulders, thorax, arms, backs of the hands and fingers, and mucous membranes of the lips and nose are less common. Rarely do they appear below the waist or on the lips, ears, nail beds, or palms.

Spider angiomas are most commonly associated with cirrhosis. They also may erupt in the second to third month of pregnancy, enlarge and multiply, then disappear about 6 weeks after delivery. Occasionally, a few lesions may persist. These lesions also may appear in normal individuals — especially elderly ones; when they do, they're smaller and fewer in number (nine or less). They may persist indefinitely or disappear spontaneously.

## History

Ask the patient how long he's had the spider angiomas and where they're located.

## Physical exam

Carefully examine the patient, noting the size and location of angiomas. Also check for other skin abnormalities, such as jaundice, dryness, and palmar erythema.

## Cause

*Cirrhosis.* Multiple spider angiomas are a hallmark of cirrhosis. Typically, they're a late sign, enlarging and multiplying as the disorder progresses. Associated signs and symptoms are widespread, varying with the degree of hepatic insufficiency and related portal hypertension. Splenomegaly and hematemesis, for example, point to portal hypertension.

Other skin effects in cirrhosis may include severe pruritus, extreme dryness, palmar erythema, and poor tissue turgor. Cardinal hepatic effects may include jaundice, hepatomegaly, ascites, and leg edema. Right upper quadrant pain that worsens when the patient sits up or leans forward is common. The patient may also display hepatic encephalopathy with such key signs as slurred speech, asterixis, fetor hepaticus, and decreased level of consciousness that progresses to coma. The male patient may have testicular atrophy, gynecomastia, and loss of chest and axillary hair. The female patient may experience menstrual irregularities.

## Nursing considerations

- Don't expect to treat spider angiomas that occur during pregnancy.
- In the patient with cirrhosis, the doctor may order cautery, electrodesiccation, or freezing to treat angiomas.

**S**

# Breast nodule

Also called a breast lump, a breast nodule has two chief causes: benign breast disease and cancer. Benign breast disease, the leading cause of nodules, can stem from cyst formation in obstructed and dilated lactiferous ducts, hypertrophy or tumor formation in the ductal system, and inflammation or infection. Fewer than 20% of breast nodules are malignant; nevertheless, they should always be evaluated in both sexes.

## History

If your patient reports a lump, ask her how and when she discovered it. Does the size and tenderness of the lump vary with her menstrual cycle? Has the lump changed since she first noticed it? Is she aware of any other unusual breast signs, such as discharge or nipple changes?

Ask if the patient has noticed a change in breast shape, size, or contour; if she's lactating; if she has fever, chills, fatigue, or other flulike symptoms; or if she has sustained a recent traumatic injury to the breast. Have her describe any pain or tenderness.

Ask about factors that increase the risk of breast cancer, such as a high-fat diet, a mother or sister with breast cancer, a history of cancer, nulliparity, a first pregnancy after age 30, and early menarche or late menopause.

## Physical exam

Pay special attention to the upper outer quadrant of each breast, the most common site of breast cancer. Carefully palpate a suspected breast nodule, noting its location, shape, size, consistency, mobility, and delineation.

Do you feel one nodule or several small ones? Inspect and palpate the skin over the nodule for warmth, redness, and edema. Palpate the lymph nodes of the breast and axilla for enlargement.

Observe the contour of your patient's breasts, looking for asymmetry, irregularities, and nipple retraction or flattening. Be alert for nipple discharge that's spontaneous, unilateral, and nonmilky.

## Causes

*Adenofibroma.* The highly mobile or "slippery" feel of this benign neoplasm helps distinguish it from other breast nodules. The nodule usually occurs singly and feels firm, elastic, and round or lobular, with well-defined margins.

*Areolar gland abscess.* Tender abscesses on the periphery of the areola follow inflammation of the sebaceous Montgomery's glands.

*Breast abscess.* A localized, hot, tender, fluctuant mass with erythema and peau d'orange typifies acute abscess. Other findings may include fever, chills, malaise, and generalized discomfort.

*Breast cancer.* A hard, poorly delineated nodule fixed to the skin or underlying tissue suggests breast cancer. Bloody nipple discharge in the presence of a nodule is a classic sign of breast cancer.

*Intraductal papilloma.* The tiny nodules of this benign lesion usually resist palpation. Nodules large enough to be palpated usually occur singly. The primary sign of this disorder is serous or bloody nipple discharge.

*Mastitis.* Breast nodules feel firm and indurated or tender, flocculent, and discrete. Gentle palpation defines the area of maximum purulent accumulation. Other findings include breast warmth, erythema, tenderness, edema, and peau d'orange; fever; chills; malaise; and fatigue.

*Proliferative (fibrocystic) breast disease.* The most common cause, it produces smooth, round, slightly elastic nodules, which increase in size and tenderness just before menstruation.

*Other causes.* Fat necrosis, mammary duct ectasia, nipple adenoma, and Paget's disease.

## Nursing considerations

- Prepare the patient for diagnostic tests.
- Teach the patient breast self-examination.
- Advise the lactating mother with mastitis to pump her breasts to prevent further milk stasis, to discard the milk, and to substitute formula until the infection responds to antibiotics.

**B**

# Skin turgor, decreased

Decreased skin turgor refers to an impairment in the skin's elasticity. After being stretched or pinched, the skin takes longer to return to its normal position. Pinched skin "holds" for up to 30 seconds, then slowly returns to its normal contour. Usually, you'll assess turgor over the arm or the sternum, areas normally free of wrinkles and wide variations in tissue thickness.

Decreased skin turgor results from dehydration (volume depletion), which moves interstitial fluid into the vascular bed to maintain circulating blood volume, leading to slackness in the skin's dermal layer. It's a normal finding in elderly people and in people who've lost weight rapidly; it also occurs in disorders affecting the GI, renal, endocrine, and other systems.

## History

Ask the patient about food and fluid intake and fluid loss. Has he had recent prolonged fluid loss from vomiting, diarrhea, draining wounds, or increased urination? Ask about a recent fever with sweating. Is he taking diuretics? If so, how often?

## Physical exam

Take the patient's vital signs. Assess for orthostatic hypotension or resting tachycardia. Note if the patient's systolic blood pressure while supine is abnormally low (90 mm Hg or less), if it drops 10 mm Hg or more when he stands, or if his pulse rate increases 10 beats/minute on standing or sitting. If you detect signs of orthostatic hypotension or resting tachycardia, call the doctor and start an I.V. line, as ordered, for fluid administration.

Assess the patient's level of consciousness (LOC) for confusion and disorientation, signs of profound dehydration. Inspect his oral mucosa, the furrows of the tongue (especially under the tongue), and the axillae for dryness. Also check his neck veins for flatness, and monitor his urine output.

## Cause

**Dehydration.** Decreased skin turgor commonly occurs in moderate to severe dehydration. Associated findings include dry oral mucosa, decreased perspiration, resting tachycardia, orthostatic hypotension, dry and furrowed tongue, increased thirst, weight loss, oliguria, fever, and fatigue. As dehydration worsens, other findings include enophthalmos, lethargy, weakness, confusion, delirium or obtundation, anuria, and shock. Hypotension persists even when the patient lies down.

## Nursing considerations

• Monitor the patient's intake and output; administer I.V. fluid replacement, if ordered; and offer frequent oral fluids. Weigh the patient daily at the same time on the same scale. If his urine output falls below 30 ml/hour or his weight loss continues, notify the doctor.

• Remember that even a small deficit in body fluid may be critical in patients with diminished total body fluid, such as young children, elderly or obese people, or patients who have lost a large amount of weight rapidly.

• Closely monitor the patient for signs of electrolyte imbalance.

• To prevent skin breakdown in a dehydrated patient with poor skin turgor, decreased LOC, and impaired peripheral circulation, turn the patient every 2 hours, and frequently massage his back and pressure points.

# Breast pain

Also called mastalgia, breast pain may be unilateral or bilateral; cyclic, intermittent, or constant; and dull or sharp. It may result from surface cuts, furuncles, contusions, and similar lesions; nipple fissures and inflammation in the papillary ducts and areolae; stromal distention in the breast parenchyma; a tumor; or inflammatory lesions.

Before menstruation, breast pain or tenderness stems from increased mammary blood flow resulting from hormonal changes. During pregnancy, breast tenderness and throbbing, tingling, or pricking sensations may occur.

In men, breast pain may stem from gynecomastia, reproductive tract anomalies, and organic disease of the pituitary, adrenal cortex, and thyroid glands.

## History
Ask the patient if breast pain is constant or intermittent. For either type, ask about onset and character. If it's intermittent, determine the relationship of pain to the phase of the menstrual cycle. Determine if the patient is a breast-feeding mother. If not, ask about nipple discharge. Ask if she's pregnant or if she has reached menopause or recently experienced flulike symptoms, sustained any injury to the breast, or noticed changes in breast shape. Have your patient describe the pain and its location.

## Physical exam
Instruct the patient to place her arms at her sides, and inspect the breasts. Note their size, symmetry, and contour and the appearance of the skin.

Note the size, shape, and symmetry of the nipples and areolae. Is ecchymosis, rash, ulceration, or discharge present? Do the nipples point in the same direction? Do you see nipple retraction?

Repeat your inspection, first with the patient's arms raised above her head, then with her hands pressed against her hips.

Palpate the breasts, first with the patient seated, then lying down with a pillow under her shoulder on the side being examined. Proceed from the sternum to the midline and from the axilla to the midline, noting warmth, tenderness, nodules, masses, or irregularities. Palpate the nipples, noting tenderness and nodules, and check for discharge. Palpate axillary lymph nodes, noting any enlargement.

## Causes
*Areolar gland abscess.* Tender, palpable abscesses on the periphery of the areola follow inflammation of the sebaceous Montgomery's glands. Fever may occur.

*Breast abscess (acute).* In the affected breast, local pain, tenderness, erythema, peau d'orange, and warmth are associated with a nodule. Malaise, fever, and chills may also occur.

*Breast cyst.* A breast cyst that enlarges rapidly may cause acute, localized, and usually unilateral pain. A palpable breast nodule may be present.

*Intraductal papilloma.* Unilateral breast pain or tenderness may accompany this condition, although the primary sign is a serous or bloody nipple discharge. Associated signs include a small (usually 2- to 3-mm), soft, poorly delineated mass in the ducts beneath the areola.

*Mastitis.* Unilateral pain may be severe. Breast skin is commonly red and warm at the inflammation site and may have an orange-peel appearance. Palpation reveals a firm area of induration.

*Proliferative (fibrocystic) breast disease.* A common cause of breast pain. The cysts feel firm, mobile, and well defined. A clear, watery nipple discharge may be present.

*Other causes.* Breast cancer, fat necrosis, mammary duct ectasia, and sebaceous cyst (infected).

## Nursing considerations
• Administer pain medication, as ordered. Suggest that the patient wear a well-fitting brassiere.
• Emphasize the importance of monthly breast self-examination. Teach the patient how to perform this examination, and instruct her to call the doctor immediately if she detects any breast changes.
• Prepare the patient for diagnostic tests.

**B**

# Skin, scaly

Scaly skin results when cells of the uppermost skin layer desiccate and shed, causing excessive accumulation of loosely adherent flakes of keratin.

## History

Ask how long the patient has had scaly skin. Has he had it before? Where did it appear first? Did a lesion or skin eruption precede it? Did he use a topical skin product recently? How often does he bathe? What kinds of soap, cosmetics, skin lotion, and shampoo does he use? Has he had recent joint pain, illness, or malaise? Ask the patient about work exposure to chemicals, use of prescribed drugs, and a family history of skin disorders.

## Physical exam

Examine the entire skin surface. Is it dry, oily, moist, or greasy? Note the location, general pattern, color, shape, and size of skin lesions. Are they thick or fine? Do they itch? Examine the patient's ears, hair, and nails and the mucous membranes of his mouth, lips, and nose.

## Causes

**Bowen's disease.** Painless, erythematous plaques are widely distributed, raised, and indurated with a thick, hyperkeratotic scale.

***Dermatitis.*** In *exfoliative dermatitis*, generalized erythema develops rapidly. Desquamation of surface skin may cause severe hypothermia. In *nummular dermatitis*, round, pustular lesions ooze purulent exudate, itch severely, and rapidly become encrusted and scaly. In *seborrheic dermatitis*, erythematous, scaly papules progress to larger scaly plaques and may involve the scalp, chest, eyebrows, back, axillae, umbilicus, and genitalia.

***Dermatophytosis.*** In *tinea capitis*, reddened lesions with elevated borders and densely scaled centers commonly become inflamed and pus-filled. In *tinea pedis*, scaling and blisters occur between the toes. In *tinea corporis*, the centers of large, crusty lesions heal, creating a ringworm shape.

***Discoid lupus erythematosus.*** Separate or coalescing lesions appear on the face or on sun-exposed areas. Ranging from pink to purple, they are covered with a yellow or brown crust. Enlarged hair follicles are filled with scale.

***Lichen planus.*** Flat, violet lesions with a fine scale may affect the lumbar region, genitalia, ankles, and anterior lower legs.

***Lymphomas.*** In *Hodgkin's disease*, scaling dermatitis with pruritus may begin in the legs and spread to the entire body. Small nodules and diffuse pigmentation may occur along with painless enlargement of the peripheral lymph nodes. In *non-Hodgkin's lymphoma*, erythematous patches with some scaling become interspersed with nodules.

***Parapsoriasis (chronic).*** Small or moderate-sized papules, with a thin, adherent scale, appear on the trunk, hands, and feet. Removal of the scale reveals a shiny brown surface.

***Pityriasis rosea.*** Widespread scaling begins with an erythematous, raised, oval herald patch anywhere on the body. Later on, yellow-tan or erythematous patches with scaly edges erupt on the trunk, limbs, face, hands, or feet.

***Psoriasis.*** Silvery white, micaceous scales cover sharply defined erythematous plaques. Scales may appear on the scalp, chest, elbows, knees, back, buttocks, and genitalia.

***Syphilis (secondary).*** A ring-shaped pattern of papulosquamous eruptions may form on the face, arms, palms, soles, chest, back, and abdomen.

***Systemic lupus erythematosus.*** A bright red maculopapular eruption with fine scales appears in a butterfly pattern on the nose and malar regions of the face.

***Tinea versicolor.*** Macular, hypopigmented, fawn-colored or brown scaly patches appear on the upper trunk, arms, and lower abdomen.

***Other causes.*** Drugs, including penicillins, sulfonamides, barbiturates, quinidine, diazepam, phenytoin, and isoniazid; and pityriasis rubra pilaris.

## Nursing considerations

• Teach the patient proper skin care, and suggest lubricating baths and emollients.

# Breast ulcer

Appearing on the nipple, the areola, or the breast itself, an ulcer indicates destruction of the skin and subcutaneous tissue. A breast ulcer is usually a late sign of cancer. However, it may be the presenting sign of breast cancer in men, who may dismiss earlier breast changes. A breast ulcer can also result from trauma, infection, or radiation.

## History
Begin by asking when the patient first noticed the ulcer and if it was preceded by other breast changes, such as nodules, edema, or nipple discharge, deviation, or retraction. Has she noticed any change in breast shape? Does the ulcer seem to be getting better or worse? Does it cause pain or produce drainage? Has the patient noticed a rash? If she has been treating the ulcer at home, find out how.

Review the patient's personal and family history for factors that raise the risk of breast cancer. For example, ask about previous cancer, especially of the breast, and mastectomy. Determine if the patient's mother or sister has had breast cancer. Ask the patient's age at menarche and menopause because more than 30 years of menstrual activity increases the risk of breast cancer. Also ask about pregnancy because nulliparity or primiparity after age 30 also increases the risk of breast cancer.

If the patient recently gave birth, ask if she breast-feeds her infant or has recently weaned him. Ask if she's currently taking any oral antibiotics and if she's diabetic. All these factors predispose the patient to *Candida* infections.

## Physical exam
Inspect the patient's breast, noting any asymmetry or flattening. Look for a rash, scaling, cracking, or red excoriation on the nipples, areola, and inframammary fold. Check especially for skin changes, such as warmth, erythema, edema, or peau d'orange. Palpate the breast for masses, noting any induration beneath the ulcer. Then carefully palpate for tenderness or nodules around the areola and the axillary lymph nodes.

## Causes
*Breast cancer.* A breast ulcer that doesn't heal within a month usually indicates cancer. Ulceration along a mastectomy scar may indicate metastatic cancer. A nodule beneath the ulcer may be a late sign of a fulminating tumor. Other signs include a palpable breast nodule, skin dimpling, nipple retraction, bloody or serous nipple discharge, erythema, peau d'orange, and enlarged axillary lymph nodes.

*Breast trauma.* Tissue destruction with inadequate healing may produce breast ulcers. Associated signs depend on the type of trauma but may include ecchymosis, lacerations, abrasions, swelling, and hematoma.

*Candida albicans infection.* Severe *Candida* infection can cause maceration of breast tissue followed by ulceration. Well-defined, bright red papular patches—usually with scaly borders—characterize the infection, which can develop in the breast folds. In breast-feeding women, cracked nipples predispose to infection.

*Paget's disease.* Bright red nipple excoriation can extend to the areola and ulcerate. Serous or bloody nipple discharge and extreme nipple itching may accompany ulceration.

*Other causes.* Radiation therapy.

## Nursing considerations
• Because breast ulcers become infected easily, teach the patient how to apply topical antifungal ointment or cream, as ordered. Instruct her to keep the ulcer dry, to minimize chafing, and to wear loose-fitting undergarments.
• If breast cancer is suspected, provide emotional support and encourage the patient to express her feelings. Prepare her for diagnostic tests, such as ultrasonography, thermography, mammography, nipple discharge cytology, and breast biopsy. If *Candida* infection is suspected, prepare her for skin or blood cultures.

# Skin, mottled

A patchy skin discoloration, mottling indicates primary or secondary changes of the deep, middle, or superficial dermal blood vessels. It may occur as a normal reaction — for example, when exposure to cold causes venous stasis in cutaneous blood vessels — or it may result from hematologic, immune, or connective tissue disorders.

Mottling that occurs with other signs and symptoms most often affects the extremities, usually indicating restricted blood flow. For instance, livedo reticularis, a characteristic network pattern of reddish blue discoloration, occurs when vasospasm of the middermal blood vessels slows local blood flow in dilated superficial capillaries and small veins. Shock causes mottling from systemic vasoconstriction.

## ▶ Emergency interventions

Be alert for acute arterial occlusion. Look for blotchy cyanosis and livedo reticularis localized in a pale, cool extremity. Ask the patient if he feels pain, numbness, or tingling. Assess for diminished or absent pulses, prolonged capillary refill time, and diminished reflexes. If you suspect occlusion, notify the doctor. Insert an I.V. line in an unaffected extremity and prepare for arteriography or immediate surgery, as ordered.

If mottling occurs in the knees and elbows, or all over, assess for hypovolemic shock. Look for sudden onset of pallor, cool skin, restlessness, tachypnea, slight tachycardia, and weak pulse. Place the patient in a supine position in bed, and notify the doctor. Administer oxygen and begin cardiac monitoring. Insert a large-bore I.V. line for fluid administration, and prepare to assist with insertion of a central line or a pulmonary artery catheter. Also prepare for catheterization to monitor urine output.

## History

Ask if the mottling began suddenly or gradually. What precipitated it? How long has the patient had it? Does anything make it go away? Does he have other symptoms, such as pain, numbness, or tingling in an extremity? If so, do they disappear with temperature changes?

## Physical exam

Observe the patient's skin color, and palpate his arms and legs for skin texture, swelling, and temperature differences. Also palpate for the presence and quality of pulses. Note breaks in the skin, muscle appearance, and hair distribution. Also assess motor and sensory functions.

## Causes

*Acute arterial occlusion.* Blotchy cyanosis and livedo reticularis may occur.

*Arteriosclerosis obliterans.* Obstructed blood flow to the extremities produces leg pallor, cyanosis, blotchy erythema, and livedo reticularis. Other findings include intermittent claudication, diminished pedal pulses, and leg coolness.

*Buerger's disease.* Unilateral or asymmetrical color changes and mottling, particularly livedo networking in the legs, may accompany intermittent claudication and erythema along extremity blood vessels.

*Cryoglobulinemia.* Along with patchy livedo reticularis, petechiae, and ecchymoses, the patient may develop fever, chills, urticaria, melena, skin ulcers, and epistaxis.

*Hypovolemic shock.* Vasoconstriction produces mottling, initially in the knees and elbows.

*Idiopathic or primary livedo reticularis.* Symmetrical, diffuse mottling may involve the hands, feet, arms, legs, buttocks, and trunk.

*Polycythemia vera.* Livedo reticularis may accompany hemangiomas, purpura, rubor, ulcerative nodules, and scleroderma-like lesions.

*Other causes.* Acrocyanosis, periarteritis nodosa, prolonged immobility, rheumatoid arthritis, systemic lupus erythematosus, and thermal exposure.

## Nursing considerations

• Teach the patient to avoid tight clothing and overexposure to cold or to heating devices.

**S**

# Breath with ammonia odor

Also known as uremic fetor, the odor of ammonia on the breath—described as urinous or "fishy" breath—typically occurs in end-stage chronic renal failure. This sign persists throughout the course of this disorder but isn't of great concern.

Ammonia breath odor reflects the long-term metabolic disturbances and biochemical abnormalities associated with uremia and end-stage chronic renal failure. Metabolic end products, blown off by the lungs, produce the ammonia odor, but a specific uremic toxin has not yet been identified. In animals, breath odor analysis has revealed toxic metabolites, such as dimethylamine and trimethylamine, which contribute to the fishy odor. The source of these amines, although still unclear, may be intestinal bacteria acting on dietary chlorine.

When you detect ammonia breath odor, the diagnosis of chronic renal failure is well established. However, you'll need to assess for associated GI symptoms so that palliative care and support can be individualized.

## History

Ask the patient if he has experienced a metallic taste, loss of smell, increased thirst, heartburn, difficulty swallowing, or loss of appetite at the sight of food. Ask about early morning vomiting. Because GI bleeding is common in chronic renal failure, ask about bowel habits, noting especially melenous stools or constipation.

## Physical exam

Inspect the patient's oral cavity for bleeding, swollen gums or tongue, and ulceration with drainage. Take the patient's vital signs. Inform the doctor of any *abnormal* hypertension (the patient with end-stage chronic renal failure is usually somewhat hypertensive) or significant hypotension. Assess for other signs of shock (such as tachycardia, tachypnea, and cool, clammy skin) and altered mental status. Any significant changes can indicate complications, such as massive GI bleeding or pericarditis with tamponade.

## Cause

*End-stage chronic renal failure.* Ammonia breath odor is a late finding. Other findings include anuria, skin pigmentation changes and excoriation, brown arcs under the nail margins, tissue wasting, Kussmaul's respirations, neuropathy, lethargy, somnolence, confusion, disorientation, behavior changes with irritability, and mood lability. Later neurologic signs that signal impending uremic coma include muscle twitching and fasciculation, asterixis, paresthesia, and footdrop. Cardiovascular findings may include hypertension and signs of congestive heart failure and pericarditis. GI findings include anorexia, nausea, heartburn, vomiting, constipation, hiccups, and a metallic taste, with oral manifestations such as stomatitis, gum ulceration and bleeding, and a coated tongue. Weight loss is common, and uremic frost, pruritus, and signs of hormonal changes (such as impotence or amenorrhea) also appear.

## Nursing considerations

• Ammonia breath odor is offensive to others, but the patient may become accustomed to it. Remind him to perform frequent mouth care, particularly before meals, because reducing foul mouth taste and odor may stimulate his appetite. A half-strength hydrogen peroxide mixture or lemon juice gargle helps neutralize the ammonia; the patient may also want to use throat lozenges or breath sprays or to suck on hard candy.

• Advise him to use a soft toothbrush or sponge to prevent trauma. If the patient can't perform mouth care, do it for him and teach his family members how to assist him.

• Maximize dietary intake by offering the patient frequent, small meals of his favorite foods, within dietary limitations. Encourage him to take the ordered antacids.

# Skin, clammy

Clammy, cool, and frequently pale skin results from a sympathetic response to stress. Stress triggers release of the hormones epinephrine and norepinephrine. These hormones cause cutaneous vasoconstriction and secretion of cold sweat from eccrine glands, particularly on the palms, forehead, and soles.

## ▶ Emergency interventions

Clammy skin accompanied by tachypnea, tachycardia, hypotension, and a weak, irregular pulse indicates shock. Notify the doctor at once, and place the patient in a supine position. Elevate his legs 20 to 30 degrees to promote perfusion to vital organs. Insert an I.V. line for administration of drugs, fluids, or blood, if ordered. Give supplemental oxygen and begin cardiac monitoring.

Suspect acute hypoglycemia if a patient with clammy skin is irritable and anxious with persistent hunger, possible tremors, and hypotension. Immediately draw blood for glucose studies, and test a drop with a glucose reagent strip. Insert an I.V. line, administer dextrose 50% solution, and begin cardiac monitoring.

Clammy skin accompanied by mental status changes, hypotension, and changes in pulse rate and rhythm indicates arrhythmias. Notify the doctor. Insert an I.V. line, and administer antiarrhythmic drugs, as ordered. Give supplemental oxygen and begin cardiac monitoring.

## History

Find out if the patient has a history of insulin-dependent diabetes mellitus or cardiac disorders. Is he currently taking any medications, especially antiarrhythmics? Is he experiencing pain, nausea, or epigastric distress? Does he feel weak? Does he have a dry mouth, diarrhea, or increased urination?

## Physical exam

Examine the pupils for dilation. Check for abdominal distention and increased muscle tension.

## Causes

*Acute hypoglycemia.* Generalized cool, clammy skin or diaphoresis may occur.

*Anxiety.* An acute anxiety attack commonly produces cold, clammy skin on the forehead, palms, and soles. Other findings may include pallor, dry mouth, tachycardia or bradycardia, palpitations, and hypertension or hypotension.

*Arrhythmias.* Besides cool, clammy skin, findings may include mental status changes, dizziness, and hypotension.

*Cardiogenic shock.* Generalized cool, moist, pale skin accompanies confusion and restlessness, hypotension, tachycardia, tachypnea, narrowing pulse pressure, cyanosis, and oliguria.

*Heat exhaustion.* In the acute stage, generalized cold, clammy skin accompanies an ashen-gray appearance, headache, confusion, syncope, giddiness, and a normal or subnormal temperature.

*Hypovolemic shock.* Generalized pale, cold, clammy skin may occur along with hypothermia, hypotension with narrowing pulse pressure, tachycardia, tachypnea, and rapid, thready pulse.

*Septic shock.* Generalized cold, clammy skin occurs during the cold shock stage. Associated findings include rapid and thready pulse, severe hypotension, persistent oliguria or anuria, and respiratory failure.

*Other causes.* Clammy skin may occur as a vasovagal reaction to severe pain.

## Nursing considerations

• Take the patient's vital signs frequently, and monitor urine output.
• If clammy skin occurs with an anxiety reaction or pain, offer the patient emotional support, administer analgesics as ordered, and provide a quiet environment.

**S**

Fecal breath odor may follow an episode of prolonged vomiting associated with a long-standing intestinal obstruction or gastrojejunocolic fistula. It represents an important late diagnostic clue to a potentially life-threatening GI disorder because complete obstruction of any part of the bowel, if untreated, can cause death within hours from vascular collapse and shock.

Fecal breath odor accompanies fecal vomiting, which results when the obstructed or adynamic intestine attempts self-decompression by regurgitating its contents; vigorous peristaltic waves propel bowel contents backward into the stomach.

▶ **Emergency interventions**
Because fecal breath odor signals a potentially life-threatening intestinal obstruction, quickly assess your patient's condition. Monitor vital signs and be alert for signs of shock.

Ask if he's experiencing nausea and vomiting. If so, have him describe the color, odor, amount, and consistency of the vomitus. Have an emesis basin nearby to collect and measure any vomitus. Immediately inform the doctor of the patient's vital signs and vomiting history.

Withhold all food and fluids. Be prepared to insert a gastric tube or assist with insertion of an intestinal tube. Insert a peripheral I.V. line for vascular access, or assist with central line insertion for large-bore access and central venous pressure monitoring. Obtain a blood sample, if ordered, and send it to the laboratory. Maintain adequate hydration and support circulatory status with additional fluids. Give a physiologic solution with a potassium supplement, as ordered, to prevent metabolic acidosis from gastric losses and metabolic alkalosis from intestinal fluid losses.

## History
Ask the patient about previous abdominal surgery and loss of appetite. Determine if the patient is experiencing abdominal pain. Have him describe its onset, duration, location, and intensity.

Ask about bowel habits, constipation, diarrhea, leakage of stool, his last bowel movement, and the stool's color and consistency.

## Physical exam
Auscultate for bowel sounds. Inspect the abdomen. Measure abdominal girth to provide baseline data for subsequent assessment of distention. Palpate for tenderness, distention, and rigidity. Percuss for tympany, indicating a gas-filled bowel, and for dullness, indicating fluid.

## Causes
***Distal small-bowel obstruction.*** In late obstruction, nausea is present although vomiting may be delayed. Vomitus consists of gastric contents initially, changing to bilious and then to fecal contents with fecal breath odor. Other findings may include achiness, malaise, polydipsia, and bowel changes with abdominal distention and persistent epigastric or periumbilical colicky pain.

***Gastrojejunocolic fistula.*** Symptoms may vary. Fecal vomiting with resulting fecal breath odor may occur. Diarrhea is the most common presenting sign. Abdominal pain commonly occurs.

***Large-bowel obstruction.*** Fecal vomiting and breath odor are a late sign. Colicky abdominal pain appears suddenly, followed by hypogastric pain and marked abdominal distention and tenderness.

## Nursing considerations
• After inserting a gastric or an intestinal tube, keep the head of the bed elevated at least 30 degrees. Turn the patient as ordered to facilitate passage of the intestinal tube through the GI tract. Ensure tube patency and irrigate as ordered. Monitor GI drainage losses. Send serum specimens to the laboratory for analysis at least once a day. Prepare the patient for any diagnostic tests.
• Encourage the patient to brush his teeth and gargle with a flavored mouthwash or half-strength hydrogen peroxide mixture to minimize offensive breath odor. Assure him that the fecal odor is temporary and will abate after treatment.

# Skin, bronze

The result of excess circulating melanin, a bronze skin tone tends to appear at pressure points—such as the knuckles, elbows, toes, and knees—and in creases on the palms and soles. Eventually, this hyperpigmentation may extend to the buccal mucosa and gums before covering the entire body. It may stem from endocrine disorders, malnutrition, biliary cirrhosis, and certain drugs.

Because bronzing develops gradually, it's sometimes mistaken for a suntan. However, hyperpigmentation can affect the entire body, not just sun-exposed areas. Sunlight deepens the bronze color of exposed areas, but this effect gradually fades.

## History

Ask the patient when the hyperpigmentation first appeared. Has its hue changed? When was he last exposed to the sun? Also ask about a history of infection, illness, surgery, or trauma. Does he have abdominal pain, weakness, fatigue, diarrhea, or constipation? Has he lost weight recently? If he is receiving maintenance drug therapy for adrenal insufficiency, has his dosage been increased?

## Physical exam

Examine the mucosa, gums, and scars for hyperpigmentation. Check for dehydration, abdominal distention, loss of body hair, and tissue and muscle wasting. Palpate for hepatosplenomegaly.

## Causes

*Adrenal hyperplasia.* The entire skin assumes a dark bronze tone within a few months. Other findings include visual field defects and headache, resulting from an expanding pituitary lesion, and signs of androgen excess in females—clitoral enlargement and male distribution patterns of hair, fat, and muscle. Congenital adrenal hyperplasia causes irregular menses.

*Adrenal insufficiency.* Bronze skin may precede other features of this disorder by many years. Other findings may include axillary and pubic hair loss, vitiligo, progressive fatigue, weakness, anorexia, nausea and vomiting, weight loss, orthostatic hypotension, weak and irregular pulse, abdominal pain, irritability, diarrhea or constipation, decreased libido, amenorrhea, and syncope. Enhanced taste, smell, and hearing may also occur.

*Biliary cirrhosis.* Bronze skin results from melanosis of exposed areas of jaundiced skin, such as the eyelids, palms, neck, chest, or back. Other findings may include generalized pruritus, weakness, fatigue, jaundice, dark urine, pale stools with steatorrhea, anorexia and weight loss, and hepatomegaly.

*Hemochromatosis.* Progressive, generalized bronzing occurs early and is accented by metallic gray-bronze skin on sun-exposed areas, genitalia, and scars. Associated effects include weakness, lethargy, weight loss, abdominal pain, loss of libido, polydipsia, and polyuria. Later findings include hepatosplenomegaly, spider angiomas, joint swelling and tenderness, ascites, jaundice, edema, arrhythmias, loss of body hair, and testicular atrophy.

*Malnutrition.* Bronzing may be accompanied by apathy, lethargy, anorexia, weakness, and slow pulse and respiratory rates. Other findings include paresthesia in the extremities; dull, sparse, dry hair; brittle nails; dark, swollen cheeks; dry, flaky skin; red, swollen lips; muscle wasting; and gonadal atrophy in males.

*Other causes.* Prolonged therapy with high doses of phenothiazines.

## Nursing considerations

• Prepare the patient for the adrenocorticotropic hormone stimulation test, thyroid function studies, a complete blood count, electrolyte analysis, electrocardiography, and a computed tomography scan of the pituitary.

Fruity breath odor results from respiratory elimination of excess acetone. This sign characteristically occurs in ketoacidosis—a potentially life-threatening condition that requires immediate treatment to prevent severe dehydration, irreversible coma, and death.

Ketoacidosis results from the excessive catabolism of fats in the absence of usable carbohydrates. This occurs when insulin levels are insufficient to transport glucose into the cells, as in diabetes mellitus, or when glucose is unavailable and hepatic glycogen stores are depleted, as in low-carbohydrate diets and malnutrition.

▶ **Emergency interventions**
When you detect fruity breath odor, quickly check for Kussmaul's respirations and assess the patient's level of consciousness. Take vital signs and check skin turgor. If stupor, poor skin turgor, and rapid, deep respirations accompany fruity breath odor, call the doctor immediately.

Try to obtain a brief history, noting especially diabetes mellitus, nutritional problems, and fad diets. Obtain venous and arterial blood samples for glucose, electrolyte, acetone, complete blood count, and arterial blood gas (ABG) studies. Also obtain a urine sample, and test for glucose and acetone. As ordered, administer I.V. fluids and electrolytes and, in diabetic ketoacidosis, regular insulin to reduce blood glucose levels.

If the patient is obtunded, assist with insertion of endotracheal and nasogastric tubes. Suction, as needed. If ordered, insert an indwelling urinary catheter and carefully monitor intake and output. Assist with insertion of central venous pressure and arterial lines to monitor the patient's fluid status and blood pressure. Place the patient on a cardiac monitor, monitor vital signs and neurologic status, and draw blood hourly for glucose, acetone, electrolyte, and ABG studies.

### History
Ask the patient and his family about the onset and duration of fruity breath odor and if and when they noticed a change in the patient's breathing pattern. Ask about increased thirst, frequent urination, weight loss, weakness, fatigue, and abdominal pain. Ask the female patient if she has had monilial vaginitis or has vaginal secretions with itching. If the patient has a history of diabetes mellitus, ask about stress, past and current infections, and noncompliance with therapy—the most common causes of ketoacidosis in the known diabetic. For the patient with suspected severe weight loss, obtain a dietary and weight history.

### Causes
*Diabetic ketoacidosis.* Fruity breath odor commonly occurs as ketoacidosis develops. Other findings include polydipsia, polyuria, weak and rapid pulse, hunger, weight loss, weakness, fatigue, nausea, vomiting, and abdominal pain. Kussmaul's respirations, orthostatic hypotension, dehydration, tachycardia, confusion, and stupor occur.

*Starvation ketoacidosis.* Fruity breath odor commonly appears in this potentially life-threatening disorder. Associated signs and symptoms include Kussmaul's respirations; anorexia; orthostatic hypotension; weight loss; bradycardia; dry, scaling skin; sore tongue; muscle and tissue wasting; weakness; fatigue; abdominal pain and distention; poor wound healing; nausea; and possible disorientation, which may progress to stupor and coma.

### Nursing considerations
• Explain to the patient and his family all tests and treatments.
• When the patient becomes more alert and his condition stabilizes, remove any nasogastric tube and start him on an appropriate diet, as ordered. The doctor will then switch the diabetic patient's insulin route from I.V. to subcutaneous.
• Provide appropriate patient teaching or referral. For example, teach the patient with uncontrolled diabetes mellitus to recognize signs of hyperglycemia. Refer the patient with starvation ketoacidosis to a psychologist or support group.

**B**

A key sign of neurologic and respiratory break-down, shallow respirations occur when a diminished volume of air enters the lungs during inspiration.

## ▶ Emergency interventions

Be alert for impending respiratory failure or arrest. Is the patient severely dyspneic? Agitated or frightened? Look for signs of airway obstruction. If obstruction is total, perform abdominal thrusts. If the airway is occluded, use suction.

If you detect wheezing, check for stridor, nasal flaring, and use of accessory muscles. Administer oxygen, as needed. Notify the doctor and administer epinephrine, as ordered.

If the patient loses consciousness, insert an artificial airway and prepare for endotracheal intubation and ventilatory support.

## History

Ask when shallow respirations began. How long do they last? What makes them subside? What aggravates them? Does the patient have asthma, allergies, or a history of heart failure or vascular disease? Does he have chronic respiratory disorders, infections, or neurologic or neuromuscular disease? Does he smoke? Obtain a medication and drug abuse history.

## Physical exam

Inspect the chest for deformities or abnormal movements. Inspect the extremities for cyanosis and digital clubbing. Palpate for lung expansion and diaphragmatic tactile fremitus, and percuss for hyperresonance or dullness. Auscultate for diminished, absent, or adventitious breath sounds and for abnormal or distant heart sounds. Note any peripheral edema.

## Causes

*Adult respiratory distress syndrome.* Early signs include rapid, shallow respirations and dyspnea.

*Asthma.* Bronchospasm and hyperinflation of the lungs cause rapid, shallow respirations. Related effects include wheezing, a productive cough, dyspnea, and prolonged expirations.

*Atelectasis.* Decreased lung expansion or pleuritic pain causes rapid, shallow respirations.

*Chronic bronchitis.* Airway obstruction causes chronic shallow respirations and a hacking cough.

*Emphysema.* Muscle fatigue from effort required to breathe leads to chronic shallow respirations, dyspnea, diminished breath sounds, cyanosis, pursed-lip breathing, and barrel chest.

*Flail chest.* Decreased air movement results in rapid, shallow respirations; paradoxical chest wall motion from rib instability; tachycardia; and pain.

*Guillain-Barré syndrome.* Progressive ascending paralysis causes shallow respirations.

*Myasthenia gravis.* Respiratory muscle weakness leads to shallow respirations and dyspnea.

*Partial airway obstruction.* Acute shallow respirations may accompany sudden gagging and dry, paroxysmal coughing.

*Pneumonia.* Pulmonary consolidation results in rapid, shallow respirations. The patient may have dyspnea, fever, chills, and chest pain.

*Pneumothorax.* Along with sudden onset of shallow respirations and dyspnea, the patient may have severe unilateral chest pain.

*Pulmonary embolism.* Anginal or pleuritic chest pain may accompany sudden rapid, shallow respirations and dyspnea.

*Other causes.* Abdominal or thoracic surgery; amyotrophic lateral sclerosis; botulism; bronchiectasis; coma; drugs, such as narcotics, sedatives and hypnotics, tranquilizers, neuromuscular blockers, magnesium sulfate, and anesthetics; kyphoscoliosis; multiple sclerosis; muscular dystrophy; Parkinson's disease; pleural effusion; pulmonary edema; spinal cord injury; and tetanus.

## Nursing considerations

• Position the patient as nearly upright as possible, ensure adequate hydration, and provide humidification.

• Have him cough and deep-breathe every hour.

# Brudzinski's sign

A positive Brudzinski's sign—flexion of the hips and knees in response to passive flexion of the neck—signals meningeal irritation from the pressure of blood or exudate collecting around the spinal nerve roots. Passive flexion of the neck stretches the nerve roots, causing pain and involuntary flexion of the knees and hips.

Brudzinski's sign is a common and important early indicator of life-threatening meningitis and subarachnoid hemorrhage. It can be elicited in children as well as in adults, although more reliable indicators of meningeal irritation exist for infants.

## ▶ Emergency interventions

Immediately report a positive Brudzinski's sign. Then, if the patient's alert, ask him about headache, neck pain, nausea, and visual disturbances. Observe for signs of increased intracranial pressure (ICP), such as altered level of consciousness (LOC), pupillary changes, bradycardia, widened pulse pressure, irregular respiratory patterns, vomiting, and moderate fever. Report any of these findings to the doctor. Keep artificial airways, intubation equipment, a manual resuscitation bag, and suction equipment on hand. Elevate the head of the patient's bed 30 to 60 degrees to promote venous drainage.

## History

Ask the patient or his family, if necessary, about a history of hypertension, spinal arthritis, or recent head trauma. Ask about dental work and any abscessed teeth and about open head injury, endocarditis, and I.V. drug abuse. Ask about sudden onset of headaches.

## Physical exam

Continue your assessment by evaluating cranial nerve function and noting any motor or sensory deficits. Assess for Kernig's sign (resistance to leg extension after flexion of the hip and knee), a further indication of meningeal irritation. Look for signs of central nervous system infection, such as fever and nuchal rigidity.

## Causes

*Arthritis.* In severe spinal arthritis, a positive Brudzinski's sign can be elicited occasionally. The patient may also report back pain (especially after weight bearing) and limited mobility.

*Meningitis.* A positive Brudzinski's sign usually can be elicited 24 hours after the onset of this life-threatening disorder. Other findings may include headache; a positive Kernig's sign; nuchal rigidity; irritability or restlessness; deep stupor or coma; vertigo; fever; chills; malaise; hyperalgesia; hypotonia; opisthotonos; symmetrical deep tendon reflexes; unequal, sluggish pupils; papilledema; photophobia; diplopia; ocular and facial palsies; nausea; and vomiting. As ICP rises, hypertension, bradycardia, widened pulse pressure, and Cheyne-Stokes or Kussmaul's respirations may appear.

*Subarachnoid hemorrhage.* Brudzinski's sign may be elicited within minutes after initial bleeding. Other findings include sudden, severe headache, nuchal rigidity, altered LOC, dizziness, photophobia, cranial nerve palsies, nausea and vomiting, fever, and a positive Kernig's sign. As ICP rises, hypertension, bradycardia, widened pulse pressure, and Cheyne-Stokes or Kussmaul's respirations may occur.

## Nursing considerations

• The patient commonly requires constant ICP monitoring, frequent neurologic checks, and intensive assessment and monitoring of vital signs, intake and output, and cardiorespiratory status. To promote comfort, maintain low lights and minimal noise, and elevate the head of the bed.
• Prepare the patient for diagnostic tests, if ordered. These may include blood, urine, and sputum cultures to identify bacteria; lumbar puncture to assess cerebrospinal fluid and relieve pressure; and computed tomography scan, cerebral angiography, and spinal X-rays to locate a hemorrhage.

**B**

# Setting-sun sign

Also called sunset eyes, the setting-sun sign describes the position of an infant's or a young child's eyes that results when pressure is placed on cranial nerves III, IV, and VI. Both eyes are forced downward so that an area of sclera shows above the irises; in some patients, the irises appear to be forced outward.

Setting-sun sign reflects increased intracranial pressure (ICP). Typically, increased ICP results from space-occupying lesions — such as tumors — or from fluid accumulation in the brain's ventricular system, as occurs in hydrocephalus. It also results from intracranial bleeding or cerebral edema.

Setting-sun sign may be intermittent — for example, it may disappear when the infant is upright because this position slightly reduces ICP. The sign may be elicited in a normal infant under age 4 weeks by suddenly changing his head position. It can also be elicited in a normal infant up to age 9 months by placing a bright light before his eyes and removing it quickly.

## History

Obtain a brief history from the parents. When did this sign appear? Has the infant fallen or had even a minor traumatic injury?

Ask about early nonspecific signs of increasing ICP. Has the infant's sucking reflex diminished? Is he irritable, restless, or unusually tired? Does he cry when moved? Is his cry high-pitched?

## Physical exam

Perform a neurologic assessment. Keep in mind that neurologic responses are primarily reflexive during early infancy. Assess level of consciousness (LOC). Is the infant awake, irritable, or lethargic? Does he reach for a bright object or turn toward the sound of a music box? Observe his posture for normal flexion and extension or opisthotonos. Examine muscle tone and observe for seizure automatisms.

Examine the infant's anterior fontanel for bulging, measure his head circumference, and observe his breathing pattern. (Cheyne-Stokes respirations may accompany increased ICP.) Also check his pupillary response to light; unilateral or bilateral dilation occurs as ICP rises. Finally, elicit reflexes — diminished in increased ICP, especially Moro's reflex. Keep endotracheal intubation equipment available.

## Cause

*Increased ICP.* Transient or intermittent setting-sun sign commonly occurs late in increased ICP. The infant may have bulging, widened fontanels; increased head circumference; and widened sutures. He also may exhibit decreased LOC, behav-ioral changes, a high-pitched cry, pupillary abnormalities, and impaired motor movement. Other findings may include increased systolic pressure, widened pulse pressure, bradycardia, changes in breathing pattern, vomiting, and seizures.

## Nursing considerations

• Monitor vital signs and neurologic status. Elevate the head of the crib, and monitor intake and output. If ordered, monitor ICP, restrict fluids, and insert an I.V. line to give diuretics and corticosteroids.

• Try to maintain a calm environment. When the infant cries, comfort him to help prevent stress-related ICP elevations. Encourage parents to help.

• Prepare to assist with measures to treat severely increased ICP. The doctor may order endotracheal intubation and mechanical hyperventilation to reduce serum carbon dioxide levels and constrict cerebral vessels, or barbiturate coma or hypothermia therapy to lower the metabolic rate.

# Bruits

Usually an indicator of life- or limb-threatening vascular disease, bruits are swishing sounds caused by turbulent blood flow. They're characterized by location, duration, intensity, pitch, and time of onset in the cardiac cycle. Loud bruits produce intense vibration and a palpable thrill.

## ▶ Emergency interventions

If you detect bruits over the abdominal aorta, check for a pulsating mass or a bluish discoloration around the umbilicus. Either sign — or severe, tearing pain in the abdomen, flank, or lower back — may signal life-threatening dissection of an aortic aneurysm. If you suspect dissection, notify the doctor immediately. Monitor the patient's vital signs constantly, and withhold food and fluids. Watch for signs of hypovolemic shock.

## History

If you detect bruits, ask the patient if he has a history of hyperthyroidism, cerebrovascular disease, or heart disease. Has the patient had any neurologic symptoms, such as dizziness, diplopia, slurred speech, or syncope? Ask if the patient has any pain in his extremities or has noticed any change in skin color.

## Physical exam

To detect bruits, auscultate all major vessels. Bruits are most significant when heard over the carotid and subclavian arteries, the thyroid gland, the abdominal aorta, and the renal, femoral, and popliteal arteries. They're also significant when heard consistently despite changes in patient position and when heard during diastole.

## Causes

*Abdominal aortic aneurysm.* A pulsating periumbilical mass and a systolic bruit over the aorta are characteristic. Associated findings may include abdominal rigidity and tenderness, mottled skin, diminished peripheral pulses, and claudication. Sharp, tearing pain in the abdomen, flank, or lower back signals imminent dissection.

*Carotid artery stenosis.* Systolic bruits can be heard over one or both carotid arteries. Other signs and symptoms may be absent. However, dizziness, vertigo, headache, syncope, aphasia, dysarthria, vision loss, hemiparesis, or hemiparalysis signals a transient ischemic attack and may herald a cerebrovascular accident.

*Peripheral vascular disease.* Bruits over the femoral artery and other arteries in the legs are characteristic. Peripheral vascular disease also can cause diminished or absent femoral, popliteal, or pedal pulses; intermittent claudication; numbness, weakness, pain, and cramping in the legs, feet, and hips; and cool, shiny skin and hair loss on the affected extremity.

*Renal artery stenosis.* Systolic bruits are heard over the abdominal midline and flank on the affected side. Hypertension commonly occurs. Headache, tachycardia, anxiety, dizziness, retinopathy, and mental sluggishness may also occur.

*Thyrotoxicosis.* A systolic bruit is commonly heard over the thyroid gland. The most characteristic accompanying signs and symptoms include thyroid enlargement, fatigue, nervousness, tachycardia, heat intolerance, sweating, tremor, diarrhea, and weight loss despite increased appetite.

*Other causes.* Abdominal aortic atherosclerosis, anemia, peripheral arteriovenous fistula, and subclavian steal syndrome.

## Nursing considerations

• Frequently check the patient's vital signs and auscultate over the affected arteries. Be especially alert for bruits that become louder or develop a diastolic component.
• Instruct the patient to inform the doctor if he develops dizziness or pain.

**B**

# Seizure, simple partial

A simple partial seizure results from an irritable focus in the cerebral cortex. It lasts about 30 to 60 seconds and doesn't alter the patient's level of consciousness (LOC). Either motor or sensory, its type and pattern reflect the location of the irritable focus.

A *simple motor seizure* involves a series of unilateral clonic (muscle jerking) and tonic (muscle stiffening) movements of one part of the body.

A jacksonian motor seizure typically begins with a tonic contraction of a finger, the corner of the mouth, or one foot. Clonic movements then spread to other muscles on the same side of the body. In the postictal phase, the patient may display paralysis (Todd's paralysis) in the affected limbs, usually resolving within 24 hours. Alternately, movements may spread to the opposite side of the body, becoming a generalized seizure and leading to a loss of consciousness.

Epilepsia partialis continua causes clonic twitching, usually in the face, arm, or leg, occurring every few seconds and persisting for hours, days, or months without spreading.

A *simple sensory seizure* affects a localized body area on one side and causes numbness, tingling, or crawling sensations.

A visual seizure involves sensations of darkness or stationary or moving lights or spots, affecting both visual fields or the visual field on the side opposite the lesion. Seizures also may involve sensations of taste or smell.

## History

Ask the patient what happened before the seizure, if he recognized its onset, and, if so, how. How does this seizure compare with others the patient has had? Check for any history of head trauma, stroke, or recent infection, especially with fever, headache, or stiff neck.

## Physical exam

If you witness a simple seizure, notify the doctor immediately so he can observe it. Record the patient's behavior in detail. Where does movement first start? Does it spread? Watch for altered consciousness, bilateral tonicity and clonicity, cyanosis, tongue biting, and urinary incontinence. During the seizure, ask the patient to describe what's happening. Afterward, check his LOC and test for sensory disturbances and muscle weakness.

## Causes

*Brain abscess.* Seizures can occur in the acute stage of abscess formation or after resolution. Decreased LOC varies from drowsiness to deep stupor. Early symptoms include nausea, vomiting, and intractable headache; later, ocular disturbances, such as nystagmus, decreased visual acuity, and unequal pupils.

*Brain tumor.* Simple seizures are commonly the earliest indicators of a brain tumor. The patient may report morning headache, dizziness, confusion, vision loss, and motor and sensory disturbances.

*Cerebrovascular accident (CVA).* A major cause of seizures in patients over age 50, a CVA may induce focal seizures within 6 months. Related effects may include decreased LOC, hemiplegia, dysphagia, ataxia, sensory loss, apraxia, agnosia, and aphasia.

*Other causes.* Multiple sclerosis, neurofibromatosis, and sarcoidosis.

## Nursing considerations

• No emergency care is necessary during a simple seizure unless it progresses to a generalized seizure. Stay with the patient during the seizure, reassuring him. Afterward, instruct him to observe and record his seizures and to contact his doctor if their character or frequency changes.
• Emphasize compliance with drug therapy.
• Prepare the patient for any diagnostic tests.
• Help minimize seizures by recommending adequate sleep, proper diet, and regular exercise.

# Buffalo hump

An accumulation of cervicodorsal fat, a buffalo hump usually indicates hypercortisolism or Cushing's syndrome. Hypercortisolism itself may result from adrenal carcinoma, adrenal adenoma, ectopic adrenocorticotropic hormone (ACTH) production, excessive pituitary secretion of ACTH (Cushing's disease), or long-term glucocorticoid therapy.

A buffalo hump doesn't help distinguish among the underlying causes of hypercortisolism, but it may help direct diagnostic testing.

## History

Ask the patient about recent weight gain and when he first noticed the buffalo hump. Typically, a history of moderate to extreme obesity, with accumulation of adipose tissue in the nape of the neck, face, and trunk and thinning of the arms and legs, indicates hypercortisolism. If the patient has an old photograph, use it to compare his current and former weight and the distribution of adipose tissue. Ask if the patient or any family member has a history of endocrine disorders, cancer, or obesity. If the patient is a female of childbearing age, ask the date of her last menses and about any changes in her normal menstrual pattern. Next, ask about any changes in diet or drug use. If the patient is receiving glucocorticoid therapy, ask about the dosage, administration route, and any recent changes in therapy.

## Physical exam

Take the patient's vital signs, height, and weight. Form an impression of his appearance, noting obvious signs such as hirsutism, diaphoresis, and moon face. Inspect the arms, legs, and trunk for striae, and note skin turgor. Assess muscle function by asking the patient to rise from a squatting position; note any difficulty because this may indicate quadriceps muscle weakness.

During your assessment, observe the patient's behavior. Extreme emotional lability along with depression, irritability, or confusion may signal hypercortisolism.

## Causes

*Hypercortisolism.* The buffalo hump varies in size depending on the severity of the disorder and the amount of weight gained. It's commonly accompanied by hirsutism, moon face, and truncal obesity with slender arms and legs. The skin may appear transparent, with purple striae and ecchymoses. Other findings may include acne, muscle weakness and wasting, fatigue, poor wound healing, elevated blood pressure, personality changes, amenorrhea or oligomenorrhea in women, and impotence in men.

*Morbid obesity.* The size of the buffalo hump depends on the amount of weight gained and the distribution of adipose tissue. Associated signs and symptoms may include generalized adiposity, silver striae, elevated blood pressure, and hypogonadism.

*Other causes.* Drugs, such as excessive dosages of glucocorticoids.

## Nursing considerations

• Prepare the patient for diagnostic tests, if ordered. Blood and urine tests can confirm hypercortisolism. Ultrasonography, computed tomography (CT) scan, or arteriography can localize adrenal tumors. Chest X-rays, bronchography, and an abdominal CT scan can determine ectopic involvement. Visual field testing and a skull CT scan can identify pituitary tumors.

**B**

# Seizure, generalized tonic-clonic

A generalized tonic-clonic seizure reflects the paroxysmal, uncontrolled discharge of central nervous system neurons, affecting the entire brain and leading to neurologic dysfunction.

This type of seizure may include an aura. The patient then loses consciousness, falls to the ground, and may utter a loud cry. His body stiffens (tonic phase), then undergoes rapid muscle jerking and hyperventilation (clonic phase). Tongue biting, incontinence, diaphoresis, profuse salivation, and signs of respiratory distress may occur.

The seizure usually lasts 2 to 5 minutes, after which the patient regains consciousness but is confused. He may complain of headache, fatigue, muscle soreness, and arm and leg weakness. Complications may include respiratory arrest, status epilepticus, and head or spinal injuries.

▶ **Emergency interventions**
If you witness a seizure, have another nurse notify the doctor while you observe the seizure and protect the patient. Place a towel under his head, loosen his clothing, and move any sharp or hard objects out of his way. Never restrain him or force a hard object into his mouth. If possible, turn him to one side to allow secretions to drain. If the seizure lasts longer than 4 minutes or if a second seizure occurs before full recovery from the first, suspect status epilepticus. Establish an airway.

Position the patient on his side in a semidependent position and periodically alter sides.

## History
Ask whether the patient has had generalized or focal seizures before. Are they frequent? Do other family members have them? Is the patient receiving drug therapy or taking medication? Ask about stress at the time the seizure occurred and any injuries caused by it.

## Causes
*Eclampsia.* Generalized seizures are a hallmark of eclampsia. Other findings include severe frontal headache, vomiting, vision disturbances, increased blood pressure, edema, and sudden weight gain.

*Encephalitis.* Seizures are an early sign of this disorder, indicating a poor prognosis. They may also occur after recovery as a result of residual damage. Other findings include fever, headache, photophobia, nuchal rigidity, vomiting, aphasia, hemiparesis, nystagmus, and irritability.

*Head trauma.* Generalized seizures may occur at the time of injury, along with decreased level of consciousness (LOC) leading to coma; soft tissue injury or bony deformity of the face, head, or neck; clear or bloody drainage from the mouth, nose, or ears; Battle's sign; and lack of response to oculocephalic and oculovestibular stimulation.

*Hypertensive encephalopathy.* This life-threatening disorder may cause seizures, severely increased blood pressure, decreased LOC, intense headache, vomiting, transient blindness, paralysis, and (later) Cheyne-Stokes respirations.

*Other causes.* Alcohol withdrawal syndrome; arsenic poisoning; barbiturate withdrawal; brain abscess; brain tumor; cerebral aneurysm; cerebral vascular accident; chronic renal failure; contrast agents used in radiologic tests; drugs, such as toxic levels of aminophylline, theophylline, lidocaine, meperidine, penicillins, and cimetidine; hepatic encephalopathy; hypoglycemia; hyponatremia; hypoparathyroidism; hypoxic encephalopathy; idiopathic epilepsy; intermittent acute porphyria; multiple sclerosis; neurofibromatosis; and sarcoidosis.

In patients with preexisting epilepsy, other causes also include such drugs as phenothiazines, tricyclic antidepressants, alprostadil, amphetamines, isoniazid, and vincristine.

## Nursing considerations
• Emphasize compliance with drug therapy and warn the patient about adverse effects. Stress the importance of follow-up appointments and having his family observe and record his seizure activity.
• Help minimize seizures by recommending adequate sleep, proper diet, and regular exercise.

**S**

A butterfly rash is a cardinal sign of systemic lupus erythematosus. However, it can also signal dermatologic disorders. Typically, a butterfly rash appears in a malar distribution across the nose and cheeks. Similar rashes may appear on the neck, scalp, and other areas. A butterfly rash is sometimes mistaken for sunburn because it can be provoked or aggravated by ultraviolet rays.

## History
Ask the patient when he first noticed the rash and if he has been exposed to the sun recently. Ask about recent weight or hair loss and about rashes elsewhere on his body. Does he have a family history of lupus erythematosus? Is he taking hydralazine or procainamide?

## Physical exam
Inspect the rash, noting any macules, papules, pustules, and scaling. Is the rash edematous? Are areas of hypopigmentation or hyperpigmentation present? Look for blisters or ulcers in the mouth, and note any inflamed lesions. Check for rashes elsewhere on the body.

## Causes
*Discoid lupus erythematosus.* This benign form of lupus erythematosus produces a unilateral or butterfly rash that consists of mildly scaly, erythematous, raised, sharply demarcated plaques with follicular plugging and central atrophy. The rash may also involve the scalp, ears, chest, or any part of the body exposed to sun. Telangiectases, scarring alopecia, and hypopigmentation or hyperpigmentation may occur later. A destructive distortion of the nose and ears may develop.

*Erysipelas.* In this streptococcal infection, a butterfly rash appears as warm, indurated, tender, pruritic, edematous, and erythematous plaques, enlarging peripherally with sharply elevated margins; vesicles and bullae may form. Commonly, the rash appears abruptly and covers the bridge of the nose and one or both cheeks, halting at the hairline of the scalp or beard. The rash may also appear on the hands and genitals. Other findings include fever, malaise, headache, vomiting, sore throat, and cervical lymphadenopathy.

*Rosacea.* Initially, the rash may appear as a prominent, nonscaling, intermittent erythema limited to the lower half of the nose or including the chin, cheeks, and central forehead. As rosacea develops, the duration of the rash increases. In advanced rosacea, the skin is oily, with papules, pustules, nodules, and telangiectases restricted to the central third of the face.

*Seborrheic dermatitis.* The butterfly rash appears as greasy, scaly, slightly yellow macules and papules of varying size. The scalp, beard, eyebrows, portions of the forehead above the bridge of the nose, nasolabial fold, and trunk may also be involved. Other findings may include crusts and fissures, pruritus, redness, blepharitis, styes, severe acne, and oily skin.

*Systemic lupus erythematosus.* Occurring in about 40% of patients with this disorder, a butterfly rash appears as a red, scaly, sharply demarcated macular eruption. It may be transient or may progress slowly to include the forehead, chin, the area around the ears, and other exposed areas. Other skin findings include photosensitivity; scaling; patchy alopecia; mucous membrane lesions; mottled erythema of the palms and fingers; periungual erythema with edema; macular, reddish purple lesions on the volar surfaces of the fingers; telangiectasia of the base of the nails or eyelids; purpura; petechiae; or ecchymoses.

*Other causes.* Drugs, such as hydralazine and procainamide, and polymorphous light eruption.

## Nursing considerations
• Withhold photosensitizing drugs, such as phenothiazines, sulfonamides, sulfonylureas, and thiazide diuretics.
• Instruct the patient to avoid exposure to the sun or to use a sunscreen.
• Suggest the use of hypoallergenic makeup to help conceal facial lesions.

Formerly known as a psychomotor seizure, a complex partial seizure may begin in multiple foci, or it may develop from a simple partial seizure, which stems from one irritable focus. In either case, this type of seizure affects only one side of the brain. A complex partial seizure can occur at any age, but incidence usually increases during adolescence and adulthood. Two-thirds of affected patients also have generalized seizures, which affect both sides of the brain.

An aura may precede a complex partial seizure; once considered a warning sign, auras now are believed to be simple partial seizures. An aura may be audiovisual (images with sounds), auditory (abnormal or normal sounds or voices from the patient's past), or olfactory (unpleasant smells, such as rotten eggs or burning materials). Other types of auras include feelings of déjà vu, unfamiliarity with surroundings, or depersonalization. Some patients become fearful or anxious or have an unpleasant feeling in the epigastric region that rises toward the chest and throat. The patient usually can recognize an aura and lie down before losing consciousness.

During a complex partial seizure, the patient has an altered level of consciousness (LOC). He may experience automatisms following an aura, appear dazed and wander aimlessly, perform inappropriate acts (such as undressing in public),

be unresponsive, utter incoherent phrases, or, rarely, go into a rage or tantrum. After the seizure, he's confused, drowsy, and can't remember the seizure or surrounding events. Behavioral automatisms rarely last longer than 5 minutes, but postseizure confusion and amnesia may persist.

## Physical exam

If you witness a complex partial seizure, notify the patient's doctor so he can observe it. Never attempt to restrain the patient. Instead, lead him gently to a safe area. (*Exception:* Don't approach him if he's angry or violent.) Calmly encourage him to sit down and remain with him until he's fully alert. After the seizure, ask the patient if he experienced an aura or any aftereffects, such as a headache or fatigue. Remember to record all your observations and findings.

## Causes

*Brain abscess.* If the brain abscess is in the temporal lobe, complex partial seizures commonly occur in the acute phase or after the abscess disappears. Related effects may include headache, nausea, vomiting, generalized seizures, and a decreased LOC. The patient may also have central facial weakness, auditory receptive aphasia, hemiparesis, and ocular disturbances.

*Brain tumor.* Complex partial seizures may be

the first sign of this disorder. Other associated signs and symptoms include headache, pupillary changes, and mental dullness. Increased intracranial pressure may cause a decreased LOC, vomiting, and possible papilledema.

*Head trauma.* Severe trauma to the temporal lobe (especially from a penetrating injury) can produce complex partial seizures months or years later. The seizures may decrease in frequency and eventually stop. Head trauma may also cause generalized seizures and behavior and personality changes.

*Herpes simplex encephalitis.* If the herpes simplex virus attacks the temporal lobe, complex partial seizures can occur. Other features include fever, headache, coma, and generalized seizures.

## Nursing considerations

• After the seizure, remain with the patient to reorient him to his surroundings and to protect him from injury. Keep him in bed until he's fully alert, and remove harmful objects. Offer emotional support to the patient and his family, and teach them how to cope with seizures.

• Prepare the patient for diagnostic tests, such as magnetic resonance imaging, electroencephalography, and computed tomography scans.

• Help minimize seizures by recommending adequate sleep, proper diet, and regular exercise.

**S**

# Café-au-lait spots

An important indicator of neurofibromatosis and other congenital melanotic disorders, café-au-lait spots appear as flat, light-brown, uniformly hyperpigmented macules on the skin surface. Typically, they arise during childhood (most often before age 10) and can be differentiated from freckles and other benign birthmarks by their larger size (ranging from a few millimeters to 1.5 cm or larger) and more irregular shape. Although one to three spots may be a normal finding, the presence of café-au-lait spots usually indicates an underlying disorder.

### History
Ask the patient or his parents when the café-au-lait spots first appeared. Also ask about a family history of these spots and of neurofibromatosis. Review the patient's history for seizures, frequent fractures, and mental retardation.

### Physical exam
Inspect the skin, noting the location and pattern of the spots. Observe for distinctive skin lesions, such as axillary freckling, mottling, small spherical patches, and areas of depigmentation. Check for subcutaneous neurofibromas along major nerve branches, especially on the trunk. Also check for bony abnormalities, such as scoliosis or kyphosis.

### Causes
*Albright's syndrome.* In this syndrome, café-au-lait spots are smaller (about 1 cm) and more irregularly shaped than those in neurofibromatosis. They may stop abruptly at the midline and seem to follow a dermatomal distribution. Usually, fewer than six spots appear, often unilaterally on the forehead, neck, and lower back. When they occur on the scalp, the hair overlying them may be more deeply pigmented. Associated signs may include skeletal deformities, frequent fractures and, in females, sexual precocity.

*Neurofibromatosis.* The most common cause of café-au-lait spots, this disorder is characterized by six or more large, smooth-bordered spots. Associated signs include axillary freckling; irregular, hyperpigmented, and mottled skin; and, most significantly, multiple skin-colored pedunculated nodules clustered along nerve sheaths. These nodules develop during childhood and proliferate throughout life, affecting all body tissues and causing marked deformity. Mental impairment, seizures, hearing loss, exophthalmos, decreased visual acuity, and GI bleeding can occur eventually.

*Tuberous sclerosis.* In this disorder, mental retardation and seizures characteristically appear first, followed several years later by cutaneous facial lesions—multiple café-au-lait spots, spher-ical areas of rough skin, and areas of yellow-red or depigmented nevi.

### Nursing considerations
• Although café-au-lait spots require no treatment, you'll need to provide emotional support for the patient and his family. Also, refer them for genetic counseling.
• If ordered, prepare the patient for diagnostic tests, such as tissue biopsy and radiographic studies.

**C**

# Seizure, absence

Absence seizures are benign, generalized seizures thought to originate subcortically. These brief episodes of unconsciousness last 10 to 20 seconds and can occur 100 or more times a day, commonly causing periods of inattention. Absence seizures most often affect children between the ages of 4 and 12 and rarely persist beyond adolescence. Their first sign may be deteriorating schoolwork and a change in behavior. Their cause isn't known.

Absence seizures occur without warning. The patient suddenly stops all purposeful activity and stares blankly ahead, unable to see, hear, or feel. These seizures may produce automatisms, such as repetitive lip smacking, or mild clonic or myoclonic movements, including mild jerking of muscles in the eyelids. The patient may drop objects he's holding, and muscle relaxation may cause him to drop his head or arms or to slump. After the attack, the patient resumes activity without confusion, typically unaware of the episode.

Absence status, a rare form of absence seizure, occurs as a prolonged absence seizure or as repeated episodes of these seizures. Usually not life-threatening, it occurs most commonly in patients with preexisting absence seizures.

## History
Find out if the family has noticed a change in behavior or deteriorating schoolwork.

## Physical exam
If you suspect a patient is having an absence seizure, assess its occurrence and duration by reciting a series of numbers, then asking him to repeat them after the attack ends. The patient will be unable to do this. Or, if the seizures are occurring within minutes of each other, ask the patient to count for about 5 minutes. He'll stop counting during a seizure, then resume when it's over. Look for accompanying automatisms.

## Cause
*Idiopathic epilepsy.* Frequently, absence seizures are accompanied by automatisms and learning disability.

## Nursing considerations
• Explain the purpose of any diagnostic tests the child has been scheduled for, such as magnetic resonance imaging, computed tomography scans, and electroencephalography.
• Teach the patient and his family about these absence seizures and how to recognize their onset, pattern, and duration. Encourage the child's parents to include his teacher and school nurse in the teaching process, if possible.
• If the seizures are being controlled with drug therapy, emphasize the importance of strict compliance.

• Teach the patient and emphasize to his parents the importance of getting adequate sleep, eating a proper diet, minimizing stress, and participating in some form of exercise on a regular basis. These activities help to reduce seizure frequency.

**S**

Capillary refill time is the time required for color to return to the nail bed of a finger or toe after application of slight pressure, which causes blanching. This duration reflects the quality of peripheral vasomotor function. Normal capillary refill time is less than 3 seconds. Prolonged refill time isn't diagnostic of any disorder but usually signals obstructive peripheral arterial disease or decreased cardiac output.

## History

Take a brief medical history, noting especially previous peripheral vascular disease. Find out which medications the patient is taking.

## Physical exam

If you detect prolonged capillary refill time, take the patient's vital signs and check pulses in the affected limb. Does the limb feel cold or look cyanotic? Does the patient report pain or any unusual sensations in his fingers or toes, especially after exposure to cold?

## Causes

*Aortic aneurysm (dissecting).* Capillary refill time is prolonged in the fingers and toes with a dissecting aneurysm in the thoracic aorta, and prolonged just in the toes with a dissecting aneurysm in the abdominal aorta. Other common findings include a pulsating abdominal mass, a systolic bruit, and substernal or abdominal pain.

*Aortic arch syndrome.* Prolonged capillary refill time in the fingers occurs early, along with absent carotid pulses and possibly unequal radial pulses. Other findings that precede loss of pulses include fever, night sweats, arthralgia, weight loss, nausea, malaise, rash, and splenomegaly.

*Arterial occlusion (acute).* Prolonged capillary refill time occurs early in the affected limb. Arterial pulses are usually absent distal to the obstruction. The affected limb appears cool and pale or cyanotic. Intermittent claudication, moderate to severe pain, numbness, and paresthesia or paralysis of the affected limb may occur.

*Buerger's disease.* Capillary refill time is prolonged in the toes. Exposure to low temperatures turns the feet cold, cyanotic, and numb. Later, the feet redden, become hot, and tingle. Other findings include intermittent claudication of the instep, weak peripheral pulses and, in later stages, ulceration, muscle atrophy, and gangrene.

*Cardiac tamponade.* Prolonged capillary refill time is a late sign of decreased cardiac output. Other findings include tachycardia, cyanosis, dyspnea, neck vein distention, and hypotension.

*Hypothermia.* Prolonged capillary refill time may appear early. Other findings, depending on the degree of hypothermia, may include shivering, fatigue, decreased level of consciousness (LOC), slurred speech, ataxia, tachycardia or bradycardia, hyporeflexia or areflexia, diuresis, oliguria, bradypnea, decreased blood pressure, and cold, pale skin.

*Peripheral arterial trauma.* Any trauma to a peripheral artery that reduces distal blood flow also prolongs capillary refill time in the affected extremity. Related findings include bruising or pulsating bleeding, weakened pulse, paresthesia, cyanosis, sensory loss, and cool, pale skin.

*Raynaud's disease.* Exposure to cold or stress produces blanching in the fingers, then cyanosis, and then erythema before fingers return to normal temperature. Warmth relieves symptoms, which may include paresthesia. Chronic disease may produce sclerodactyly, ulcerations, or paronychia.

*Other causes.* Aortic bifurcation occlusion (acute); diagnostic tests, such as cardiac catheterization; drugs that cause vasoconstriction; peripheral vascular disease; shock; treatments, such as an arterial or umbilical line or an improperly fitted cast; and Volkmann's contracture.

## Nursing considerations

• Frequently assess the patient's vital signs, LOC, and affected extremity, and report any changes, such as progressive cyanosis or loss of an existing pulse.

Scrotal swelling occurs when a condition affecting the testicles, epididymis, or scrotal skin produces edema or a mass. It can be unilateral or bilateral, painful or painless, and may or may not involve the penis. It can affect males of any age.

The sudden onset of painful scrotal swelling suggests torsion of a testicle or testicular appendages, especially in the prepubescent male. This emergency requires immediate surgery.

## ▶ Emergency interventions

If severe pain accompanies scrotal swelling, find out when the swelling began. If it began suddenly, notify a urologist immediately. Use a Doppler stethoscope to assess blood flow to the scrotum. If it's decreased or absent, suspect testicular torsion and prepare the patient for surgery. Apply an ice pack to the scrotum to reduce pain and swelling.

## History

Ask the patient about injury to the scrotum, urethral discharge, cloudy urine, increased urinary frequency, and dysuria. Is the patient sexually active? When was his last sexual contact? Find out about recent illnesses, particularly mumps. Does he have a history of prostate surgery or prolonged catheterization? Does changing his body position or level of activity affect the swelling?

## Physical exam

Take the patient's vital signs, noting especially any fever, and palpate his abdomen for tenderness. Assess the scrotum with the patient supine and standing, noting its size and color. Is the swelling unilateral or bilateral? Do you see signs of trauma or bruising? Gently palpate the scrotum for a cyst or a lump, noting tenderness or increased firmness. Check the testicles' position in the scrotum. Transilluminate the scrotum to distinguish a fluid-filled cyst from a solid mass.

## Causes

*Epididymitis.* Key features are pain, extreme tenderness, and swelling in the groin and scrotum. Other findings may include a high fever, malaise, urethral discharge, cloudy urine, and lower abdominal pain.

*Hernia.* Herniation of bowel into the scrotum can cause swelling and a soft or unusually firm scrotum.

*Hydrocele.* Fluid accumulation produces gradual, usually painless scrotal swelling. The scrotum may be soft and cystic or firm and tense. Palpation reveals a round, nontender scrotal mass.

*Idiopathic scrotal edema.* Swelling occurs quickly and usually disappears within 24 hours. The affected testicle is pink.

*Orchitis (acute).* Mumps may precipitate this disorder, which causes sudden painful swelling of one or both testicles. Related findings include a hot, reddened scrotum; fever of up to 104° F (40° C); lower abdominal pain; vomiting; and extreme weakness. Urinary signs are usually absent.

*Spermatocele.* This painless or painful cystic mass lies above and behind the testicle and contains opaque fluid and sperm. Its onset may be acute or gradual. Less than 1 cm in diameter, the mass is movable and may be transilluminated.

*Testicular torsion.* Most common before puberty, this urologic emergency causes scrotal swelling, sudden and severe pain, and possible elevation of the affected testicle within the scrotum.

*Testicular tumor.* Typically painless, smooth, and firm, a testicular tumor produces swelling and a sensation of excessive weight in the scrotum.

*Other causes.* Elephantiasis of the scrotum, epididymal cysts, epididymal tuberculosis, gumma, scrotal burns, scrotal trauma, surgery, and torsion of a hydatid of Morgagni.

## Nursing considerations

• As ordered, keep the patient on bed rest and give antibiotics. Provide adequate fluids, fiber, and stool softeners. Place a rolled towel between the patient's legs and under the scrotum to help reduce swelling. Encourage sitz baths, and apply heat or ice packs to decrease inflammation.

# Carpopedal spasm

A carpopedal spasm is the violent, painful contraction of the muscles in the hands and feet. It's an important sign of tetany, a potentially life-threatening condition commonly associated with hypocalcemia and characterized by increased neuromuscular excitation and sustained muscle contraction.

A carpopedal spasm requires prompt evaluation and intervention; if untreated, it can cause laryngospasm, seizures, cardiac arrhythmias, and cardiac and respiratory arrest.

### ▶ Emergency interventions

If you detect a carpopedal spasm, quickly assess the patient for signs of respiratory distress (laryngospasm, stridor, loud crowing noises, cyanosis) and cardiac arrhythmias, which indicate hypocalcemia. If you detect these signs, call a doctor immediately, administer an I.V. calcium preparation as ordered, and give emergency respiratory and cardiac support as needed. If calcium infusion doesn't control seizures, administer a sedative, such as chloral hydrate or phenobarbital, as ordered.

### History

If the patient isn't in distress, obtain a detailed history. Ask about the onset and duration of the spasms and the degree of pain they produce. Also ask about related signs and symptoms of hypocalcemia, such as numbness and tingling of the fingertips and feet; other muscle cramps or spasms; and nausea, vomiting, and abdominal pain. Check for previous neck surgery, calcium or magnesium deficiency, and hypoparathyroidism.

While taking the history, try to form a general impression of the patient's mental status and behavior. If possible, ask the patient's family members or friends if they've noticed changes in the patient's behavior. Mental confusion or even personality changes may occur with hypocalcemia.

### Physical exam

Inspect the patient's skin and fingernails, noting any dryness or scaling and the presence of ridged, brittle nails.

### Causes

*Hypocalcemia.* A carpopedal spasm is an early sign of hypocalcemia. It's usually accompanied by paresthesia of the fingers, toes, and perioral area; muscle weakness, twitching, and cramping; hyperreflexia; chorea; fatigue; and palpitations. Positive Chvostek's and Trousseau's signs can be elicited. Laryngospasm, stridor, and seizures may appear in severe hypocalcemia.

Chronic hypocalcemia may be accompanied by mental status changes; cramps; dry, scaly skin; brittle nails; and thin, patchy hair and eyebrows.

*Other causes.* Surgical procedures that impair calcium absorption, such as ileostomy formation and gastric resection with gastrojejunostomy; and treatments, such as multiple blood transfusions and parathyroidectomy.

### Nursing considerations

- A carpopedal spasm can cause severe pain and anxiety, leading to hyperventilation. If this occurs, help the patient slow his breathing through your relaxing touch, reassuring attitude, and clear directions for what he should do.
- Provide a quiet, dark environment to reduce the patient's anxiety.
- As ordered, prepare the patient for laboratory tests, such as complete blood count and serum calcium, phosphorus, and parathyroid hormone studies.

# Scotoma

A scotoma is an area of partial or complete blindness within an otherwise normal or slightly impaired visual field. Usually located within the central 30-degree area, the defect ranges from absolute blindness to a barely detectable loss of visual acuity. Typically, the patient can pinpoint the scotoma's location in the visual field.

Resulting from retinal, choroid, or optic nerve disorders, a scotoma can be absolute, relative, or scintillating. An *absolute scotoma* is the total inability to see all sizes of test objects used in mapping the visual field. A *relative scotoma* refers to the ability to see only large test objects. A *scintillating scotoma* refers to the flashes or bursts of light commonly seen before a migraine headache.

## History

Explore the patient's history for eye disorders, vision problems, or chronic systemic disorders. Does the patient take medications or use eyedrops?

## Physical exam

Test for a scotoma using such visual field tests as the tangent screen examination and the automated perimetry test. Next, test the patient's visual acuity and inspect his pupils for size, equality, and reaction to light. If requested, assist with an ophthalmoscopic examination and measurement of intraocular pressure (IOP).

## Causes

*Chorioretinitis.* Inflammation of the choroid produces a paracentral scotoma. Ophthalmoscopic examination reveals clouding and cells in the vitreous humor, subretinal hemorrhage, and neovascularization.

*Glaucoma.* Prolonged elevation of IOP can cause an arcuate scotoma. Poorly controlled glaucoma can also cause cupping of the optic disk, loss of peripheral vision, and reduced visual acuity. The patient may also see rainbow-colored halos around lights.

*Macular degeneration.* Any degenerative process or disorder affecting the fovea centralis results in a central scotoma. Ophthalmoscopic examination reveals changes in the macular area. The patient may notice subtle changes in visual acuity, color perception, and the size and shape of objects.

*Migraine headache.* Transient scintillating scotomas, usually bilateral and often homonymous, can occur with a classic migraine aura. Besides pain, characteristic associated symptoms include paresthesia of the lips, face, or hands; slight confusion; dizziness; and photophobia.

*Optic neuritis.* Inflammation, degeneration, or demyelination of the optic nerve produces central, circular, or centrocecal scotoma. The scotoma may be unilateral with involvement of one nerve or bilateral with involvement of both nerves. It can vary in size, density, and symmetry. The patient may have severe visual loss or blurring lasting up to 3 weeks, and pain—especially with eye movement. Common ophthalmoscopic findings include hyperemia of the optic disk, retinal vein distention, blurred disk margins, and filling of the physiologic cup.

*Retinal pigmentary degenerations.* Premature retinal cell changes lead to cell death. Retinitis pigmentosa—a degenerative disorder—initially involves loss of peripheral rods. The resulting annular scotoma progresses concentrically until only a central field of vision (tunnel vision) remains. Impaired night vision is the earliest symptom and appears during adolescence. Associated signs include narrowing of the retinal blood vessels and pallor of the optic disk. Eventually, with invasion of the macula, blindness may occur.

## Nursing considerations

• For the patient with an arcuate scotoma associated with glaucoma, emphasize regular testing of IOP and visual fields. In addition, teach the patient with a disorder involving the fovea centralis (or the area surrounding it) to periodically use the Amsler grid to detect progression of macular degeneration.

**S**

The uneven extension of portions of the chest wall during inspiration, asymmetrical chest expansion may develop suddenly or gradually and may affect one or both sides of the chest wall. It may occur as *delayed expiration* (chest lag); as *abnormal movement during inspiration* (for example, intercostal retractions, paradoxical movement, or chest-abdomen asynchrony); or as *unilateral absence of movement*. It usually results from pleural disorders but can also result from musculoskeletal or neurologic disorders, airway obstruction, or trauma.

## ▶ Emergency interventions

If you detect asymmetrical chest expansion, first consider traumatic chest injury, which can cause flail chest (paradoxical chest movement). Take vital signs and look for signs of acute respiratory distress. If these signs are present, have another nurse call the doctor immediately. Then splint the unstable flail segment. Give oxygen and start an I.V. line.

## History

If the patient isn't in acute respiratory distress, find out if he's experiencing dyspnea or pain during breathing. Is dyspnea constant or intermittent? Does repositioning, coughing, or any other activity relieve or worsen it? Can he inhale deeply?

Ask about respiratory or systemic illness, tho-racic surgery, and blunt or penetrating chest trauma. Ask the patient if he could have inhaled or aspirated a toxic substance.

## Physical exam

Palpate the trachea for midline positioning. Then examine the posterior chest wall for tenderness or deformity. Evaluate the extent of chest expansion. Next, use the ulnar surface of your hand to palpate for vocal or tactile fremitus. Percuss and auscultate to detect air and fluid in the lungs and pleural spaces, and auscultate for breath sounds.

## Causes

*Bronchial airway obstruction.* Lack of chest movement indicates complete airway obstruction; chest lag signals partial obstruction. Other signs: dyspnea, accessory muscle use, retractions, and decreased or absent breath sounds.

*Flail chest.* In this life-threatening injury to the ribs or sternum, the unstable portion of the chest wall collapses and causes paradoxical movement.

*Hemothorax.* Life-threatening bleeding into the pleural space causes chest lag during inspiration. Other findings may include signs of traumatic chest injury, pain at the injury site, dullness on percussion, tachypnea, and tachycardia.

*Myasthenia gravis.* Loss of ventilatory muscle function produces chest-abdominal asynchrony that can lead to acute respiratory distress.

*Pleural effusion.* Chest lag at end-inspiration occurs gradually in this life-threatening condition. Usually, a combination of dyspnea, tachypnea, and tachycardia precedes chest lag.

*Pneumonia.* Asymmetrical chest expansion occurs as inspiratory chest lag or as chest-abdomen asynchrony, depending on where consolidation occurs. The patient will typically have fever, chills, tachycardia, and tachypnea.

*Pneumothorax.* Entrapment of air in the pleural space can cause chest lag at end-inspiration. Sudden, stabbing chest pain may radiate to the arms, face, back, or abdomen.

*Pulmonary embolism.* This life-threatening disorder causes chest lag, stabbing chest pain, tachycardia, dyspnea, blood-tinged sputum, and pleural friction rub.

*Other causes.* Accidental intubation of a mainstem bronchus, cerebral palsy, diaphragmatic hernia, kyphoscoliosis, phrenic nerve dysfunction, pneumonectomy, poliomyelitis, and surgical removal of several ribs.

## Nursing considerations

• Regularly auscultate breath sounds in an intubated patient to detect a misplaced tube. If confirmed, prepare the patient for a chest X-ray to allow repositioning of the tube.

# Salt craving

Craving salty foods is a compensatory response to the body's failure to adequately conserve sodium. Normally, the renal tubules reabsorb almost all sodium, allowing less than 1% of it to be excreted in the urine. This reabsorption is regulated by aldosterone, a hormone synthesized in the adrenal gland. However, adrenal dysfunction can reduce aldosterone levels, thereby impairing reabsorption and increasing sodium excretion.

## History
Because normal salt intake varies widely, depending on dietary preferences and cultural differences, find out how much salt the patient typically uses. Has he increased this amount recently? Has he also experienced weakness, fatigue, anorexia, or weight loss? Has he felt dizzy or fainted? Check for a history of adrenal insufficiency or diabetes mellitus and for recent onset of polydipsia or polyuria.

## Physical exam
Inspect the patient's skin for hyperpigmentation or hypopigmentation. Take his vital signs, too, noting postural hypotension. Remember that sudden or rapidly worsening salt craving may indicate adrenal crisis if it's accompanied by hypotension, tachycardia, oliguria, and cool, clammy skin.

## Cause
*Primary adrenal insufficiency.* Often called Addison's disease, this disorder reduces aldosterone secretion. As a result, the patient may exhibit an intense craving for salty food. He may display diffuse brown, tan, or bronze-to-black hyperpigmentation of exposed areas (such as the face, knees, and knuckles) and of nonexposed areas (such as palmar creases, the tongue, or buccal mucosa) and darkening of normally pigmented areas, moles, and scars. In about 15% of cases, the patient also displays hypopigmentation. Related findings include weakness, anorexia, nausea, irritability, vomiting, weight loss, abdominal pain, and slowly progressive fatigue.

## Nursing considerations
• Prepare the patient for laboratory tests, such as serum aldosterone and electrolytes, plasma cortisol and glucose, and urine 17-ketogenic steroids and 17-hydroxycorticosteroids. Special provocative studies may include the metyrapone test or the rapid adrenocorticotropic hormone test. Collect a urine specimen and use a reagent strip to test for glucose and acetone.
• To check for volume depletion, monitor and record the patient's intake, output, and weight. Promote fluid intake and arrange for a diet that helps maintain adequate sodium and potassium levels. Be alert for signs of hyponatremia, such as hypotension, muscle twitching and weakness, and abdominal cramps. Also be alert for signs of hyperkalemia, such as muscle weakness, tachycardia, nausea, vomiting, and characteristic ECG changes—tented and elevated T waves, widened QRS complex, prolonged PR interval, flattened or absent P waves, and depressed ST segment.
• If diagnostic tests confirm primary adrenal insufficiency, emphasize the importance of complying with lifelong steroid therapy, including glucocorticoids and mineralocorticoids. Teach the patient the signs and symptoms of steroid toxicity and underdosage. Also explain that his dosage may need to be increased during stress (infection, injury, even profuse sweating) to prevent adrenal crisis.
• Instruct him to carry a medical identification card at all times, stating that he takes a steroid and giving the drug's name and dosage. Teach him how to give himself a hydrocortisone injection, and tell him to keep hydrocortisone available in a prepared syringe for emergency use.

S

Usually a result of thoracic or abdominal disorders, chest pain can also result from musculoskeletal and hematologic disorders, anxiety, and drug therapy. It can be provoked by stress, anxiety, exertion, deep breathing, or eating certain foods.

### ▶ Emergency interventions

If your patient reports sudden crushing, shooting, ripping or tearing chest pain, or chest pain that radiates to the left arm, jaw, or shoulder blades, suspect a pulmonary embolism, dissecting aortic aneurysm, or myocardial infarction. Assess for diaphoresis, dyspnea, hemoptysis, tachycardia, and weak pulses. Take vital signs, and have another nurse call the doctor immediately. Give oxygen, insert an I.V. line, and begin cardiac monitoring.

If your patient reports diffuse chest tightness and you detect wheezing and tachypnea, suspect an asthmatic attack. Have another nurse call the doctor. Give oxygen, insert an I.V. line, and prepare to give epinephrine and a bronchodilator.

### History

Ask the patient when his chest pain began and if it developed suddenly or gradually. Is the pain sharp or knifelike? Constant or intermittent? Ask him what aggravates or alleviates the pain. Is the pain getting worse? Ask him to indicate the painful area. Does the pain radiate to the neck, jaw, arms, or back? Review the history for cardiac or respiratory disease, chest trauma, or intestinal disease. Obtain a drug history.

### Physical exam

Take vital signs. Assess for jugular vein distention and peripheral edema, observe breathing pattern, and inspect the chest for asymmetrical expansion. Auscultate the heart and lungs. Palpate for lifts, heaves, thrills, gallops, tactile fremitus, abdominal masses, and tenderness.

### Causes

*Angina.* This pain usually occurs in the retrosternal region and radiates to the neck, jaw, and arms. It lasts 2 to 10 minutes, during which you may hear an atrial gallop ($S_4$) or murmur.

*Aortic aneurysm (dissecting).* Sudden, excruciating, tearing pain in the chest and neck radiates to the upper back, abdomen, and lower back.

*Asthma.* Diffuse, painful chest tightness arises suddenly with a dry cough and mild wheezing.

*Cholecystitis.* Epigastric or right upper quadrant pain may be steady or intermittent and may radiate to the back.

*Hiatal hernia.* Typically, this disorder produces an angina-like sternal burning, ache, or pressure that may radiate to the left shoulder and arm.

*Mitral prolapse.* A prolapsed mitral valve causes sharp, stabbing precordial chest pain or ache.

*Myocardial infarction.* Crushing substernal pain lasts from 15 minutes to hours and may radiate to the left arm, jaw, neck, or shoulder blades. Other findings: dyspnea, pallor, diaphoresis, anxiety, atrial gallop, and blood pressure changes.

*Peptic ulcer.* Sharp, burning pain arises in the epigastric region, usually hours after food intake.

*Pericarditis.* Precordial or retrosternal pain worsens with deep breathing, coughing, and movement.

*Pneumothorax.* Spontaneous pneumothorax causes sudden, sharp, severe chest pain that increases with chest movement.

*Other causes.* Abrupt withdrawal of beta blockers, acute bronchitis, anxiety, blastomycosis, cardiomyopathy, Chinese restaurant syndrome, coccidioidomycosis, costochondral inflammation, distention of the colon's splenic flexure, esophageal spasm, herpes zoster, interstitial lung disease, Legionnaires' disease, lung abscess, lung cancer, mediastinitis, muscle strain, nocardiosis, pancreatitis, pleurisy, pneumonia, psittacosis, pulmonary actinomycosis, pulmonary embolism or hypertension, rib fracture, sickle cell crisis, thoracic outlet syndrome, and tuberculosis.

### Nursing considerations

• Because the patient may deny his discomfort, stress the importance of reporting symptoms.

Also known as polysialia or ptyalism, this uncommon symptom may result from GI disorders, especially of the mouth. Increased salivation also accompanies certain systemic disorders and may result from the effects of drugs and toxins. Saliva may also accumulate because of difficulty swallowing.

## History
Ask the patient about related signs and symptoms, such as fatigue, fever, headache, or a sore throat. Ask about exposure to industrial toxins, such as mercury. Is the patient currently taking any medications? Note especially use of iodides, cholinergics, and miotics.

## Physical exam
A patient who complains of increased salivation may have overproductive salivary glands or difficulty swallowing. To distinguish these, first test for a gag reflex and observe the patient's ability to swallow and chew. Is he drooling? Is his chewing uncoordinated? An impaired gag reflex, drooling, and chewing incoordination suggest difficulty swallowing.

Inspect the mouth and mucous membranes for lesions. If present, are they painful? Put on gloves and palpate the lesions, which may be suppurative or infectious. Describe them in your notes. Next, inspect the uvula, gingivae, and pharynx. Palpate the lymph nodes, and determine if the parotid glands are swollen or sore.

## Causes
*Arsenic poisoning.* Increased salivation infrequently occurs in this disorder. More common effects are diarrhea, diffuse skin hyperpigmentation, and edema of the eyelids, face, and ankles. The patient may have a garlicky breath odor, pruritus, alopecia, irritated mucous membranes, headache, drowsiness, and confusion. He may also have muscle aching, weakness, paresthesia, and seizures.

*Drugs.* Increased salivation may occur in iodide toxicity, but the earliest symptoms are a brassy taste and a burning sensation in the mouth and throat. Other findings include sneezing, irritated eyelids, and, commonly, pain in the frontal sinuses.

Pilocarpine and other miotics used to treat glaucoma may be absorbed systemically, increasing salivation. Cholinergics, such as bethanechol and neostigmine, may also cause increased salivation.

*Mercury poisoning.* Stomatitis—involving increased salivation and a metallic taste—commonly occurs in mercury poisoning. The patient's teeth may be loose; his gums are painful, swollen, and prone to bleeding. A blue line appears on the gingivae. The patient may also have personality changes, abdominal cramps, diarrhea, paresthesia, and tremors of the eyelids, lips, tongue, and fingers.

*Stomatitis.* Mucosal ulcers may be accompanied by moderately increased salivation, mouth pain, fever, and erythema. Spontaneous healing usually occurs in 7 to 10 days, but scarring and recurrence are possible.

*Syphilis.* In secondary syphilis, mucosal ulcers cause increased salivation that may persist for up to a year. Related findings include fever, malaise, headache, anorexia, weight loss, nausea, vomiting, sore throat, and generalized lymphadenopathy. A rash appears on the arms, trunk, palms, soles, face, and scalp.

*Tuberculosis.* Certain forms of tuberculosis may produce solitary, irregularly shaped mouth or tongue ulcers, covered with exudate, that cause increased salivation. Other findings include weight loss, anorexia, fever, fatigue, malaise, dyspnea, cough, night sweats (a common sign), and hemoptysis.

## Nursing considerations
• Although annoying to the patient, increased salivation doesn't require treatments beyond those needed to correct the underlying disorder.

The most common pattern of periodic breathing, Cheyne-Stokes respirations are characterized by a waxing and waning period of hyperpnea that alternates with a shorter period of apnea. This pattern can occur normally in people who live at high altitudes and in elderly people during sleep. Usually, though, it indicates increased intracranial pressure (ICP) from a deep cerebral or brain stem lesion (usually bilateral) or a metabolic disturbance in the brain.

Cheyne-Stokes respirations always indicate a major change in the patient's condition—usually for the worse. For example, in a patient who has had head trauma or brain surgery, Cheyne-Stokes respirations may signal increasing ICP.

### ▶ Emergency interventions
If you detect Cheyne-Stokes respirations in a patient with a history of head trauma, recent brain surgery, or other brain insult, quickly take his vital signs and immediately notify the doctor. Keep the patient's head elevated 30 degrees, and perform a rapid neurologic assessment to obtain baseline data. Reassess his neurologic status often. If ICP continues to rise, you'll detect changes in his level of consciousness (LOC), pupillary reactions, and ability to move his extremities. Be prepared to assist with ICP monitoring, as ordered.

Be alert for prolonged periods of apnea. Frequently check blood pressure; also check skin color to detect signs of hypoxemia. Maintain airway patency and administer oxygen as needed. If the patient's condition worsens, assist with endotracheal intubation.

### History
When the patient's condition permits, obtain a brief history. Ask especially about drug use—large doses of narcotics, hypnotics, or barbiturates can precipitate Cheyne-Stokes respirations.

### Physical exam
Time the periods of hyperpnea and apnea for 3 or 4 minutes to evaluate respirations and to obtain baseline data.

### Causes
*Heart failure.* In left ventricular failure, Cheyne-Stokes respirations may occur with exertional dyspnea and orthopnea. Related findings include fatigue, weakness, tachycardia, tachypnea, and crackles. A cough, usually nonproductive but occasionally producing clear or blood-tinged sputum, may also occur.

*Hypertensive encephalopathy.* In this life-threatening disorder, severe hypertension precedes Cheyne-Stokes respirations. The patient's LOC will be decreased, and he may experience vomiting, seizures, severe headaches, visual disturbances (including transient blindness), and transient paralysis.

*Increased ICP.* As ICP rises, Cheyne-Stokes is the first irregular respiratory pattern to occur. It's preceded by decreased LOC and accompanied by hypertension, headache, vomiting, impaired or unequal motor movement, and visual disturbances (blurring, diplopia, photophobia, and pupillary changes). In late stages of increased ICP, bradycardia and widened pulse pressure occur.

*Renal failure.* In end-stage chronic renal failure, Cheyne-Stokes respirations may occur along with bleeding gums, oral lesions, ammonia breath odor, and marked changes in every body system.

*Stokes-Adams attacks.* Cheyne-Stokes respirations may follow a Stokes-Adams attack—a syncopal episode associated with atrioventricular block. The patient is hypotensive, with a heart rate between 20 and 50 beats/minute. He may also appear pale, shaking, and confused.

*Other causes.* Drugs, such as large doses of hypnotics, narcotics, or barbiturates.

### Nursing considerations
• When evaluating Cheyne-Stokes respirations, be careful not to mistake periods of hypoventilation or decreased tidal volume for apnea.

# Salivation, decreased

Also known as dry mouth or xerostomia, decreased salivation is a common but minor complaint that usually results from mouth breathing. However, this symptom can also result from salivary duct obstruction, Sjögren's syndrome, the use of anticholinergics and other drugs, and the effects of radiation. It can even result from vigorous exercise or from autonomic stimulation — for example, triggered by fear.

## History

Evaluate the patient's complaint of dry mouth by asking him when he first noticed the symptom. Was he exercising at the time? Is he currently taking any medication? Is his sensation of dry mouth intermittent or continuous? Is it related to or relieved by a particular activity? Ask about related symptoms, such as burning or itchy eyes, or changes in his sense of smell or taste.

## Physical exam

Inspect the patient's mouth, including the mucous membranes, for any abnormalities. Observe his eyes for problems that could be caused by lack of moisture, such as conjunctival irritation, matted lids, and corneal epithelial thickening. Perform simple tests of smell and taste to detect possible impairment of these senses. Next, check to see if the patient has enlarged parotid and submaxillary glands. Palpate for tender or enlarged areas along the neck, too.

## Causes

***Salivary duct obstruction.*** Usually associated with a salivary stone, this obstruction causes reduced salivation and local pain and swelling.

***Sjögren's syndrome.*** Diminished secretions from the lacrimal, parotid, and submaxillary glands produce the hallmarks of this disorder: decreased or absent salivation, and dry eyes with a persistent burning, gritty sensation. The patient may also have dryness that involves the respiratory tract, vagina, and skin. Related oral signs and symptoms include difficulty chewing, talking, and swallowing, as well as ulcers and soreness of the lips and mucosa. The parotid and submaxillary glands may be enlarged. Nasal crusting, epistaxis, fatigue, lethargy, nonproductive cough, abdominal discomfort, and polyuria may be present.

***Other causes.*** Drugs, such as anticholinergics, antihistamines, tricyclic antidepressants, phenothiazines, clonidine hydrochloride, and narcotic analgesics; and radiation, from antineoplastic treatments or dental X-rays.

## Nursing considerations

• If markedly reduced salivation interferes with speaking, eating, or swallowing, allow the patient extra time for these activities.
• Encourage him to increase his fluid intake during meals and to brush his teeth, floss, and use mouthwash. Also encourage him to suck sour hard candies to relieve his dry mouth.

**S**

Also known as rigors, chills are extreme, involuntary muscle contractions with characteristic paroxysms of violent shivering and teeth chattering. Chills are commonly accompanied by fever and tend to develop suddenly, usually as a warning of infection. Depending on the disorder, they may be brief, intermittent, or continuous for up to 1 hour.

## History

Ask the patient when the chills began and if they're continuous or intermittent. Also ask about headache, confusion, abdominal pain, nausea, and muscle disturbances. Does he have any known allergies? Find out which medications he's taking and if any drug has improved or worsened his symptoms. Ask about recent exposure to animals, including birds. Also ask about recent insect or animal bites and travel to foreign countries.

## Physical exam

Because fever commonly accompanies chills, monitor the patient's rectal temperature carefully.

## Causes

*Cholangitis.* Charcot's triad—chills with spiking fever, abdominal pain, and jaundice—characterizes sudden obstruction of the common bile duct.

*Gram-negative bacteremia.* This infection causes sudden chills and fever as well as nausea, vomiting, diarrhea, and prostration.

*Hemolytic anemia.* Fulminating chills occur with fever, abdominal pain, and hepatomegaly.

*Infective endocarditis.* Intermittent, shaking chills and fever occur abruptly along with petechiae, Janeway's spots on hands and feet, and Osler's nodes on palms and soles.

*Influenza.* This is marked by abrupt onset of chills, high fever, malaise, headache, myalgias, and a nonproductive cough.

*Legionnaires' disease.* This is marked by sudden onset of chills, high fever, and a cough with mucoid or mucopurulent sputum and possibly hemoptysis.

*Lymphogranuloma venereum.* Along with chills and lymphadenopathy, fever, headache, anorexia, myalgias, arthralgias, and weight loss may occur.

*Malaria.* Initially, chills last 1 to 2 hours, followed by 3 to 4 hours of high fever, and then 2 to 4 hours of profuse diaphoresis.

*Pelvic inflammatory disease.* Chills and fever are accompanied by lower abdominal pain and tenderness as well as purulent vaginal discharge.

*Pneumonia.* A single shaking chill usually heralds the onset of pneumococcal pneumonia; other pneumonias commonly cause intermittent chills. Related findings include fever, a productive cough with bloody sputum, chest pain, and dyspnea.

*Pyelonephritis.* The acute form of this disorder causes chills, high fever, and possibly nausea and vomiting over several hours to days.

*Rocky Mountain spotted fever.* This disorder begins with sudden onset of chills, fever, malaise, excruciating headache, and muscle, bone, and joint pain. The tongue is covered with a thick white coating that gradually turns brown.

*Septic shock.* Early symptoms include chills, fever, and flushed, warm, dry skin; blood pressure is normal or slightly low. Later, the arms and legs become cool and cyanotic.

*Typhoid fever.* Body temperature gradually increases for 5 to 7 days with accompanying chilliness or frank chills. Rose spots develop on the upper abdomen and anterior thorax.

*Other causes.* Acute suppurative otitis media; drugs, such as amphotericin B, I.V. bleomycin, and oral antipyretics; hemolytic or nonhemolytic transfusion reactions; Hodgkin's disease; I.V. insertion site infection; kidney abscess; liver abscess; lung abscess; lymphangitis; miliary tuberculosis; pit viper snakebite; postabortal or puerperal sepsis; psittacosis; septic arthritis; sinusitis; and violin spider bite.

## Nursing considerations

• Provide adequate hydration and nutrients, and give antipyretics as needed. Remember that irregular use of antipyretics can trigger compensatory chills. Give antibiotics, as ordered.

# Romberg's sign

Relatively uncommon, Romberg's sign refers to a patient's inability to maintain his balance when standing erect with his feet together and his eyes closed. It indicates a proprioceptive disorder or a disorder of the spinal tracts (the posterior columns) that carry proprioceptive information—the perception of one's position in space, joint movements, and pressure sensations—to the brain. A person with insufficient proprioceptive information cannot execute precise movements and maintain his balance without visual cues.

### History
Ask the patient if he's noticed sensory changes, such as numbness and tingling in his limbs. If so, when did they begin?

### Physical exam
Test the patient's proprioception. If he can maintain his balance with his eyes open, ask him to hop on one foot, then on the other. Next, ask him to do a knee bend, then to walk a straight line, placing heel to toe. Lastly, ask him to walk a short distance so you can evaluate his gait.

Test the patient's awareness of body-part position by changing the position of one of his fingers, or any other joint, while his eyes are closed. Ask him to describe the change you've made.

Test the patient's direction of movement. Ask him to close his eyes and touch his nose with the index finger of one hand, then with the other. Ask him to repeat this movement several times, gradually increasing his speed. Then have him rapidly touch each finger of one hand to the thumb. Next, using a pin, test sensation in all dermatomes. Test two-point discrimination by touching two pins (one in each hand) to his skin simultaneously. Test the patient's deep tendon reflexes.

Test the patient's vibratory sense by asking him to close his eyes, then applying a vibrating tuning fork to his clavicles, spinous processes, elbows, finger joints, knees, ankles, and toes. Hold it in each location until it stops vibrating. Tell the patient to report when the vibrations start and stop.

### Causes
*Multiple sclerosis.* Early features may include blurred vision, diplopia, and paresthesia. Besides a positive Romberg's sign, other findings may include nystagmus, constipation, muscle weakness and spasticity, hyperreflexia, dysphagia, dysarthria, incontinence, and impotence.

*Peripheral nerve disease.* Besides a positive Romberg's sign, advanced disease may produce impotence, fatigue, and paresthesia, hyperesthesia, or anesthesia in the hands and feet. Related findings include incoordination, ataxia, burning pain in the affected area, progressive muscle weak-ness and atrophy, and loss of vibration sense.

*Pernicious anemia.* A positive Romberg's sign and loss of proprioception in the lower limbs reflect peripheral nerve and spinal cord damage. Gait changes, muscle weakness, impaired coordination, paresthesia, and sensory loss may be present. Deep tendon reflexes may be hypoactive or hyperactive. Other findings include a sore tongue, a positive Babinski's reflex, fatigue, blurred vision, diplopia, and light-headedness.

*Spinal cerebellar degeneration.* A positive Romberg's sign accompanies decreased visual acuity, paresthesia, loss of vibration sense, ataxic gait, incoordination, and muscle weakness and atrophy.

*Spinal cord disease.* A positive Romberg's sign may accompany fasciculations, muscle weakness and atrophy, and loss of proprioception, vibration, and other senses. Deep tendon reflexes may be hypoactive at the level of the lesion and hyperactive above it.

*Other causes.* Tabes dorsalis and vestibular disorders.

### Nursing considerations
- Help the patient walk, especially in poorly lit areas. Also keep a night-light on in his room, and raise the side rails of the bed. Encourage him to use visual cues to maintain his balance.

**R**

# Chorea

Brief, unpredictable bursts of rapid, jerky motion, chorea interrupts normal coordinated movement. Also called choreiform movements, chorea indicates dysfunction of the extrapyramidal system. Choreiform movements are seldom repetitive; they tend to appear purposeful despite their involuntary nature. Although any muscle can be affected, chorea usually involves the face, head, lower arms, and hands. It can affect one or both sides of the body but, when it affects the face, both sides are always involved. Chorea may worsen with excitement or fatigue and may disappear during sleep.

## History

Ask the patient and his family when they first noticed the choreiform movements. Do the movements disappear when the patient is asleep? Find out if anyone in the patient's family has the same type of movements and ask about a family history of such diseases as Huntington's chorea. Also ask which medications the patient is taking. Obtain an occupational history, noting especially prolonged exposure to manganese dioxide or lead.

## Physical exam

Observe the patient for excessive restlessness and periodic facial grimaces that may interrupt his speech. Ask the patient to stick out his tongue and keep it out. Typically, his tongue will dart in and out of his mouth. Observe the patient's arms and legs for involuntary jerky movements. Ask him to extend and flex his hand as if halting traffic, and note the choreiform movements. Also check for related signs: athetosis, rigidity, or tremors.

To assess for choreoathetoid gait, ask the patient to walk. He may change the positions of his trunk and upper body with each step and jerk and tilt his head to one side. Because of superimposed involuntary movements and postures, the patient's legs may move only slowly and awkwardly.

## Causes

*Cerebral infarction.* An infarction that involves the thalamic area produces unilateral or bilateral chorea. The patient may also experience dysarthria, tremors, rigidity, weakness, and sensory disturbances, such as paresthesia.

*Encephalitis.* Chorea occurs in the recovery phase of this disorder. Low-grade fever and athetosis may be present, along with hemiparesis, hemiplegia, and facial droop.

*Huntington's chorea.* Chorea may be the first sign or may occur with intellectual decline that leads to emotional disturbances and dementia. The patient's movements tend to be choreoathetoid and may be accompanied by dysarthria, dystonia, prancing gait, dysphagia, and facial grimacing.

*Lead poisoning.* In later stages, chorea occurs along with seizures, headache, memory lapses, and severe mental impairment. The patient may have a masklike face, footdrop, wristdrop, ataxia, weakness, abdominal pain, vomiting, lead line on the gums, and a metallic taste in his mouth.

*Manganese poisoning.* In miners who've been exposed to manganese dioxide for prolonged periods, chorea occurs with propulsive gait, dystonia, and rigidity. Initially, the patient may have a masklike face, resting tremor, and personality changes; later, muscle weakness and lethargy.

*Wilson's disease.* Chorea is an early indicator, along with dystonia of the arms and legs. The patient experiences dysarthria, tremors, hoarseness, dysphagia, and slowed body movements; he may also have emotional and behavioral disturbances, drooling, rigidity, and mental deterioration. The Kayser-Fleischer ring in the cornea appears as the disease progresses.

*Other causes.* Carbon monoxide poisoning; and drugs, such as phenothiazines, haloperidol, thiothixene, loxapine, metoclopramide, metyrosine, oral contraceptives, levodopa, and phenytoin.

## Nursing considerations

• Pad the side rails of the patient's bed, and keep sharp objects away from him. Help him minimize physical activity and emotional upset, and provide adequate periods of rest and sleep.

# Rhonchi

Continuous adventitious breath sounds detected by auscultation, rhonchi are usually louder and lower-pitched than crackles. More like a hoarse moan or deep snore, they may also be described as rattling, sonorous, bubbling, rumbling, or musical. Sibilant rhonchi, or wheezes, are high-pitched.

Rhonchi are heard over large airways when air flows through passages that have been narrowed by secretions, a tumor or foreign body, bronchospasm, or mucosal thickening. The resulting vibration of airway walls produces the rhonchi.

## History

Ask the patient if he smokes. If so, obtain a history in pack years. Has he recently lost weight or felt tired or weak? Does he have asthma or other pulmonary disorders? Is he currently taking any prescribed or over-the-counter drugs?

Keep in mind that thick or excessive secretions, bronchospasm, or inflammation of mucous membranes may lead to airway obstruction. If necessary, suction the patient and keep bronchodilators and equipment for inserting an airway available.

## Physical exam

Take the patient's vital signs and be alert for signs of respiratory distress. Characterize the patient's respirations as rapid or slow, shallow or deep, and regular or irregular. Inspect the chest, noting accessory muscle use. Auscultate for abnormal breath sounds. If detected, note the location. Are breath sounds diminished or absent? Next, percuss the chest. If the patient has a cough, note its frequency and characterize its sound. If it's productive, examine the sputum for color, odor, consistency, and blood.

## Causes

*Adult respiratory distress syndrome.* Fluid accumulation in this life-threatening disorder produces rhonchi and crackles. Initial features include rapid, shallow respirations and dyspnea, sometimes after the patient appears stable. Developing hypoxemia leads to intercostal and suprasternal retractions, diaphoresis, and fluid accumulation. As hypoxemia worsens, the patient displays increased breathing difficulty, apprehension, decreased level of consciousness, cyanosis, and motor dysfunction.

*Asthma.* An asthmatic attack can cause rhonchi, crackles, and wheezes. Other features include apprehension, a dry cough that later becomes productive, prolonged expirations, and intercostal and supraclavicular retractions on inspiration.

*Bronchitis.* Acute tracheobronchitis produces sonorous rhonchi and wheezes. Related findings include chills, sore throat, a low-grade fever, and substernal tightness. A cough becomes productive as secretions increase. Chronic bronchitis may produce scattered rhonchi, coarse crackles, wheezing, high-pitched piping sounds, and prolonged expirations. An early hacking cough later becomes productive. The patient also displays exertional dyspnea, increased accessory muscle use, barrel chest, cyanosis, and tachypnea.

*Pneumonia.* Bacterial pneumonias can cause rhonchi and a dry cough that later becomes productive. Related signs and symptoms develop suddenly and include shaking chills, high fever, myalgias, headache, pleuritic chest pain, tachypnea, tachycardia, dyspnea, cyanosis, diaphoresis, decreased breath sounds, and fine crackles.

*Other causes.* Aspiration of a foreign body; bronchiectasis; diagnostic tests, such as pulmonary function tests or bronchoscopy; emphysema; pulmonary coccidioidomycosis; and respiratory therapy.

## Nursing considerations

• Place the patient in semi-Fowler's position, and reposition him every 2 hours. Or, if appropriate, encourage increased activity to promote drainage of secretions. Teach deep-breathing and coughing techniques and splinting, if necessary.

• Provide humidification and encourage fluid intake. Pulmonary physiotherapy with postural drainage and percussion can also help loosen secretions.

# Chvostek's sign

Chvostek's sign is an abnormal spasm of the facial muscles elicited by lightly tapping the patient's facial nerve near his lower jaw. This sign usually suggests hypocalcemia but can occur normally in about 25% of patients. Typically, it precedes other signs of hypocalcemia and persists until the onset of tetany. It can't be elicited during tetany because of strong muscle contractions.

Normally, eliciting Chvostek's sign is attempted only in patients with suspected hypocalcemic disorders. But because the parathyroid gland regulates calcium balance, Chvostek's sign may also be tested in patients before neck surgery, to provide a baseline.

## History

Obtain a brief history. Find out if the patient has had surgical removal of the parathyroid glands or has a history of hypoparathyroidism, hypomagnesemia, or malabsorption disorder. Ask the patient or his family if he has experienced any mental changes, such as depression or slowed responses, which can accompany chronic hypocalcemia.

## Physical exam

If you elicit Chvostek's sign, notify the doctor. Then test for Trousseau's sign, a more reliable indicator of hypocalcemia. Closely monitor the patient for signs of tetany, such as carpopedal spasms or circumoral and extremity paresthesia.

## Causes

*Hypocalcemia.* The intensity of Chvostek's sign reflects the patient's serum calcium level. Initially, hypocalcemia produces paresthesia in the fingers, toes, and circumoral area that progresses to muscle tension and carpopedal spasms. The patient may also complain of muscle weakness, fatigue, and palpitations. Muscle twitching, hyperactive deep tendon reflexes, choreiform movements, and muscle cramps may also occur. The patient with chronic hypocalcemia may have mental status changes; diplopia; difficulty swallowing; abdominal cramps; dry, scaly skin; brittle nails; and thin, patchy scalp and eyebrow hair.

Hypocalcemia may result from inadequate intake of calcium and vitamin D, hypoparathyroidism, malabsorption or loss of calcium from the GI tract, severe infections or burns, overcorrection of acidosis, pancreatic insufficiency, renal failure, or hypomagnesemia.

*Other causes.* Massive blood transfusions can lower serum calcium levels and allow Chvostek's sign to be elicited.

## Nursing considerations

• As ordered, collect serum samples for serial calcium studies to evaluate the severity of hypocalcemia and the effectiveness of therapy. Such therapy involves oral or I.V. calcium supplements.
• Watch for hypocalcemia in patients receiving massive transfusions of citrated blood and in those with chronic diarrhea, severe infections, and insufficient dietary intake of calcium and protein (especially elderly patients).

Also called nasal discharge, rhinorrhea is the free discharge of thin nasal mucus. Common but rarely serious, it can be self-limiting or chronic. Rhinorrhea can result from nasal, sinus, or systemic disorders, a basilar skull fracture, sinus or cranial surgery, excessive use of vasoconstricting nose drops or sprays, or other irritants. Depending on the cause, the discharge may be clear, purulent, bloody, or serosanguineous.

## History

Ask the patient if the discharge runs from both nostrils. Is it intermittent or persistent? Did it begin suddenly or gradually? Does the position of his head affect it? Is the discharge watery, bloody, purulent, or foul-smelling? Is it copious or scanty? Does it worsen or improve with the time of day? Find out if the patient is taking any medications, especially nose drops or sprays. Has he been exposed to nasal irritants at home or at work? Has he had a recent head injury?

## Physical exam

Examine the patient's nose, assessing airflow from each nostril. Evaluate the size, color, and condition of the turbinate mucosa. Examine the area beneath each turbinate and the sinus opening into each meatus, and trace purulent discharge to the involved sinus. Palpate over the frontal, ethmoid, and maxillary sinuses for tenderness. Transilluminate the maxillary and frontal sinuses; then, using a nonirritating substance, test for anosmia.

## Causes

*Basilar skull fracture.* A tear in the dura can lead to cerebrospinal rhinorrhea, which increases when the patient lowers his head. Associated findings may include epistaxis, otorrhea, and a bulging tympanic membrane. It may also cause impaired eye movement, depressed level of consciousness, Battle's sign, and raccoon's eyes.

*Ethmoiditis.* In acute bacterial ethmoiditis, nasal discharge is yellow-gray and purulent; in acute viral ethmoiditis, it's mucoid. Other findings include nasal congestion, headache, fever, malaise, postnasal drip, an impaired sense of smell and taste, and pain, erythema, and tenderness over bone in the upper lateral areas of the nose.

*Rhinitis.* *Allergic rhinitis* produces an episodic, profuse watery discharge along with increased lacrimation; nasal congestion; itchy eyes, nose, and throat; postnasal drip; and frontal or temporal headache. The turbinates are pale and engorged; the mucosa, pale and boggy.

In *atrophic rhinitis,* nasal discharge is scanty, purulent, and foul-smelling. The mucosa is pale pink and shiny.

In *vasomotor rhinitis,* a profuse and watery nasal discharge accompanies chronic nasal obstruction, recurrent postnasal drip, and pale, swollen turbinates. The nasal septum is pink, the mucosa blue.

*Sinusitis.* *Acute sphenoid sinusitis* produces purulent nasal discharge that leads to nasal obstruction, along with fever, malaise, and deep pain behind the eyes that's referred to the top or back of the head or to the mastoid area.

In *chronic frontal sinusitis,* intermittent and purulent discharge may lead to obstruction. Other findings include postnasal drip, a constant headache, and dull tenderness over the affected sinus.

In *chronic maxillary sinusitis,* mucopurulent discharge is intermittent and ipsilateral and may lead to unilateral nasal obstruction. Related features include facial aching, pain in the upper teeth, swelling and tenderness in the anterior maxilla, and postnasal drip.

*Other causes.* Cluster headache; common cold; drugs, such as nasal sprays or drops containing vasoconstrictors; mucormycosis; nasal or sinus tumors; scleroma; sinus or cranial surgery; and Wegener's granulomatosis.

## Nursing considerations

• Promote fluid intake. Warn the patient to avoid using over-the-counter nasal sprays for longer than 5 days, unless ordered.

A nonspecific sign of respiratory and cyanotic cardiovascular disorders, clubbing is the painless, usually bilateral increase in soft tissue around the terminal phalanges of the fingers or toes. It does not involve changes in the underlying bone. In early clubbing, the normal 160-degree angle between the nail and the nail base approximates 180 degrees. As clubbing progresses, the angle widens and the base of the nail becomes visibly swollen. In late clubbing, the angle where the nail meets the now-convex nail base extends more than halfway up the nail.

## History
Ask the patient about smoking, difficulty breathing, and edema, particularly swelling of the feet. Ask about a history of cardiovascular or respiratory disorders.

## Physical exam
You'll probably detect clubbing while assessing for other signs of known respiratory or cardiovascular disease. Review the patient's current plan of treatment because clubbing may resolve with correction of the underlying disorder. Evaluate the extent of clubbing in both the fingers and toes.

## Causes
*Bronchiectasis.* Clubbing occurs commonly in the late stage of this disorder. You may also see this classic sign: a cough producing copious, foul-smelling, and mucopurulent sputum. Hemoptysis and coarse crackles heard over the affected area during inspiration are also characteristic. The patient may complain of weight loss, fatigue, weakness, and dyspnea on exertion. He may also have rhonchi, fever, malaise, and halitosis.

*Bronchitis.* In chronic bronchitis, clubbing may occur as a late sign and is unrelated to the severity of the disease. The patient has a chronic productive cough. He may display barrel chest, dyspnea, wheezing, increased use of accessory muscles, cyanosis, tachypnea, crackles, scattered rhonchi, and prolonged expiration.

*Congestive heart failure.* Clubbing occurs as a late sign along with wheezing, dyspnea, and fatigue. Other findings may include neck vein distention, hepatomegaly, tachypnea, palpitations, dependent edema, unexplained weight gain, nausea, anorexia, chest tightness, slowed mental response, hypotension, diaphoresis, narrowed pulse pressure, pallor, oliguria, a ventricular gallop ($S_3$), and crackles on inspiration.

*Emphysema.* Clubbing occurs late in this disease. The patient may have anorexia, malaise, dyspnea, tachypnea, diminished breath sounds, peripheral cyanosis, and pursed lip breathing. He may also display accessory muscle use, barrel chest, and a productive cough.

*Endocarditis.* In subacute infective endocarditis, clubbing may be accompanied by fever, anorexia, pallor, weakness, night sweats, fatigue, tachycardia, and weight loss. The patient may also have arthralgia, petechiae, Osler's nodes, splinter hemorrhages, Janeway's spots, splenomegaly, and Roth's spots. Cardiac murmurs are usually present.

*Interstitial fibrosis.* Clubbing occurs in almost all patients with advanced interstitial fibrosis. The patient typically will also have intermittent chest pain, dyspnea, crackles, fatigue, and weight loss, and may have cyanosis.

*Lung abscess.* Initially produces clubbing, which may reverse with resolution of the abscess. It can also produce pleuritic chest pain; dyspnea; crackles; a productive cough with purulent, foul-smelling, often bloody sputum; and halitosis.

*Lung and pleural cancer.* Clubbing is common. Associated findings may include hemoptysis, dyspnea, wheezing, chest pain, weight loss, anorexia, fatigue, and fever.

## Nursing considerations
• Don't mistake curved nails—a normal variation—for clubbing. Remember that the angle between the nail and its base remains normal in curved nails, but not in clubbing.

A cardinal sign of respiratory distress in infants and children, retractions are visible indentations of the soft tissue covering the chest wall. They may be suprasternal (directly above the sternum and clavicles), intercostal (between the ribs), subcostal (below the lower costal margin of the rib cage), or substernal (just below the xiphoid process). Retractions may be mild or severe, producing barely visible to deep indentations.

## ▶ Emergency interventions
If the child displays retractions, quickly check for other signs of respiratory distress, such as cyanosis, tachypnea, and tachycardia. Have another nurse notify the doctor immediately, while you monitor the child's respiratory status. Prepare for suctioning, insertion of an artificial airway, and administration of oxygen.

## History
Ask the child's parents about his medical history. Was he born prematurely? Was the delivery complicated? Has he had an upper respiratory infection recently? How often has he had respiratory problems in the past year? Has he been in contact with anyone who has had a cold, the flu, or other respiratory ailments? Did he aspirate any food, liquid, or foreign body? Inquire about any personal or family history of allergies or asthma.

## Physical exam
Observe the depth and location of the retractions. Also note the rate, depth, and quality of respirations. Assess for accessory muscle use, nasal flaring during inspiration, or grunting during expiration. If the child has a cough, record the color, consistency, and odor of any sputum. Note if the child appears restless or lethargic. Auscultate his lungs to detect abnormal breath sounds.

## Causes
*Asthmatic attack.* Intercostal and suprasternal retractions may accompany an attack. They're preceded by dyspnea, wheezing, a hacking cough, and pallor. Related features may include cyanosis or flushing, crackles, rhonchi, diaphoresis, tachycardia, and tachypnea.

*Bronchiolitis.* Most common in children under age 2, this acute lower respiratory tract infection may cause intercostal and subcostal retractions, nasal flaring, tachypnea, dyspnea, cough, restlessness, and possibly a slight fever. Periodic apnea may occur in infants under 6 months old.

*Congestive heart failure.* Usually linked to a congenital heart defect, this disorder may cause intercostal and substernal retractions along with nasal flaring and progressive tachypnea. In severe respiratory distress, it may cause grunting respirations, edema, and cyanosis.

*Epiglottitis.* This life-threatening bacterial infection may precipitate severe respiratory distress with suprasternal, substernal, and intercostal retractions; stridor; nasal flaring; cyanosis; and tachycardia. Initially, it causes a sudden barking cough and high fever, along with sore throat, hoarseness, dysphagia, drooling, and dyspnea. The child becomes panicky as edema makes breathing difficult. Total airway occlusion may occur in 2 to 5 hours.

*Respiratory distress syndrome.* Affecting premature infants shortly after birth, substernal and subcostal retractions signal this life-threatening syndrome, along with tachypnea, tachycardia, and respiratory grunting. Later, intercostal and suprasternal retractions occur, and apnea or irregular respirations replace grunting.

*Other causes.* Laryngotracheobronchitis (acute), pneumonia (bacterial), and spasmodic croup.

## Nursing considerations
• Monitor the child's vital signs. Keep suction equipment and an appropriate-size airway at the bedside.
• If the infant weighs less than 15 lb, place him in an oxygen hood, as ordered. If he weighs more, place him in a cool mist tent instead.

R

This cardinal sign of Parkinson's disease is characterized by muscle rigidity that abates in a series of jerking movements when the muscle is passively stretched.

## History

After you've elicited cogwheel rigidity, take the patient's history to determine when he first noticed associated signs of Parkinson's disease. For example, how long has he experienced tremors? Did he notice tremors of his hands first? Does he have "pill-rolling" hand movements? When did he first notice that his movements were becoming slower? How long has he experienced stiffness in his arms and legs? While taking the history, observe for signs of pronounced parkinsonism, such as drooling, a masklike face, dysphagia, speaking in a monotone, and altered gait.

Find out which medications the patient is taking, and ask if they've helped relieve some of his symptoms. If he's taking levodopa and symptoms have worsened, find out if he has exceeded the prescribed dosage. If you suspect an overdose, inform the doctor and withhold the drug, as ordered.

If the patient is taking a phenothiazine or another antipsychotic and has no history of Parkinson's disease, he may be having an adverse reaction to his medication. Inform the doctor and withhold the drug, as ordered.

## Physical exam

Cogwheel rigidity can be elicited by stabilizing the patient's forearm, then moving his hand through the range of motion. This sign usually appears in the arms, but it can sometimes be elicited in the ankle. Both the patient and the examiner can see and feel these characteristic movements, thought to be a combination of rigidity and tremor.

## Causes

*Parkinson's disease.* In this disorder, cogwheel rigidity occurs together with an insidious tremor, which usually begins in the fingers (unilateral pill-roll tremor), increases during stress or anxiety, and decreases with purposeful movement and sleep.

Bradykinesia (slowness of voluntary movements and speech) also occurs. The patient walks with difficulty; his gait lacks normal parallel motion and may be retropulsive or propulsive. He has a high-pitched, monotonal way of speaking and a masklike facial expression. He may experience drooling; loss of posture control, so that he walks with his body bent forward; dysphagia; or dysarthria. An oculogyric crisis (eyes fixed upward and involuntary tonic movements) or blepharospasm (complete eyelid closure) may also occur.

*Other causes.* Drugs, such as phenothiazines and other antipsychotics (haloperidol, thiothixene, and loxapine) can cause cogwheel rigidity. Metoclopramide and metyrosine infrequently cause it.

## Nursing considerations

• If the patient has associated muscular dysfunction, assist him with ambulation, feeding, and other activities of daily living, as needed. Provide symptomatic care, as appropriate. For example, administer stool softeners if the patient has constipation, or offer a soft diet with small, frequent feedings if he has dysphagia.

• Refer the patient to the National Parkinson Foundation or the American Parkinson Disease Association for educational materials and support.

# Rectal pain

A common symptom of anorectal disorders, rectal pain is discomfort in the anal-rectal area. Although the anal canal is separated from the rest of the rectum by the internal sphincter, the patient may refer to all local pain as rectal pain. Because the mucocutaneous border of the anal canal and the perianal skin contain somatic nerve fibers, lesions in this area are especially painful.

The pain may result from or be aggravated by diarrhea, constipation, or passage of hardened stools. It may also be aggravated by intense pruritus and continued scratching associated with drainage of mucus, blood, or fecal matter that irritates the perianal skin and nerve endings.

## History

Ask the patient to describe the pain. Is it sharp or dull, burning or knifelike? How often does it occur? Ask if the pain is worse during or immediately after defecation. Does he avoid having bowel movements because of anticipated pain? Also find out what alleviates the pain. Ask about associated signs and symptoms. Does the patient experience bleeding along with rectal pain? If so, find out how frequently and whether the blood is on the toilet tissue, on the surface of the stool, or in the toilet bowl. Is the blood bright or dark red? Ask about other drainage, such as mucus or pus, and if the patient has constipation or diarrhea.

## Physical exam

Inspect for rectal bleeding; abnormal drainage, such as pus; or protrusions, such as skin tags or thrombosed hemorrhoids. Also observe the patient's perianal skin for inflammation and other lesions. Notify the doctor right away if you detect any of these findings because he may want to perform an immediate rectal examination.

## Causes

*Anal fissure.* This longitudinal crack in the anal lining causes sharp rectal pain on defecation. The patient experiences a burning sensation and gnawing pain that can continue up to 4 hours after defecation. Fear of provoking this pain may lead to acute constipation. Other findings may include anal pruritus, extreme tenderness, and spots of blood on the toilet tissue after defecation.

*Anorectal abscess.* A superficial abscess produces constant, throbbing local pain that is exacerbated by sitting or walking. The local pain associated with a deeper abscess may begin insidiously, commonly occurring high in the rectum or in the lower abdomen, and is accompanied by an indurated anal mass. The patient may also develop fever, malaise, anal swelling and inflammation, purulent drainage, and local tenderness.

*Anorectal fistula.* Pain develops when a tract formed between the anal canal and skin temporarily seals. It persists until drainage resumes. Other chief complaints include pruritus and drainage of pus, blood, mucus, and occasionally stool.

*Cryptitis.* This disorder results when particles of stool lodged in the anal folds decay and cause infection, which may produce dull anal pain or discomfort and anal pruritus.

*Hemorrhoids.* Thrombosed or prolapsed hemorrhoids cause rectal pain that may worsen during defecation and abate after it. Usually, rectal pain is accompanied by severe itching. Internal hemorrhoids may produce intermittent bleeding that occurs as spotting on the toilet tissue or on the stool surface. External hemorrhoids are visible outside the anal sphincter.

*Other causes.* Anal carcinoma, proctalgia fugax, and prostatic abscess.

## Nursing considerations

- Apply analgesic ointment or suppositories, as ordered, and administer stool softeners, if needed. Stress to the patient the importance of proper diet to maintain soft stools.
- Teach the patient how to apply hot compresses and give himself a sitz bath. If he has prolapsed hemorrhoids, apply cold compresses.

**R**

This increased sensitivity to cold temperatures usually develops gradually, reflecting damage to the body's temperature-regulating mechanism or a decreased basal metabolic rate (BMR). Typically, this symptom results from tumors or hormonal deficiency. In elderly patients, it usually reflects normal age-related decreases in BMR and muscle mass.

## History

Find out when the patient first noticed cold intolerance. When did he begin using more blankets? Wearing heavier clothing? Ask about associated signs and symptoms, such as changes in vision or in the texture or amount of body hair. If the patient is female, ask about changes in her normal menstrual pattern.

Before proceeding with the physical examination, obtain a brief history. Does the patient have a history of hypothyroidism or hypothalamic disease? Is he currently taking any medications? If so, is he complying with the prescribed dosage? Has the regimen been changed recently?

## Physical exam

Take the patient's vital signs, and check for dry skin and hair loss. Then ask the patient to straighten and extend his arms. Are his hands shaking? During the examination, note if the patient shivers or complains of chills. Provide a blanket, if necessary.

## Causes

*Hypopituitarism.* Clinical features usually develop slowly and vary with the disorder's severity. Cold intolerance and shivering typically accompany fine wrinkles around the mouth and skin that's cold, dry, and thin with a waxy pallor. Other findings may include fatigue, lethargy, menstrual disturbances, impotence, decreased libido, nervousness, irritability, headache, and hunger. If hypopituitarism results from a pituitary tumor, expect neurologic signs and symptoms, such as headache, bilateral temporal hemianopia, loss of visual acuity, and possibly blindness.

*Hypothalamic lesion.* A patient with hypothalamic damage may show unexplained fluctuations from cold intolerance to heat intolerance. Cold intolerance develops suddenly. The patient typically complains of feeling chilled, shivering, and wearing extra clothes to keep warm. Related findings may include amenorrhea, sleep pattern disturbances, increased thirst and urination, vigorous appetite with weight gain, loss of visual acuity, headache, and personality changes, such as attacks of rage, laughing, and crying.

*Hypothyroidism.* Cold intolerance develops early in this disorder and progressively worsens. Other early findings include fatigue, anorexia with weight gain, constipation, and menorrhagia. Later, the patient has loss of libido and slowed intellectual and motor activity. The hair becomes dry and sparse, the nails thick and brittle, and the skin dry, pale, cool, and doughy. Eventually, the patient displays a characteristic dull expression with periorbital and facial edema and puffy hands and feet. Deep tendon reflexes are delayed. Bradycardia, abdominal distention, and ataxia may also occur.

## Nursing considerations

• Help increase the patient's comfort by regulating his room temperature and providing extra clothing and blankets. Instruct the patient and his family to adapt the patient's environment to meet his needs.

• Prepare the patient for diagnostic tests, as ordered, to determine the cause of cold intolerance. Once the cause is known, explain the disease process to the patient and his family to help alleviate their anxiety. Also explain that, with proper treatment, he can expect relief from his symptoms.

# Rebound tenderness

Also called Blumberg's sign, rebound tenderness—an intense, elicited abdominal pain caused by rebound of palpated tissue—is a reliable indicator of peritonitis. It may be localized, as in an abscess, or generalized, as in perforation of an intra-abdominal organ. Rebound tenderness usually occurs with abdominal pain, tenderness, and rigidity. When a patient has sudden, severe abdominal pain, this symptom is usually elicited to detect peritoneal inflammation.

## ▶ Emergency interventions

If you elicit rebound tenderness in a patient who's experiencing constant, severe abdominal pain, quickly take his vital signs and have another nurse notify the doctor immediately. Insert a large-bore I.V. catheter and begin administering I.V. fluids. Also insert an indwelling urinary catheter, and monitor fluid intake and output. Give supplemental oxygen, as needed, and continue to monitor the patient for signs of shock.

## History

When the patient's condition permits, ask him to describe the events that led up to the tenderness. Does movement, exertion, or other activity relieve or aggravate the tenderness? Also ask about other signs and symptoms.

## Physical exam

Inspect the abdomen for distention, visible peristaltic waves, or scars. Then auscultate for bowel sounds and characterize their motility. Finally, palpate for associated rigidity or guarding.

## Cause

*Peritonitis.* In this life-threatening disorder, rebound tenderness is accompanied by sudden and severe abdominal pain, which may be either diffuse or localized. Because movement worsens the patient's pain, he'll usually lie still. Typically, he'll display weakness, pallor, excessive sweating, and cold skin. He may also display hypoactive or absent bowel sounds; tachypnea; nausea and vomiting; abdominal distention, rigidity, and guarding; and a fever of 103° F (39.4° C) or higher. Inflammation of the diaphragmatic peritoneum may cause shoulder pain and hiccups.

## Nursing considerations

• Promote comfort by having the patient flex his knees or assume semi-Fowler's position. Administer analgesics carefully because these drugs can mask associated symptoms. Administer antiemetics and antipyretics, as ordered. However, because of decreased intestinal motility and the probability of surgery, don't give the patient oral drugs or fluids.

• As ordered, obtain samples of blood, urine, and feces for laboratory testing, and prepare the patient for chest and abdominal X-rays, sonograms, and computed tomography scans.

• Perform or assist the doctor with a rectal or pelvic examination.

R

# Confusion

An umbrella term for puzzling or inappropriate behavior or responses, confusion reflects the inability to think quickly and coherently. Depending on its cause, confusion may arise suddenly or gradually and may be temporary or irreversible. Aggravated by stress and sensory deprivation, confusion tends to be more common in hospitalized patients, especially elderly people.

When severe confusion arises suddenly with hallucinations and psychomotor hyperactivity, the condition is called delirium. Long-term, progressive confusion with deterioration of all cognitive functions is called dementia.

## History

Ask the patient to describe what's bothering him. He may complain of memory loss, a nagging sense of apprehension, or an inability to concentrate. Ask when this feeling began and if he feels this way all the time or just occasionally. Find out if the patient has a history of head trauma or a cardiopulmonary, metabolic, cerebrovascular, or neurologic disorder. What medication is he taking, if any? Ask about any changes in eating or sleeping habits and in drug or alcohol use.

## Physical exam

Perform a neurologic assessment to establish the patient's level of consciousness.

## Causes

*Fluid and electrolyte imbalance.* The extent of imbalance determines the severity of confusion. Typically, the patient will show signs of dehydration along with hypotension and a low-grade fever.

*Head trauma.* Concussion, contusion, and brain hemorrhage may produce confusion at the time of injury, shortly afterward, or months or years afterward. The patient may be delirious, with periodic loss of consciousness. Vomiting, severe headache, pupillary changes, and sensory and motor deficits are also common.

*Heat stroke.* This disorder causes pronounced confusion that gradually worsens as body temperature rises. Initially, the patient may be irritable and dizzy; later, he may become delirious, have seizures, and lose consciousness.

*Hypothermia.* Confusion may be an early sign. The patient displays slurred speech, cold and pale skin, hyperactive deep tendon reflexes, rapid pulse, and decreased blood pressure and respiratory rate. As his body temperature drops further, his confusion progresses to stupor and coma, his muscles become rigid, and his respiratory rate becomes depressed further.

*Hypoxemia.* Acute pulmonary disorders that result in hypoxemia produce confusion that can range from mild disorientation to delirium. Chronic pulmonary disorders produce persistent confusion.

*Low perfusion states.* Mild confusion is an early sign of decreased cerebral perfusion. Associated findings usually include hypotension, tachycardia or bradycardia, irregular pulse, ventricular gallop, edema, and cyanosis.

*Metabolic encephalopathy.* Hyperglycemia and hypoglycemia can produce sudden onset of confusion. Hypoglycemia may also cause transient delirium and seizures. Uremic and hepatic encephalopathies produce gradual confusion that may progress to seizures and coma.

*Other causes.* Alcohol intoxication; brain tumor; cerebrovascular disorders; dementia; drugs, such as central nervous system depressants, lidocaine, digitalis, indomethacin, cycloserine, chloroquine, atropine, and cimetidine, as well as narcotic and barbiturate withdrawal; heavy metal poisoning; infection; nutritional disorders; seizure disorders; and thyroid hormone disorders.

## Nursing considerations

• Never leave a confused patient unattended. Keep the patient calm and quiet, and plan uninterrupted rest periods. Keep a large calendar and a clock visible. Always reintroduce yourself to the patient each time you enter his room.

# Raccoon's eyes

Raccoon's eyes refer to bilateral periorbital ecchymoses that do not result from facial trauma. Usually an indicator of basilar skull fracture, this sign develops when damage at the time of fracture tears the meninges and causes the venous sinuses to bleed into the arachnoid villi and the cranial sinuses. Raccoon's eyes may be the only indicator of a basilar skull fracture, which isn't always visible on skull X-rays. Their appearance signals the need for careful assessment to detect any underlying trauma because a basilar skull fracture can injure cranial nerves, blood vessels, and the brain stem. Raccoon's eyes can also occur after a craniotomy if the surgery causes a meningeal tear.

### History
Try to find out when the head injury occurred.

### Physical exam
After detecting raccoon's eyes, check the patient's vital signs and assess the extent of the underlying trauma. Start by evaluating the patient's level of consciousness (LOC) with the Glasgow Coma Scale. Next, assess function of the cranial nerves, especially nerves I (olfactory), III (oculomotor), IV (trochlear), VI (abducens), and VII (facial).

If the patient's condition permits, test his visual acuity and gross hearing. Note any irregularities in the facial or skull bones, as well as any swelling, localized pain, or lacerations of the face and scalp. Check for ecchymoses over the mastoid bone. Inspect for hemorrhage or cerebrospinal fluid (CSF) leakage from the nose or ears. Collect any drainage with a sterile 4" × 4" gauze pad, and note if you find a halo sign—a circle of clear fluid that surrounds the drainage, indicating CSF. Also, use a glucose reagent strip to test any clear drainage for glucose. A positive test indicates CSF because mucus doesn't contain glucose. Inform the doctor of your findings.

### Causes
**Basilar skull fracture.** This injury produces raccoon's eyes following a head trauma that doesn't involve orbital fracture. Associated signs and symptoms vary with the fracture site and may include pharyngeal hemorrhage, epistaxis, rhinorrhea, otorrhea, or a bulging tympanic membrane from blood or CSF. The patient may experience hearing difficulty, headache, nausea, vomiting, and altered LOC. He may also have Battle's sign. In addition, most patients experience cranial nerve palsies.

**Surgery.** Raccoon's eyes that occur after a craniotomy may indicate a meningeal tear and bleeding into the sinuses.

### Nursing considerations
• Keep the patient on complete bed rest, and position him as ordered. Perform a neurologic assessment every hour to reevaluate his LOC. Also check vital signs hourly; be alert for such changes as bradypnea, bradycardia, hypertension, and fever.
• To avoid the worsening of a dural tear, instruct the patient not to blow his nose, cough vigorously, or strain. If otorrhea or rhinorrhea is present, don't attempt to stop the flow. Instead, place a sterile, loose gauze pad under the nose or ear to absorb the drainage. Monitor the amount and test it with a glucose reagent strip to confirm or rule out CSF leakage.
• Never suction or pass a nasogastric tube through the patient's nose, to prevent further tearing of the mucous membranes and infection. Observe the patient for signs and symptoms of meningitis, such as fever and nuchal rigidity, and expect to administer prophylactic antibiotics.
• Prepare the patient for diagnostic tests, such as a skull X-ray and possibly a computed tomography scan. If the dural tear does not heal spontaneously, contrast cisternography may be performed to locate the tear, possibly followed by corrective surgery.

R

# Conjunctival injection

A common sign indicating inflammation, conjunctival injection is nonuniform redness of the conjunctiva from hyperemia. This redness can be diffuse, localized, or peripheral, or it may encircle a clear cornea. Conjunctival injection usually results from bacterial or viral conjunctivitis. It can also signal a severe ocular disorder such as trachoma, which could lead to blindness if untreated. Conjunctival injection can also result from minor eye irritation caused by inadequate sleep, overuse of contact lenses, or environmental irritants.

▶ **Emergency interventions**
If the patient reports a chemical splash to the eye, immediately irrigate the eye with copious amounts of normal saline solution. Evert the lids and wipe the fornices with a cotton-tipped applicator to remove any foreign body particles and as much of the chemical solution as possible.

**History**
Ask if the patient has eye pain. If so, when did it begin, and where is it located? Ask about itching, burning, or a foreign body sensation. Does he have photophobia, halo vision, or excessive tearing. Does he have a history of eye disease or trauma?

**Physical exam**
If the patient has suffered ocular trauma, avoid touching the affected eye. Test his visual acuity and intraocular pressure (IOP) only if his eyelids can be opened without applying pressure. If appropriate, determine the location and severity of conjunctival injection. Note conjunctival or lid edema, ocular deviation, conjunctival follicles, ptosis, or exophthalmos. Note any discharge. Test the patient's visual acuity and pupillary reaction to light. Assist with IOP measurements.

**Causes**
*Chemical burns.* In this ocular emergency, diffuse conjunctival injection occurs along with severe pain. The patient also has photophobia, blepharospasm, and decreased visual acuity in the affected eye. The cornea may appear gray and the pupil may be unilaterally smaller.

*Conjunctivitis.* Allergic conjunctivitis produces a milky, diffuse, peripheral conjunctival injection. The patient complains of photophobia and a feeling of fullness around the eyes. He'll have a watery, stringy eye discharge; increased tearing; itching; and palpebral conjunctival follicles.

*Bacterial conjunctivitis* causes diffuse peripheral conjunctival injection and a thick, purulent eye discharge with mucous threads. Other findings include excessive tearing, photophobia, burning, and itching.

*Fungal conjunctivitis* causes photophobia and increased tearing, itching, and burning. The discharge is thick and purulent. Corneal involvement causes pain.

In *viral conjunctivitis,* the conjunctival injection is brilliant red, diffuse, and peripheral. The patient may have conjunctival edema, follicles on the palpebral conjunctiva, lid edema, itching, increased tearing, and a foreign body sensation.

*Glaucoma.* In acute closed-angle glaucoma, conjunctival injection is circumcorneal. The patient has severe eye pain along with nausea and vomiting. His IOP is severely elevated, his vision blurred. He sees rainbow-colored halos around lights, and his corneas appear steamy. The pupil of the affected eye will be moderately dilated and unresponsive.

*Other causes.* Astigmatism, blepharitis, conjunctival foreign bodies and abrasions, corneal abrasion, corneal erosion, corneal ulcer, dacryoadenitis, episcleritis, hyphema, iritis, keratoconjunctivitis sicca, ocular lacerations and intraocular foreign bodies, ocular tumors, scleritis, Stevens-Johnson syndrome, and uveitis.

**Nursing considerations**
• If the patient has photophobia, darken the room, or suggest that he wear sunglasses.
• Stress the importance of hand washing and of not touching the affected eye to prevent contagion.

# Pyrosis

Also called heartburn, pyrosis is a substernal burning sensation that rises in the chest and may radiate to the neck or throat. It's caused by reflux of gastric contents into the esophagus and usually is accompanied by regurgitation. Because increased intra-abdominal pressure contributes to reflux, pyrosis commonly occurs with pregnancy, ascites, or obesity. It also accompanies various GI disorders, connective tissue disease, and use of numerous drugs.

Usually, pyrosis develops after meals or when the patient lies down, bends over, lifts heavy objects, or exercises vigorously. Typically, pyrosis worsens with swallowing and improves when the patient sits upright or takes antacids.

A patient experiencing a myocardial infarction (MI) may mistake chest pain for pyrosis. However, he'll probably have other signs and symptoms, such as dyspnea, palpitations, nausea, and vomiting, that will help distinguish MI from pyrosis. Antacids won't relieve the pain of MI.

## History

Ask the patient if he's experienced heartburn before, whether certain foods or beverages trigger it, and if stress or fatigue aggravate it. Also ask if movement, certain body positions, or ingestion of very hot or cold liquids worsens or relieves his heartburn. Ask about the location of the pain and determine if it radiates to other areas. Also find out if the patient regurgitates sour or bitter-tasting fluids along with the pyrosis.

## Causes

*Esophageal cancer.* Pyrosis may be a sign of this cancer, depending on tumor size and location. The first symptom is usually painless dysphagia that progressively worsens. Eventually, partial obstruction and rapid weight loss occur. The patient may complain of steady pain in the front and back of the chest. He may also experience hoarseness, sore throat, nausea, vomiting, and a feeling of substernal fullness.

*Gastroesophageal reflux disease.* Pyrosis, frequently severe, is the most common symptom. The pyrosis tends to be chronic, occurs 30 to 60 minutes after eating, and may be triggered by certain foods or beverages. It worsens with lying down or bending and abates with sitting, standing, or after antacid ingestion. Other findings include postural regurgitation, dysphagia, flatulent dyspepsia, and dull retrosternal pain that may radiate.

*Peptic ulcer disease.* Pyrosis and indigestion usually signal the start of a peptic ulcer attack. Most patients experience a gnawing, burning pain in the left epigastrium, although some may report sharp pain. Typically, the pain arises when the stomach is empty and is relieved by eating or taking antacids. The pain may also occur after ingestion of coffee, aspirin, or alcohol.

*Scleroderma.* This connective tissue disease may cause esophageal dysfunction resulting in reflux with pyrosis, the sensation of food sticking behind the breastbone, odynophagia, bloating after meals, and weight loss. Other GI effects include abdominal distention, constipation or diarrhea, and malodorous floating stools. Early signs include blanching, cyanosis, and stress- or cold-induced erythema of the fingers and toes. Later developments include finger and joint pain, stiffness, and swelling; skin thickening on the hands and forearms; and masklike facies.

*Other causes.* Drugs, including acetohexamide, tolbutamide, lypressin, aspirin, anticholinergic agents, and those having anticholinergic effects; esophageal diverticula; and obesity.

## Nursing considerations

• Prepare the patient for diagnostic tests, such as barium swallow, upper GI series, esophagoscopy, and laboratory studies.

• After the causative disorder is determined, teach the patient how to avoid pyrosis.

• If the patient's pyrosis is severe, instruct him to sleep with extra pillows or to raise the head of the bed by placing 6" wooden blocks under the legs at the head end.

Defined as small, infrequent, difficult bowel movements, constipation must be determined in relation to the patient's normal elimination pattern. Constipation may be a minor annoyance or, uncommonly, a sign of a life-threatening disorder. Untreated, constipation can lead to headache, anorexia, and abdominal discomfort. Most often, constipation occurs when the urge to defecate is suppressed and the muscles associated with bowel movements remain contracted.

## History
Ask the patient to describe the frequency of his bowel movements and the size and consistency of his stools. How long has he experienced constipation? Does he have pain related to constipation? If so, when did he first notice the pain, and where is it located? Ask the patient if elimination worsens or helps relieve the pain. Ask the patient to describe a typical day's menu; estimate his daily fiber and fluid intake. Ask him about any changes in eating habits, in medication or alcohol use, or in physical activity. Has he experienced recent emotional distress?

Inquire about a history of GI, rectoanal, neurologic, or metabolic disorders; abdominal surgery; or radiation therapy. Ask about medication use, including over-the-counter drugs.

## Physical exam
Inspect the abdomen for distention or scars from previous surgery. Then auscultate for bowel sounds. Percuss all four quadrants and palpate for abdominal tenderness, a mass, and hepatomegaly. Examine the patient's rectum for inflammation, lesions, scars, fissures, and external hemorrhoids. Use a disposable glove and lubricant to palpate the anal sphincter for laxity or stricture. Also palpate for rectal masses and fecal impaction. Obtain a stool sample and test it for occult blood.

## Causes
*Diverticulitis.* Constipation occurs with left lower quadrant pain and tenderness and possibly a palpable abdominal mass. The patient may have mild nausea, flatulence, or a low-grade fever.

*Intestinal obstruction.* Constipation varies in severity and onset with the location and extent of the obstruction. In a partial obstruction, constipation may alternate with leakage of liquid stool. In a complete obstruction, obstipation may occur. Constipation can be the earliest sign of partial colon obstruction, but it usually occurs later if the level of the obstruction is more proximal. Associated findings may include colicky abdominal pain, abdominal distention, nausea, and vomiting.

*Irritable bowel syndrome.* Usually, this common syndrome produces chronic constipation, although patients may have intermittent, watery diarrhea or alternating constipation and diarrhea. Stress may trigger nausea and abdominal distention and tenderness, but defecation relieves these symptoms. The stools are scybalous and contain visible mucus.

*Mesenteric artery ischemia.* This life-threatening disorder produces sudden constipation with failure to expel stool or flatus. Initially, it also produces severe abdominal pain, tenderness, vomiting, and anorexia. Later, abdominal guarding, rigidity, and distention; tachycardia; tachypnea; fever; and signs of shock. A bruit may be heard.

*Other causes.* Anal fissure; anorectal abscess; cirrhosis; Crohn's disease; diabetic neuropathy; diagnostic tests, such as certain GI studies; drugs, such as codeine, meperidine, methadone, morphine, vinca alkaloids, antacids containing aluminum or calcium, anticholinergics, and drugs with anticholinergic effects; hemorrhoids; hepatic porphyria; hypercalcemia; hypothyroidism; multiple sclerosis; rectoanal surgery; spinal cord lesion; tabes dorsalis; ulcerative colitis; and ulcerative proctitis.

## Nursing considerations
• Stress the importance of a high-fiber diet, and encourage the patient to drink sufficient fluids.
• Warn against overuse of laxatives or enemas.

# Pustular rash

A pustular rash is made up of crops of pustules—vesicles and bullae that fill with purulent exudate. These lesions vary in size and shape and can be generalized or localized to the hair follicles or sweat glands. Pustules appear in skin and systemic disorders, with the use of certain drugs, and with exposure to skin irritants. Although many pustular lesions are sterile, a pustular rash usually indicates infection. Any vesicular eruption can become pustular if a secondary infection occurs.

## History
Have the patient describe the appearance, location, and onset of the first pustular lesion. Ask him if another type of skin lesion preceded the pustule. Find out how the lesions spread. Ask what medications the patient takes and if he has applied any topical medication to his rash. If so, ask him what type and when it was last applied. Find out if he has a family history of skin disorders.

## Physical exam
Examine the entire skin surface, noting if it's dry, oily, moist, or greasy. Record the exact location and distribution of the skin lesions and their color, shape, and size.

## Causes
*Acne vulgaris.* Pustules typify inflammatory lesions of this disorder, accompanied by papules, nodules, cysts, and open comedones. Lesions appear on the face, shoulders, back, and chest. Other findings may include pain on pressure, pruritus, or burning of the affected area. Chronic recurrent lesions produce scars.

*Blastomycosis.* This fungal infection produces small, painless, nonpruritic macules or papules that can enlarge to well-circumscribed, verrucous, crusted, or ulcerated lesions edged by pustules. Localized infection may cause only one lesion; systemic infection may produce many lesions on the hands, feet, face, and wrists. Blastomycosis also produces signs of pulmonary infection.

*Folliculitis.* This bacterial infection of hair follicles produces individual pustules, each pierced by a hair and possibly attended by pruritus. Hot-tub folliculitis produces pustules on areas covered by a bathing suit.

*Furunculosis.* Crops of furuncles begin as small, tender red pustules at the bases of hair follicles. They're likely to occur on the face, neck, forearms, groin, axillae, buttocks, and legs, and to produce local pain, swelling, and redness. The pustules remain tense for 2 to 4 days, then become fluctuant. Rupture discharges pus and necrotic material. The pain subsides, but erythema and edema may persist.

*Gonococcemia.* A rash of scanty, pinpoint erythematous macules rapidly becomes vesiculopustular, maculopapular and, in many cases, hemorrhagic. Bullae may form. Mature lesions are elevated, with gray necrotic centers and surrounding erythema. The rash appears on the distal parts of the arms and legs, usually during the first day that other findings, such as fever and joint pain, occur. The rash disappears after 3 or 4 days but may recur with each episode of fever.

*Pompholyx.* This common recurrent disorder produces symmetrical vesicular lesions that can become pustular. The lesions appear on the palms and, less often, on the soles and may be accompanied by minimal erythema and pruritus.

*Other causes.* Drugs, such as bromides, iodides, adrenocorticotropic hormone, corticosteroids, dactinomycin, trimethadione, lithium, phenytoin, phenobarbital, isoniazid, oral contraceptives, androgens, and anabolic steroids; nummular or annular dermatitis; pustular miliaria; pustular psoriasis; rosacea; and scabies.

## Nursing considerations
• Observe wound and skin isolation procedures until infection is ruled out. If the organism is infectious, do not allow any drainage to touch unaffected skin. Instruct the patient to keep toilet articles and linen separate from those of other family members.

The corneal reflex is tested bilaterally by drawing a fine-pointed wisp of sterile cotton from a corner of each eye to the cornea. Normally, the patient blinks bilaterally each time either cornea is touched. When this reflex is absent, neither eyelid closes when the cornea of one is touched.

The site of the afferent fibers for this reflex is in the ophthalmic branch of the trigeminal nerve (cranial nerve V). The efferent fibers are located in the facial nerve (cranial nerve VII). Unilateral or bilateral absence of the corneal reflex may result from damage to these nerves.

## History

Because an absent corneal reflex may signify such progressive neurologic disorders as Guillain-Barré syndrome, ask the patient about facial pain, dysphagia, and limb weakness.

## Physical exam

If you can't elicit the corneal reflex, assess the patient for other signs of trigeminal nerve dysfunction. To test the three sensory portions of the nerve, touch each side of the patient's face on the brow, cheek, and jaw with a cotton wisp, and ask him to compare the sensations.

If you suspect facial nerve involvement, note if both the upper and lower face are weak bilaterally.

## Causes

*Acoustic neuroma.* This tumor affects the trigeminal nerve, causing a diminished or absent corneal reflex, tinnitus, and unilateral hearing impairment. Facial palsy and anesthesia, palate weakness, and signs of cerebellar dysfunction may result if the tumor impinges on the adjacent cranial nerves, brain stem, and cerebellum.

*Bell's palsy.* A common cause of diminished or absent corneal reflex, this disorder causes paralysis of cranial nerve VII. It can also produce complete hemifacial weakness or paralysis, and drooling on the affected side. The affected side sags and appears masklike. The eye on the affected side can't be shut and tears constantly.

*Brain stem infarction or injury.* Absent corneal reflex can occur on the side opposite the lesion when infarction or injury affects cranial nerve V or VII, or their connection in the central trigeminal tract. The patient's level of consciousness may be decreased. He may have dysphagia, dysarthria, and contralateral limb weakness, and may show early signs of increased intracranial pressure. In massive brain stem infarction or injury, other findings include apneustic breathing or periods of apnea; bilateral pupillary dilation or constriction with decreased responsiveness to light; rising systolic blood pressure; widening pulse pressure; bradycardia; and coma.

*Guillain-Barré syndrome.* In this disorder, a diminished or absent corneal reflex accompanies ipsilateral loss of facial muscle control. The patient may also have dysarthria, nasality, and dysphagia. Muscle weakness typically starts in the legs, then extends to the arms and facial nerves within 72 hours. Other findings may include paresthesia, respiratory muscle paralysis, respiratory insufficiency, postural hypotension, incontinence, diaphoresis, and tachycardia.

*Trigeminal neuralgia (tic douloureux).* A diminished or absent corneal reflex may stem from a superior maxillary lesion that affects the ophthalmic branch. The patient experiences sudden bursts of intense pain or shooting sensations, lasting 1 to 15 minutes, in one of the divisions of the trigeminal nerve, primarily the superior mandibular or maxillary division. Local stimulation, such as a light touch to the cheeks, may trigger an attack. An attack may also follow exposure to hot or cold, or eating or drinking hot or cold food or beverages.

## Nursing considerations

• When the corneal reflex is absent, take measures to protect the patient's affected eye from injury. For example, lubricate the eye with artificial tears to prevent drying. Cover the cornea with a shield and avoid excessive corneal reflex testing.

Purpura—extravasation of red blood cells from blood vessels into the skin, subcutaneous tissue, or mucous membranes—is marked by purplish or brownish-red discoloration that's visible through the epidermis. Purpura differs from erythema in that it doesn't blanch with pressure. Purpuric lesions include petechiae, ecchymoses, and hematomas.

## History

Ask the patient when he first noticed the lesion and if he has noticed other lesions on his body. Does he or his family have a history of bleeding disorders or easy bruising? Obtain a medication history and ask him to describe his diet. Ask about recent trauma or transfusions and the development of associated signs, such as epistaxis, bleeding gums, hematuria, and rectal bleeding. Ask the female patient about menstrual flow.

## Physical exam

Inspect the patient's entire skin surface and mucous membranes to determine the type, size, location, distribution, and severity of purpuric lesions.

## Causes

*Disseminated intravascular coagulation.* Varying degrees of purpura may occur, depending on the syndrome's severity and underlying cause. Other findings may include acrocyanosis; dyspnea; seizures; severe muscle, back, and abdominal pain; and signs of acute tubular necrosis.

*Ehlers-Danlos syndrome (EDS).* Besides petechiae, this syndrome features easy bruising, epistaxis, gum bleeding, hematuria, melena, menorrhagia, and excessive bleeding after surgery. EDS characteristically produces soft, velvety, hyperelastic skin; hyperextensible joints; and dislocations of the temporomandibular joint.

*Folic acid deficiency.* In this disorder, the patient may complain of fatigue, weakness, dyspnea, palpitations, nausea, and anorexia. He may be irritable and forgetful and report headaches.

*Idiopathic thrombocytopenic purpura (ITP).* Chronic ITP typically begins insidiously, with scattered petechiae that are most common on the distal arms and legs.

*Leukemia.* Persistent widespread petechiae appear on the skin, mucous membranes, retina, and serosal surfaces. The patient may also have swollen and bleeding gums, epistaxis, and other bleeding tendencies. Lymphadenopathy and splenomegaly are common.

*Liver disease.* Hepatic disease may cause purpura, particularly ecchymoses, and other bleeding tendencies. Associated findings may include hepatomegaly, ascites, right upper quadrant pain, jaundice, nausea, vomiting, and anorexia.

*Thrombotic thrombocytopenic purpura.* Generalized purpura is usually a presenting sign in this disorder. Other findings usually include fever, hematuria, vaginal bleeding, jaundice, and pallor.

*Other causes.* Allergic purpura, amyloidosis, anticoagulants (coumadin, heparin), arterial catheterization, autoerythrocyte sensitivity, B-cell lymphoma, chemotherapy, congenital factor deficiencies, cryoglobulinemia, easy bruising syndrome, Gaucher's disease, hemodialysis, hemophilia, Hodgkin's disease, hyperglobulinemia, multiple blood transfusions with platelet-poor blood, plasma expanders, polycythemia vera, pseudoxanthoma elasticum, radiation therapy, Schamberg's disease, septicemia, stasis, surgery (cardiac, pulmonary), systemic lupus erythematosus, thrombasthenia, venipuncture, vitamin deficiencies ($B_{12}$, C, and K), von Willebrand's disease, and Wiskott-Aldrich syndrome.

## Nursing considerations

- Prepare the patient for any diagnostic tests.
- Advise the patient not to use cosmetic fade creams or other products to try to reduce pigmentation. If the patient has a hematoma, apply pressure and cold compresses initially to help reduce bleeding and swelling. After the first 24 hours, advise the patient to apply warm compresses.

This elicited symptom indicates sudden distention of the renal capsule. It almost always accompanies unelicited, dull, constant flank pain in the costovertebral angle (CVA) just lateral to the sacrospinal muscle and below the 12th rib. This associated pain typically travels anteriorly in the subcostal region toward the umbilicus.

Percussing the CVA elicits tenderness. A patient who doesn't have this symptom will perceive a thudding, jarring, or pressure-like sensation when tested, but no pain. A patient with a disorder that distends the renal capsule will experience intense pain as the renal capsule stretches and stimulates the afferent nerves, which emanate from the spinal cord at levels T11 through L2 and innervate the kidney.

## History

After detecting CVA tenderness, assess the possible extent of renal damage. First, find out if the patient has other symptoms of renal or urologic dysfunction. Ask about his voiding habits. How frequently does he urinate and in what amounts? Has he noticed any change in intake or output? If so, when did he notice the change? (Be sure to ask about fluid intake before judging his output abnormal.) Ask about nocturia, pain or burning during urination, and difficulty starting a stream. Does the patient strain to urinate without being able to do so (tenesmus)? Ask about urine color; brown or bright red urine may contain blood.

Explore other signs and symptoms. For example, if the patient's experiencing pain in his flank, abdomen, or back, when did he first notice the pain? How severe is it and where is it located?

Find out if the patient or a family member has a history of urinary tract infections, congenital anomalies, calculi, or other obstructive nephropathies or uropathies. Ask about a history of renovascular disorders, such as occlusion of the renal arteries or veins.

## Physical exam

Take the patient's vital signs. Fever and chills in a patient with CVA tenderness may indicate acute pyelonephritis. If the patient has hypertension and bradycardia, be alert for other autonomic effects of renal pain, such as diaphoresis and pallor. Inspect, auscultate, and gently palpate the abdomen for clues to the underlying cause of CVA tenderness. Be alert for abdominal distention, hypoactive bowel sounds, and palpable masses.

## Causes

*Calculi.* Infundibular and ureteropelvic junction calculi produce CVA tenderness, flank pain, and possibly nausea, vomiting, severe abdominal pain, abdominal distention, and decreased bowel sounds.

*Perirenal abscess.* Causing exquisite CVA tenderness, this disorder may also produce severe unilateral flank pain, dysuria, persistent high fever, chills, and sometimes a palpable abdominal mass.

*Pyelonephritis (acute).* Perhaps the most common cause of CVA tenderness, acute pyelonephritis is commonly accompanied by persistent high fever, chills, flank pain, weakness, dysuria, hematuria, nocturia, and urinary urgency, frequency, and tenesmus.

*Renal artery occlusion.* The patient experiences flank pain as well as CVA tenderness. Other findings may include severe, continuous upper abdominal pain; nausea; vomiting; decreased bowel sounds; and a high fever after 1 or 2 days.

*Renal vein occlusion.* The patient with this disorder has CVA tenderness and flank pain. He also may have fever, hematuria, and sudden, severe back pain.

## Nursing considerations

• Administer pain medication, as ordered, and continue to monitor vital signs and intake and output. As ordered, collect serum and urine samples and prepare the patient for radiologic studies, such as intravenous pyelography, renal arteriography, and a computed tomography scan.

# Purple striae

Thin, purple streaks on the skin, purple striae are a common result of pregnancy or significant weight gain. These streaks also characteristically occur in hypercortisolism along with other cushingoid signs, such as a buffalo hump and moon face. Although hypercortisolism can result from adrenocortical carcinoma, adrenal adenoma, and pituitary adenoma, it usually results from excessive use of glucocorticoid drugs.

The catabolic action of excess glucocorticoids on skin, fat, and muscle produces purple striae by inhibiting fibroblast activity, resulting in loss of collagen and connective tissue. This causes extreme thinning of the skin, which, along with erythrocytosis, is responsible for the striae's purple color.

Purple striae are most common over the abdominal area, but they may also occur over the breasts, hips, buttocks, thighs, and axillae. Developing gradually, purple striae may, with treatment, gradually fade or decrease in size. When they result from pregnancy or weight gain, striae typically fade to silvery streaks without treatment.

## History

Ask the patient when—and on what part of his body—he first noticed purple striae. To help determine the rate of progression, find out if he has photographs of himself before and over the course of striae development. Next, obtain a complete medication history. If the patient is receiving glucocorticoid therapy, find out the drug's name, the daily dosage, and the reason for treatment. Ask if the dosage has been altered recently and if the drug is given intramuscularly. Find out if the patient uses topical corticosteroid preparations, especially fluorinated products. Ask about concomitant use of occlusive dressings and, with large skin surface areas, the amount of corticosteroid applied.

## Physical exam

Examine the patient, noting all areas where purple striae appear. When checking for striae, remember that the patient's skin is extremely thin and susceptible to bruising.

## Causes

*Hypercortisolism.* In this disorder, purple striae (usually more than 1 cm wide) develop gradually over the abdomen and possibly the breasts, hips, buttocks, thighs, and axillae. Inspection also reveals moon face, buffalo hump, and truncal obesity—the cardinal signs of hypercortisolism. Other findings may include acne, ecchymoses, petechiae, muscle weakness and wasting, poor wound healing, excessive perspiration, hypertension, fatigue, and personality changes. Women may develop hirsutism, menstrual irregularities, and loss of ability to achieve orgasm. Men may have impotence.

*Other causes.* Excessive use of glucocorticoids, pregnancy, and significant weight gain.

## Nursing considerations

- Prepare the patient for diagnostic tests to confirm hypercortisolism and determine its cause.
- Expect to collect 24-hour urine samples before and during the 2-day low-dose and 2-day high-dose dexamethasone tests. Explain that follow-up tests may be performed.
- Help the patient cope with changes in his body image by clearly explaining the disease process and allowing him to express his concerns openly.

# Cough, barking

Resonant, brassy, and harsh, a barking cough is part of a complex of signs and symptoms that characterize croup syndrome—a group of pediatric disorders marked by varying degrees of respiratory distress. Croup syndrome is most common in boys and most prevalent in winter, and it may recur in the same child. Because infants' and children's airways are smaller in diameter than adults', pediatric patients can rapidly develop airway occlusion from edema. A barking cough indicates edema of the larynx and surrounding tissue and may signal a life-threatening emergency.

### ▶ Emergency interventions

Quickly assess the child's respiratory status, and have another nurse notify the doctor. Take the child's vital signs, being especially alert for tachycardia and signs of hypoxemia. Check for decreased level of consciousness (LOC).

Find out if the child has been playing with a small object that he may have aspirated. Check for cyanosis of the lips and nail beds. Observe for sternal or intercostal retractions or nasal flaring. Note the rate and depth of respirations; they may become shallow as respiratory distress worsens. Observe the child's position: Is he sitting up, leaning forward, struggling to breathe? Observe his activity level, facial expression, and LOC. With increasing respiratory distress from airway edema, the child will become restless, with a frightened, wide-eyed expression. As air hunger continues, he'll become lethargic and difficult to arouse.

If the child shows signs of severe distress, maintain airway patency and provide oxygen. Prepare to assist with endotracheal intubation or tracheotomy.

### History

When the child's condition permits, ask his parents when the barking cough began and which signs or symptoms accompanied it. When did the child first seem ill? Has he had croup before?

### Causes

*Aspiration of a foreign body.* Partial upper airway obstruction first causes sudden hoarseness, then a barking cough and inspiratory stridor. Other effects of this life-threatening condition include gagging, tachycardia, dyspnea, decreased breath sounds, wheezing, and possibly cyanosis.

*Epiglottitis.* Typically, this life-threatening disorder arises during the night, heralded by a barking cough and high fever. The child is hoarse, dysphagic, dyspneic, and restless and appears extremely ill and panicky. His barking cough may progress to severe respiratory distress with sternal and intercostal retractions, nasal flaring, cyanosis, and tachycardia. Total airway occlusion may occur in 2 to 5 hours.

*Laryngotracheobronchitis (acute).* Most common in infants and young children, this viral infection initially causes low to moderate fever, rhinitis, and cough. Descending infection leads to barking cough, hoarseness, and inspiratory stridor. Worsening distress brings on substernal and intercostal retractions, tachycardia, and shallow, rapid respirations.

*Spasmodic croup.* A barking cough typically awakens the child from sleep. Usually, he will not have a fever, but he may be hoarse, restless, and dyspneic. Worsening distress brings on the same signs as acute laryngotracheobronchitis. These signs commonly subside within a few hours, but attacks tend to recur.

### Nursing considerations

- If respiratory distress isn't severe, X-rays may be ordered to rule out epiglottal edema and lower respiratory tract infection.
- Depending on the child's age and extent of distress, provide a mist tent, oxygen hood, or bedside humidifier.
- Check the child frequently, provide periods of uninterrupted rest, and encourage the parents to stay with him.

C

An abnormally slow response to light, sluggish pupillary reaction can occur in one pupil or both. It can accompany degenerative disease of the central nervous system and diabetic neuropathy or can simply be a normal sign of aging.

## Physical exam

First, test the patient's direct light reflex. Darken the room, cover one of the patient's eyes, and ask him to keep the other eye open. Hold it open for him if necessary. Approaching from the side, shine a bright penlight directly into his open eye. If normal, the pupil will promptly constrict. Now test the consensual light reflex. With both of the patient's eyelids open, shine the light into one eye. If normal, both pupils will promptly constrict. Repeat both procedures in the opposite eye. A sluggish reaction in one or both pupils indicates dysfunction of cranial nerves II and III, which mediate the pupillary light reflex.

Test the patient's visual acuity in both eyes. Then test the pupillary reaction to accommodation: Pupils should constrict equally as the patient shifts his gaze from a distant to a near object. Next, hold a penlight at the side of each eye and examine the cornea and iris. As ordered, assist the doctor in measuring intraocular pressure (IOP) with a tonometer. Or you can estimate IOP without a tonometer by placing your fingers over the patient's closed eyelid. If the eyeball feels rock hard, suspect elevated IOP.

## Causes

*Adie's syndrome.* After an abrupt onset of unilateral mydriasis and sluggish pupillary response, pupils may become nonreactive. The patient may complain of blurred vision and cramplike eye pain. Eventually, both eyes may be affected. Other findings include hypoactive or absent deep tendon reflexes in the arms and legs.

*Diabetic neuropathy.* Besides sluggish pupillary response, a patient with long-standing diabetes may have orthostatic hypotension and syncope. Other findings may include dysphagia, episodic constipation or diarrhea, painless bladder distention with overflow incontinence, retrograde ejaculation, and impotence.

*Encephalitis.* After an initially bilateral sluggish pupillary response, pupils become dilated and nonreactive; decreased accommodation may occur, along with other cranial nerve palsies. Within 48 hours, encephalitis causes a decreased level of consciousness, headache, high fever, vomiting, and nuchal rigidity.

*Herpes zoster.* This virus may cause a sluggish pupillary response by affecting the nasociliary nerve. The conjunctiva will have follicles. Other findings include a serous discharge, absence of tears, ptosis, and extraocular muscle palsy.

*Iritis (acute).* The affected eye exhibits a sluggish pupillary response and conjunctival injection; the pupil may also be irregularly shaped. Other findings include sudden eye pain, photophobia, and blurred vision.

*Multiple sclerosis.* This disorder may produce small, irregularly shaped pupils that react better to accommodation than to light. Additional findings may include ptosis, nystagmus, diplopia, and blurred vision. Visual problems and sensory impairment are usually the earliest findings. Later, various features may develop, including muscle weakness and paralysis, intention tremor, spasticity, and gait ataxia.

*Wernicke's disease.* Initial signs include intention tremor and sluggish pupillary reaction. Later, pupils may become nonreactive. Additional findings include diplopia, gaze paralysis, nystagmus, ptosis, decreased visual acuity, conjunctival injection, postural hypotension, tachycardia, ataxia, apathy, and confusion.

*Other causes.* Familial amyloid polyneuropathy, myotonic dystrophy, and tertiary syphilis.

## Nursing considerations

• Sluggish pupillary reaction isn't diagnostically significant, although it occurs in a variety of disorders.

A noisy, forceful expulsion of air from the lungs that doesn't yield sputum or blood, a nonproductive cough is one of the most common respiratory complaints. A nonproductive cough that becomes productive is a classic sign of progressive respiratory disease. A patient may disregard a chronic nonproductive cough, or he may consider it normal, not seeking treatment until other symptoms arise.

## History

Ask the patient when his cough began and whether any body position, time of day, or specific activity affects it. How does the cough sound? Is it related to smoking or a chemical irritant? Does the patient cough often or paroxysmally? Does he feel pain?

Obtain a medical, surgical, allergy, and drug history. Ask about recent changes in appetite, weight, exercise tolerance, or energy and about recent exposure to fumes, chemicals, or smoke.

## Physical exam

Is the patient agitated, restless, or lethargic; pale, diaphoretic, or flushed; anxious, confused, or nervous? Take vital signs, check respiratory depth and rhythm, and note if wheezing or "crowing" noises occur with breathing. Is the patient's skin cold or warm, clammy or dry? Check his nose and mouth for congestion, inflammation, drainage, or signs of infection. Inspect his neck for distended veins and tracheal deviation, and palpate for masses or enlarged lymph nodes.

Examine chest configuration and chest wall motion. Percuss for dullness, tympany, or flatness. Auscultate for wheezes, crackles, rhonchi, pleural friction rubs, and decreased or absent breath sounds. Examine the abdomen.

## Causes

*Asthma.* Attacks typically occur at night and start with a nonproductive cough and mild wheezing.

*Bronchitis (chronic).* A nonproductive, hacking cough later becomes productive.

*Bronchogenic carcinoma.* The earliest indicators of this disorder can be a chronic nonproductive cough, dyspnea, and vague chest pain.

*Common cold.* This disorder commonly starts with a nonproductive, hacking cough.

*Laryngeal tumor.* Mild, nonproductive cough is an early sign along with sore throat and hoarseness.

*Laryngitis.* Acute laryngitis causes a nonproductive cough, local pain, fever, and malaise.

*Lung abscess.* This disorder typically begins with nonproductive coughing, weakness, dyspnea, and pleuritic pain. Later, the cough produces large amounts of purulent, possibly bloody sputum.

*Pneumonia. Bacterial pneumonia* usually starts with a nonproductive, hacking, painful cough that rapidly becomes productive. In *mycoplasmal pneumonia,* a nonproductive cough arises 2 to 3 days after other signs. *Viral pneumonia* causes a nonproductive, hacking cough.

*Pneumothorax.* This life-threatening disorder causes a dry cough and respiratory distress.

*Pulmonary edema.* Initially, this disorder causes a dry cough, exertional dyspnea, paroxysmal nocturnal dyspnea, orthopnea, tachycardia, tachypnea, dependent crackles, and ventricular gallop.

*Tracheobronchitis (acute).* Initially, this disorder produces a dry cough that later becomes productive as secretions increase.

*Other causes.* Acute bronchiolitis, airway occlusion, atelectasis, cystic fibrosis, esophageal disorders, Hodgkin's disease, hypersensitivity pneumonitis, incentive spirometry, intermittent positive pressure breathing, interstitial lung disease, Legionnaires' disease, mediastinal tumor, pericardial effusion, pleural effusion, psittacosis, pulmonary embolism, sarcoidosis, sinusitis, and suctioning.

## Nursing considerations

• A nonproductive, paroxysmal cough may induce life-threatening bronchospasm. If bronchospasm occurs, give a bronchodilator. Unless the patient has chronic obstructive pulmonary disease, give antitussives and sedatives to suppress the cough.
• Humidify the air. Tell the patient to avoid smoking and use of aerosols and powders.

Nonreactive (fixed) pupils fail to respond to light. The development of a unilateral or bilateral nonreactive response could signal a life-threatening emergency or brain death. It also occurs with certain optic drugs.

▶ **Emergency interventions**

If the patient is unconscious and develops unilateral or bilateral nonreactive pupils, take his vital signs while another nurse immediately informs the doctor. Be alert for decerebrate or decorticate posture, bradycardia, elevated systolic blood pressure, and widened pulse pressure. A unilateral dilated, nonreactive pupil may be an early sign of uncal brain herniation.

## History

If possible, ask the patient what type of eyedrops, if any, he's using, and when they were last instilled. Ask if he has any pain and, if so, try to determine its location, intensity, and duration.

## Physical exam

To assess pupillary reaction, first test the patient's direct light reflex. Darken the room; cover one of the patient's eyes and have him hold the other open. Hold it open for him if necessary. Moving from the side, shine a bright penlight directly into his open eye. If normal, the pupil will promptly constrict. To test consensual light reflex, shine a light into one eye while both eyes remain open. If normal, both pupils will promptly constrict. Repeat in the opposite eye. No reaction indicates dysfunction of cranial nerves II and III.

Assess the patient's visual acuity in both eyes. Test pupillary reaction to accommodation: Both pupils should constrict equally as the patient shifts his gaze from a distant to a near object. Hold a penlight at the side of each eye and examine the cornea and iris. As ordered, assist in measuring intraocular pressure (IOP) with a tonometer, or estimate the pressure by placing your second and third fingers over the patient's closed eyelid. If the eyeball feels rock hard, suspect elevated IOP. If the patient has had ocular trauma, don't manipulate the affected eye.

## Causes

*Botulism.* Bilateral mydriasis and nonreactive pupils appear 12 to 36 hours after ingestion of tainted food. Other findings are blurred vision, diplopia, ptosis, strabismus, extraocular muscle palsies, vomiting, and diarrhea. Vertigo, deafness, hoarseness, nasal voice, dysarthria, and dysphagia follow. Progressive muscle weakness and absent deep tendon reflexes evolve over 2 to 4 days, causing severe constipation and respiratory paralysis.

*Encephalitis.* Initially sluggish pupils become dilated and nonreactive. Decreased accommodation and other symptoms of cranial nerve palsies develop. Within 48 hours, encephalitis causes a decreased level of consciousness, high fever, headache, vomiting, and nuchal rigidity.

*Glaucoma (acute closed-angle).* In this ophthalmic emergency, examination reveals a moderately dilated, nonreactive pupil. Conjunctival injection, corneal clouding, and decreased visual acuity also occur. The patient experiences sudden blurred vision and severe pain in and around the eye.

*Oculomotor nerve palsy.* Often, the first signs are a dilated, nonreactive pupil and loss of accommodation in one or both eyes. Life-threatening brain herniation can cause total paralysis of cranial nerve III; central herniation causes bilateral midposition nonreactive pupils; uncal herniation initially causes a unilateral dilated, nonreactive pupil.

*Other causes.* Adie's syndrome; drugs, such as topical mydriatics and cycloplegics, glutethimide, deep ether anesthesia, opiates, and atropine poisoning; familial amyloid polyneuropathy; iris disease; midbrain lesions; ocular trauma; uveitis; and Wernicke's disease.

## Nursing considerations

• If the patient is conscious, monitor his pupillary light reflex. If he's unconscious, close his eyes to prevent corneal exposure.

# Cough, productive

Productive coughing clears airway passages of accumulated secretions that normal mucociliary action doesn't remove. It's a sudden, forceful, noisy expulsion of air that contains sputum, blood, or both. Usually caused by a cardiopulmonary disorder, productive coughing typically stems from acute or chronic infection that causes inflammation, edema, and increased mucus production in the airways. This sign can also result from inhalation of antigenic or irritating substances. In fact, its most common cause is cigarette smoking.

## History

Ask when the cough began, and find out how much sputum the patient coughs up each day. Does sputum production have any relationship to time of day, meals, activities, or environment? Has sputum production increased since coughing began? Ask about sputum color, odor, and consistency.

How does the cough sound and feel? Ask about cigarette, drug, and alcohol use and changes in weight or appetite. Obtain a medical, surgical, allergy, and drug history. Does the patient work around chemicals or respiratory irritants?

## Physical exam

Examine the patient's mouth and nose for congestion, drainage, or inflammation. Note breath odor. Inspect the neck for distended veins, and palpate for tenderness, masses, or enlarged lymph nodes. Observe the chest for accessory muscle use, retractions, and uneven expansion. Percuss for dullness, tympany, or flatness. Auscultate for pleural friction rub and abnormal breath sounds.

## Causes

*Asthma.* A severe attack typically starts with a dry cough, progressing to severe dyspnea, audible wheezing, tight chest, and productive cough.

*Bacterial pneumonia.* An initially dry cough becomes productive. Rust-colored sputum occurs in pneumococcal pneumonia; brick red or "currant jelly" sputum in *Klebsiella* pneumonia; salmon-colored sputum in staphylococcal pneumonia; and mucopurulent sputum in streptococcal pneumonia.

*Bronchitis (chronic).* This disorder causes a cough that may be nonproductive initially. Eventually, though, it causes mucopurulent sputum.

*Common cold.* When a cold causes productive coughing, sputum is mucoid or mucopurulent.

*Lung abscess (ruptured).* The cardinal sign is coughing that produces copious amounts of purulent, foul-smelling, possibly blood-tinged sputum.

*Lung cancer.* An early sign of bronchogenic carcinoma, chronic cough produces small amounts of purulent (or mucopurulent), blood-streaked sputum. In bronchoalveolar cancer, coughing raises large amounts of frothy sputum.

*Pulmonary edema.* Patients with a severe case of this life-threatening disorder have a cough that produces frothy, bloody sputum.

*Pulmonary emphysema.* This disorder causes minimal chronic productive coughing with scant, mucoid, translucent, grayish white sputum that can become mucopurulent.

*Pulmonary tuberculosis.* Besides a mild to severe productive cough, pleuritic pain, hemoptysis, malaise, and dyspnea may occur.

*Other causes.* Actinomycosis, acute bronchiolitis, aspiration and chemical pneumonitis, blastomycosis, bronchiectasis, coccidioidomycosis, cystic fibrosis, expectorants, incentive spirometry, intermittent positive-pressure breathing, Legionnaires' disease, nocardiosis, pertussis, psittacosis, pulmonary embolism, silicosis, and tracheobronchitis.

## Nursing considerations

- Give mucolytics and expectorants, and increase oral fluids to thin secretions. Give a bronchodilator and antibiotics as ordered.
- Humidify the air around the patient and, as ordered, provide chest physiotherapy.
- Provide uninterrupted rest periods. Keep the patient from using aerosols, powders, or other respiratory irritants. Encourage him not to smoke.
- Prepare the patient for diagnostic tests.

Pulsus paradoxus (paradoxical pulse) is a decline in blood pressure of more than 10 mm Hg during inspiration. When systolic pressure falls more than 20 mm Hg, the peripheral pulses may be barely palpable or disappear during inspiration. Pulsus paradoxus is thought to result from an inspirational increase in negative intrathoracic pressure.

▶ **Emergency interventions**

Pulsus paradoxus may signal cardiac tamponade. After you detect this pulse pattern, quickly take the patient's other vital signs while another nurse notifies the doctor immediately. Check for dyspnea, tachypnea, diaphoresis, distended neck veins, tachycardia, narrowed pulse pressure, and hypotension. If necessary, assist with emergency pericardiocentesis, after which the degree of pulsus paradoxus should decrease.

### History

If the patient doesn't have cardiac tamponade, find out if he has a history of chronic cardiac or pulmonary disease. Ask about associated signs and symptoms, such as a cough or chest pain. Then auscultate for abnormal breath sounds.

### Physical exam

To detect and measure pulsus paradoxus, inflate a blood pressure cuff 10 to 20 mm Hg beyond the peak systolic pressure. Deflate the cuff 2 mm Hg/second until you hear the first Korotkoff sound during expiration. Note the systolic pressure. Continue to deflate the cuff slowly. If pulsus paradoxus exists, the Korotkoff sounds will disappear with inspiration and return with expiration. Continue to deflate the cuff until you hear Korotkoff sounds during both inspiration and expiration. Note the systolic pressure and subtract this reading from the first one. A difference of more than 10 mm Hg is abnormal. Also try palpating the radial pulse. Marked pulse diminution during inspiration indicates pulsus paradoxus.

### Causes

*Cardiac tamponade.* Pulsus paradoxus commonly occurs in this disorder but may be difficult to detect. In severe tamponade, findings include hypotension, muffled heart sounds, and jugular vein distention. Related findings include chest pain, pericardial friction rub, narrowed pulse pressure, restlessness, clammy skin, hepatomegaly, dyspnea, tachypnea, and cyanosis. The patient typically sits up and leans forward to facilitate breathing. If tamponade develops gradually, pulsus paradoxus may accompany weakness, anorexia, and possibly chest pain, but the patient won't have muffled heart sounds or severe hypotension.

*Chronic obstructive pulmonary disease.* Wide fluctuations in intrathoracic pressure produce pulsus paradoxus and possibly tachycardia. Other findings may include dyspnea, tachypnea, wheezing, productive or nonproductive cough, accessory muscle use, barrel chest, and clubbing. The patient may show labored breathing.

*Pericarditis (chronic constrictive).* Pulsus paradoxus occurs in up to 50% of cases. Other findings include pericardial friction rub, chest pain, exertional dyspnea, orthopnea, hepatomegaly, ascites, peripheral edema, and Kussmaul's sign.

*Pulmonary embolism (massive).* Decreased left ventricular filling and stroke volume produces pulsus paradoxus along with syncope and severe apprehension, dyspnea, tachypnea, pleuritic chest pain, cyanosis, and distended neck veins.

*Right ventricular infarction.* This infarction may produce pulsus paradoxus and elevated jugular venous or central venous pressure. Other findings are similar to those of myocardial infarction.

### Nursing considerations

• Prepare the patient for an echocardiogram. Monitor the patient's vital signs, and frequently check the degree of paradox. Inform the doctor immediately if you note a steady increase in the degree of paradox.

Also known as rales and crepitations, crackles are nonmusical clicking or rattling noises heard during auscultation of breath sounds. A common finding in certain cardiovascular and respiratory disorders, they indicate abnormal movement of air through fluid-filled airways. Crackles usually occur during inspiration and recur constantly from one respiratory cycle to the next. They're characterized by their pitch, loudness, occurrence in the respiratory cycle, and location.

## ▶ Emergency interventions

If you detect crackles, take vital signs and assess for respiratory distress or airway obstruction. Also check for increased accessory muscle use and chest wall motion, retractions, stridor, or nasal flaring. Give oxygen, and be prepared to assist with endotracheal intubation.

## History

If the patient has a cough, ask when it began and if it's constant or intermittent. Have him describe any sputum. Ask about pain, where it's located, when he noticed it, if it radiates to other areas, and if movement, coughing, or breathing worsens or helps it. Ask about tobacco and alcohol use, recent weight loss, fatigue, weakness, vertigo, syncope, and exposure to chemical irritants.

## Physical exam

Examine the nose and mouth for infection. Check the neck for masses, tenderness, swelling, lymphadenopathy, or venous distention. Inspect the chest for abnormal configuration or uneven expansion. Percuss for dullness, tympany, or flatness. Auscultate the lungs for other abnormal, diminished, or absent breath sounds. Listen to the heart for abnormal sounds. Check the hands and feet for edema or clubbing.

## Causes

*Adult respiratory distress syndrome.* Diffuse crackles are usually heard in the dependent portions of the lungs. Other findings include cyanosis, nasal flaring, tachypnea, grunting respirations, rhonchi, and decreased level of consciousness.

*Asthma.* An attack typically causes a dry to productive cough, dyspnea, chest tightness, prolonged expirations, intercostal and supraclavicular retractions on inspiration, accessory muscle use, and flaring nostrils. A severe attack causes dry, whistling crackles.

*Bronchiectasis.* Persistent coarse crackles accompany a chronic cough that produces mucopurulent sputum.

*Bronchitis (chronic).* This disorder produces coarse crackles at lung bases, prolonged expiration, wheezing, rhonchi, and a productive cough.

*Pneumonia.* Medium to fine diffuse crackles accompany fever, a cough that may become productive, decreased breath sounds, and myalgias.

*Pulmonary edema.* Early signs include moist, bubbling crackles on inspiration; dyspnea on exertion; and a cough that may produce frothy, bloody sputum. Related effects include tachypnea and a ventricular gallop ($S_3$).

*Pulmonary embolism.* Associated signs include fine to coarse crackles, a cough that may be dry or produce blood-tinged sputum, severe dyspnea, and possibly pleuritic chest pain.

*Pulmonary tuberculosis.* Fine crackles occur after coughing. Other findings include hemoptysis and chest pain.

*Tracheobronchitis (acute).* Moist or coarse crackles occur along with a productive cough, chills, sore throat, rhonchi, and wheezing.

*Other causes.* Chemical pneumonitis, cystic fibrosis, interstitial lung fibrosis, Legionnaires' disease, lung abscess, psittacosis, sarcoidosis, sickle cell anemia, silicosis, and tracheoesophageal fistula.

## Nursing considerations

• Elevate the head of the patient's bed to facilitate his breathing, and give fluids, humidified air, or oxygen, as ordered. Turn the patient every 1 to 2 hours, and encourage him to breathe deeply.

# Pulsus bisferiens

Pulsus bisferiens is a hyperdynamic, double-beating pulse characterized by two systolic peaks separated by a midsystolic dip. Both peaks may be equal or one may be larger than the other; usually, the first peak is taller or more forceful than the second. The first peak (percussion wave) is believed to be the pulse pressure and the second (tidal wave), reverberation from the periphery. Pulsus bisferiens occurs in conditions such as aortic insufficiency, in which a large volume of blood is rapidly ejected from the left ventricle. The pulse can be palpated in peripheral arteries or observed on an arterial pressure wave recording.

## History

After you detect pulsus bisferiens, review the patient's history for cardiac disorders. Next, find out what medication he's taking, if any, and ask if he has any other illnesses. Also ask about the development of any associated signs and symptoms, such as dyspnea, chest pain, or fatigue. Find out how long he's had these symptoms and if they change with activity or rest.

## Physical exam

To detect pulsus bisferiens, lightly palpate the carotid, brachial, radial, or femoral artery. (The pulse is easiest to palpate in the carotid artery.) At the same time, listen to the patient's heart sounds to determine if the two palpable peaks occur during systole. If they do, you'll feel the double pulse between the first and second heart sounds.

Take the patient's vital signs and auscultate for abnormal heart or lung sounds.

## Causes

*Aortic insufficiency.* This heart defect is the most common organic cause of pulsus bisferiens. Most patients with chronic aortic insufficiency are asymptomatic until age 40 or 50. However, exertional dyspnea, worsening fatigue, orthopnea and, eventually, paroxysmal nocturnal dyspnea may develop.

Acute aortic insufficiency may produce signs and symptoms of left ventricular failure and cardiovascular collapse, such as weakness, severe dyspnea, hypotension, ventricular gallop ($S_3$), and tachycardia. Additional findings may include chest pain, palpitations, pallor, and strong, abrupt carotid pulsations. The patient may also have widened pulse pressure and one or more murmurs, especially an apical diastolic rumble (Austin Flint murmur).

*Aortic stenosis with aortic insufficiency.* Pulsus bisferiens is commonly seen in aortic stenosis when stenosis is accompanied by moderately severe aortic insufficiency. In aortic stenosis, the pulse rises slowly and the second wave of the double beat is the more forceful one. This is commonly accompanied by dyspnea and fatigue. Chest pain and syncope suggest aortic stenosis alone rather than stenosis combined with aortic insufficiency.

*High cardiac output states.* Pulsus bisferiens commonly occurs in high-output states, such as anemia, thyrotoxicosis, fever, or exercise. Associated findings vary with the underlying cause and may include moderate tachycardia, a cervical venous hum, and widened pulse pressure.

*Hypertrophic obstructive cardiomyopathy.* About 40% of patients with this disorder have pulsus bisferiens because of a pressure gradient in the left ventricular outflow tract. Recorded more often than it's palpated, the pulse rate rises rapidly, and the first wave is the more forceful one. Associated findings may include a systolic murmur, dyspnea, angina, fatigue, and syncope.

## Nursing considerations

• Prepare the patient for diagnostic tests, such as an ECG, chest X-ray, cardiac catheterization, or angiography, to help determine the underlying cause of the abnormal pulse.

Also called bony crepitus, bony crepitation is a palpable vibration or an audible crunching sound that occurs when one bone grates against another. It can result from a fracture or when bones stripped of their protective articular cartilage grind against each other as they articulate, as in advanced arthritic or degenerative joint disorders.

Eliciting bony crepitation can help confirm diagnosis of a fracture. But it can also cause further soft tissue, nerve, or vessel injury. What's more, rubbing fractured bone ends together can convert a closed fracture into an open fracture if a bone end penetrates the skin. Therefore, after initial detection of crepitation in a patient with a fracture, avoid subsequent elicitation of this sign.

## History

If you detect bony crepitation in a patient with a suspected fracture, ask him if he feels any pain and, if so, if he can point to the painful area. Ask how and when the injury occurred. If the patient doesn't have a suspected fracture, ask about a history of osteoarthritis or rheumatoid arthritis. Ask what medications he takes and if any medication helps ease arthritic discomfort.

## Physical exam

If the patient has a suspected fracture, immobilize the affected area by applying a splint to prevent lacerating nerves, blood vessels, or other structures. Elevate the affected area, if possible, and apply cold packs. Inspect the affected area for abrasions or lacerations. Palpate pulses distal to the injury site and check the skin for pallor or coolness. Also test motor and sensory function distal to the injury site. If the patient does not have an injury, take his vital signs and test range of motion.

## Causes

*Fracture.* Besides bony crepitation, a fracture also causes acute local pain, edema, and decreased range of motion. Other findings may include deformity, point tenderness, discoloration of the limb, and loss of limb function. Neurovascular damage may cause prolonged capillary refill time, diminished or absent pulses, mottled cyanosis, paresthesia, and decreased sensation (all distal to the fracture site). An open fracture, of course, produces an obvious skin wound.

*Osteoarthritis.* In advanced cases of this disorder, joint crepitation may be elicited by range-of-motion testing. The cardinal symptom of osteoarthritis is joint pain, especially during motion and weight bearing. Other findings include joint stiffness that typically occurs after resting and subsides within a few minutes after the patient begins moving.

*Rheumatoid arthritis.* In advanced cases of this disorder, bony crepitation is heard when the affected joint is rotated. However, rheumatoid arthritis usually develops insidiously, producing nonspecific signs and symptoms such as fatigue, malaise, anorexia, a persistent low-grade fever, weight loss, lymphadenopathy, and vague arthralgias and myalgias. Then more specific and localized articular signs develop, frequently at the proximal finger joints. These signs usually occur bilaterally and symmetrically and may extend to the wrists, knees, elbows, and ankles. The affected joints stiffen after inactivity. The patient also has increased warmth, swelling, and tenderness of affected joints, and limited range of motion.

## Nursing considerations

• If you suspect a fracture, prepare the patient for X-rays of the affected area, and reassess his neurovascular status frequently.
• Keep the affected part immobilized and elevated until treatment is begun.
• Give analgesics, as ordered, to relieve pain.

# Pulsus alternans

A sign of severe left ventricular failure, pulsus alternans is a beat-to-beat change in the size and intensity of a peripheral pulse. Although the pulse rhythm remains regular, strong and weak contractions alternate. A change in the intensity of heart sounds and of existing heart murmurs may accompany this sign.

Pulsus alternans is thought to result from the change in stroke volume that occurs with beat-to-beat alteration in the left ventricle's contractility. Recumbency or exercise increases venous return and reduces the abnormal pulse. Treatment for heart failure usually resolves the problem. Rarely, a patient with normal left ventricular function has pulsus alternans, but the abnormal pulse seldom persists for more than 10 to 12 beats.

## ▶ Emergency interventions
Pulsus alternans indicates a critical change in the patient's status. After you detect it, quickly check other vital signs and have another nurse notify the doctor immediately. Closely assess the patient's heart rate, respiratory pattern, and blood pressure. Auscultate for a ventricular gallop ($S_3$) and increased crackles.

## History
After detecting pulsus alternans, review the patient's history for cardiac disorders. Find out what medication he's taking, if any, and ask if he has any other illnesses. Ask about associated signs and symptoms, such as dyspnea, tachypnea, fatigue, and weakness. Find out how long he's had these symptoms and if they change with activity or rest.

## Physical exam
Although most easily detected by sphygmomanometry, pulsus alternans can be detected by palpating the brachial, radial, or femoral artery when systolic pressure varies from beat to beat by more than 20 mm Hg. Because the small changes in arterial pressure that occur during normal respirations may obscure this abnormal pulse, you'll need to have the patient hold his breath during palpation. Apply light pressure to avoid obliterating the weaker pulse.

When using a sphygmomanometer to detect pulsus alternans, inflate the cuff to 10 to 20 mm Hg above the systolic pressure as determined by palpation, then slowly deflate it. At first, you'll hear only the strong beats. With further deflation, all beats will become audible and palpable, and then equally intense. (The difference between this point and the peak systolic level is often used to determine the degree of pulsus alternans.) When the cuff is removed, pulsus alternans returns.

Occasionally, the pulsation is so weak that no palpable pulse is detected at the periphery. This produces total pulsus alternans, an apparent halving of the pulse rate.

## Cause
*Left ventricular failure.* In this disorder, pulsus alternans is commonly initiated by a premature beat. It's almost always associated with a ventricular gallop. Other findings may include hypotension and cyanosis. Possible respiratory findings include exertional and paroxysmal nocturnal dyspnea, orthopnea, tachypnea, Cheyne-Stokes respirations, hemoptysis, and crackles. Fatigue and weakness are common.

## Nursing considerations
• If left ventricular failure develops suddenly, prepare the patient for transfer to an intensive or cardiac care unit. Meanwhile, elevate the head of his bed to promote respiratory excursion and increase oxygenation. The doctor may adjust the patient's current treatment plan to improve cardiac output, reduce the heart's work load, and promote diuresis.

When bubbles of air or other gases are trapped in subcutaneous tissue, palpation or stroking of the skin produces a crackling sound called subcutaneous crepitation or crepitus. The bubbles feel like small unstable nodules and aren't painful, even though subcutaneous crepitation is often associated with painful disorders. Usually, the affected tissue is visibly edematous—this can lead to airway occlusion if the neck or upper chest is involved.

The air or gas bubbles enter the tissues through open wounds, from the action of anaerobic microorganisms, or from rupture or perforation of pulmonary or GI organs.

## ▶ Emergency interventions

Because subcutaneous crepitation can indicate a life-threatening disorder, perform a rapid initial assessment.

## History

Ask the patient if he's experiencing any pain. If he is, find out where the pain is located, how severe it is, and when it began. Ask about recent thoracic surgery, diagnostic tests, respiratory therapy, or a history of trauma or chronic pulmonary disease.

## Physical exam

Palpate the affected skin to evaluate the location and extent of subcutaneous crepitation. Repalpate frequently to determine if the subcutaneous crepitation is increasing.

## Causes

*Gas gangrene.* Subcutaneous crepitation is the hallmark of this rare but commonly fatal infection. It's accompanied by local pain, swelling, and discoloration; formation of bullae; and necrosis. The skin over the wound may rupture, revealing dark red or black necrotic muscle and producing foul-smelling watery or frothy discharge.

*Orbital fracture.* This fracture allows air from the nasal sinuses to escape into subcutaneous tissue, causing subcutaneous crepitations of the eyelid and orbit. The most common sign of orbital fracture is periorbital ecchymosis. The patient has facial edema, diplopia, a hyphema or, occasionally, a dilated or unreactive pupil on the affected side.

*Pneumothorax.* Severe pneumothorax produces subcutaneous crepitation in the upper chest and neck. Many patients have unilateral chest pain that increases on inspiration. Dyspnea, anxiety, restlessness, tachypnea, cyanosis, tachycardia, accessory muscle use, asymmetrical chest expansion, and a nonproductive cough can also occur. Findings on the affected side include absent or decreased breath sounds, hyperresonance or tympany, and decreased vocal fremitus.

*Rupture of the esophagus.* A ruptured esophagus produces subcutaneous crepitation in the neck, chest wall, or supraclavicular fossa. In rupture of the cervical esophagus, the patient has severe pain in the neck or supraclavicular area, his neck resists passive motion, and he has local tenderness, soft tissue swelling, dysphagia, odynophagia, and orthostatic vertigo. Life-threatening rupture of the intrathoracic esophagus can produce mediastinal emphysema; severe retrosternal, epigastric, neck, or scapular pain; edema of the chest wall and neck; dyspnea; asymmetrical chest wall expansion; cyanosis; diaphoresis; hypotension; dysphagia; and fever.

*Rupture of the trachea or major bronchus.* This life-threatening injury produces abrupt subcutaneous crepitation of the neck and anterior chest wall. The patient has severe dyspnea with nasal flaring, tachycardia, accessory muscle use, hypotension, cyanosis, extreme anxiety, and possibly hemoptysis and mediastinal emphysema.

*Other causes.* Endoscopic tests, as a result of rupture or perforation of pulmonary or GI organs; mechanical ventilation and intermittent positive pressure breathing; and thoracic surgery.

## Nursing considerations

• Monitor the patient's vital signs frequently. Be alert for signs of respiratory distress.

# Pulse rhythm abnormality

An abnormal pulse rhythm is an irregular expansion and contraction of the peripheral arterial walls. It may be persistent or sporadic, and rhythmic or arrhythmic. Detected by palpating the radial or carotid pulse, an abnormal pulse rhythm is typically reported by the patient as palpitations and reflects an underlying cardiac arrhythmia, which may range from benign to life-threatening. Arrhythmias are commonly associated with cardiovascular, renal, respiratory, metabolic, and neurologic disorders as well as the effects of drugs, diagnostic tests, and treatments.

## ▶ Emergency interventions

Quickly assess the patient for signs of reduced cardiac output, such as decreased level of consciousness (LOC), hypotension, or dizziness. If you detect these signs, immediately notify the doctor. Obtain an ECG and possibly a chest X-ray, and begin cardiac monitoring. Insert an I.V. line and give oxygen by nasal cannula or mask. Monitor the patient's vital signs, pulse quality, and cardiac rhythm. Keep emergency intubation and suction equipment handy.

## History

If the patient's condition permits, ask if he's experiencing any pain. If so, find out when the pain started, where it's located, and whether it radiates. Ask about a history of heart disease and treatments for arrhythmias. Find out which medications the patient is currently taking and if he's complying with the prescribed dosage.

## Physical exam

Check the patient's apical and peripheral arterial pulses. An apical rate exceeding a peripheral arterial rate indicates a pulse deficit. Evaluate heart sounds: A long pause between $S_1$ and $S_2$ may indicate a conduction defect; a faint or absent $S_1$ and an easily audible $S_2$ may indicate atrial fibrillation or flutter. You may hear the two heart sounds close together on certain beats, possibly indicating premature atrial contractions or other variations in heart rate or rhythm.

Take the patient's apical and radial pulses while you listen for heart sounds. In some arrhythmias, such as premature ventricular contractions, you may hear the beat with your stethoscope but not feel it over the radial artery. This indicates an ineffective contraction that failed to produce a peripheral pulse. Now count the apical pulse for 60 seconds, noting the frequency of skipped peripheral beats. Report your findings to the doctor.

## Cause

*Arrhythmias.* An abnormal pulse rhythm may be the only sign. The patient may complain of palpitations, a fluttering heartbeat, or weak and skipped beats. Pulses may be weak and rapid or slow. Depending on the arrhythmia, dull chest pain or discomfort and hypotension may occur. Associated findings—if there are any—reflect decreased cardiac output and may include confusion, dizziness, decreased LOC, decreased urine output, dyspnea, pallor, and diaphoresis.

## Nursing considerations

• If ordered, prepare the patient for transfer to a cardiac or intensive care unit. Raise the side rails of the patient's bed, and don't leave him unattended while he's sitting or walking. Check his vital signs frequently, and monitor intake and output and the patient's daily weight.

• If ordered, collect blood samples for serum electrolyte, cardiac enzyme, and drug level studies. Prepare the patient for a chest X-ray and a 12-lead ECG. If possible, obtain a previous ECG to compare with current findings. If ordered, prepare the patient for 24-hour Holter monitoring.

• Stress to the patient the importance of keeping a diary of his activities and any symptoms that develop, to correlate with the incidence of arrhythmias.

• Instruct the patient to avoid smoking and caffeine.

# Cyanosis

A bluish or bluish black discoloration of the skin and mucous membranes, cyanosis results from excessive unoxygenated hemoglobin in the blood. *Central cyanosis* reflects inadequate oxygenation of systemic arterial blood caused by cardiac shunting, pulmonary disease, or hematologic disorders. It may occur anywhere on the skin and mucous membranes of the mouth, lips, and conjunctiva.

*Peripheral cyanosis* reflects sluggish peripheral circulation caused by vasoconstriction, reduced cardiac output, or vascular occlusion. It may be widespread or may occur locally in one extremity. It doesn't affect mucous membranes.

Cyanosis is usually undetectable until the oxygen saturation of hemoglobin falls below 80%. A nonpathologic cyanosis may result from environmental factors, such as exposure to cold.

## ▶ Emergency interventions

If the patient displays sudden localized cyanosis and other signs of arterial occlusion, protect the affected limb from injury, but don't massage it. If you see central cyanosis stemming from a pulmonary disorder or shock, perform a rapid assessment. Then take steps to maintain an airway, assist breathing, and monitor circulation.

## History

Review the patient's history, focusing on cardiac, respiratory, and hematologic disorders. Ask the patient when he first noticed cyanosis. Does it subside and recur? Is it aggravated by cold, smoking, or stress? Is it alleviated by massage or rewarming? Ask about headache, dizziness, blurred vision, chest pain, coughing, nocturnal dyspnea, orthopnea, nausea, anorexia, and weight loss.

## Physical exam

Take the patient's vital signs. Inspect the skin and mucous membranes to determine the extent of cyanosis. Check for redness, ulceration, and cool, pallid skin. Also note clubbing. Next, assess the patient's level of consciousness. Test his motor strength and ask about pain or abnormal sensations in his arms and legs. Palpate peripheral pulses, test capillary refill time, and note edema. Auscultate heart rate and rhythm and the abdominal aorta and femoral arteries. Check for nasal flaring, accessory muscle use, asymmetrical chest wall expansion, or barrel chest. Auscultate the lungs and percuss for dullness or hyperresonance. Inspect the abdomen for ascites. Percuss and palpate for liver enlargement and tenderness.

## Causes

*Deep-vein thrombosis.* Acute peripheral cyanosis occurs in the affected extremity along with tenderness, edema, warmth, prominent superficial veins, and a positive Homans' sign.

*Peripheral arterial occlusion (acute).* Acute cyanosis occurs in one arm or leg along with sharp or aching pain that worsens with movement. The affected extremity will be weak, pale, and cool, and have paresthesia. Examination reveals decreased or absent pulse and prolonged capillary refill time.

*Pneumothorax.* A cardinal sign is acute central cyanosis accompanied by sharp chest pain that's exacerbated by movement, deep breathing, and coughing. Asymmetrical chest wall expansion and shortness of breath also occur.

*Pulmonary embolism.* Acute central cyanosis occurs when a large embolus obstructs the pulmonary circulation. Syncope and neck vein distention may occur. Other findings include dyspnea, chest pain, tachycardia, dry cough or cough with blood-tinged sputum, low-grade fever, and restlessness.

*Other causes.* Arteriosclerotic occlusive disease; bronchiectasis; Buerger's disease; chronic obstructive pulmonary disease (COPD); congestive heart failure; lung cancer; methemoglobinemia; pneumonia; polycythemia vera; pulmonary edema; Raynaud's disease; and shock.

## Nursing considerations

- Provide supplemental oxygen; give small doses (2 liters/minute) to patients with COPD.

Pulse pressure is the difference between systolic and diastolic blood pressures. Normally, systolic pressure is about 40 mm Hg higher than diastolic.

Widened pulse pressure—a difference greater than 50 mm Hg—commonly occurs as a physiologic response to fever, hot weather, or exercise. It can also result from certain neurologic and cardiovascular disorders that reduce arterial compliance or cause backflow of blood into the heart with each contraction; chief among these disorders is a life-threatening increase in intracranial pressure (ICP). Widened pulse pressure can be identified easily by monitoring arterial blood pressure and is commonly detected during routine sphygmomanometric recordings.

▶ **Emergency interventions**

If the patient's level of consciousness (LOC) is decreased, and you suspect that his widened pulse pressure results from increased ICP, check his vital signs and have another nurse notify the doctor immediately. Maintain a patent airway, and prepare to hyperventilate the patient with a manual resuscitation bag to help reduce partial pressure of carbon dioxide and, thus, ICP.

Perform a thorough neurologic examination to serve as a baseline for assessing subsequent changes. Use the Glasgow Coma Scale to evaluate the patient's LOC. Check cranial nerve function—especially nerves III, IV, and VI—and assess pupillary reactions, reflexes, and muscle tone. If ordered, assist with insertion of an ICP monitor and begin monitoring ICP.

## History

If you don't suspect increased ICP, ask about associated symptoms, such as chest pain, shortness of breath, weakness, fatigue, or syncope.

## Physical exam

Check for edema and auscultate for murmurs.

## Causes

*Aortic insufficiency.* In acute aortic insufficiency, pulse pressure widens progressively as the valve deteriorates, and a bounding pulse and an atrial gallop ($S_4$) develop. Other possible findings include chest pain; palpitations; pallor; strong, abrupt carotid pulsations; pulsus bisferiens; and signs of congestive heart failure, such as crackles, dyspnea, and distended neck veins. Auscultation may reveal several murmurs, such as an early systolic murmur (common) and an apical diastolic rumble (Austin Flint murmur).

*Arteriosclerosis.* Reduced arterial compliance causes progressive widening of pulse pressure, which becomes permanent without treatment of the underlying disorder. It's preceded by moderate hypertension and accompanied by signs of vascular insufficiency, such as claudication and speech disturbances.

*Febrile disorders.* Fever can cause widened pulse pressure. Accompanying symptoms vary, depending on the specific disorder.

*Increased ICP.* Pulse pressure widens as ICP rises, making widened pulse pressure an intermediate to late sign of increased ICP. The earliest indicator of increased ICP is decreased LOC. Assessment reveals Cushing's triad: bradycardia, hypertension, and respiratory pattern changes. Other findings may include headache, vomiting, and impaired or unequal motor movement. The patient may also have visual disturbances, such as blurring or photophobia, and pupillary changes.

## Nursing considerations

• If the patient has increased ICP, continually reassess his neurologic status, and compare your findings carefully with those of previous assessments. Immediately notify the doctor if you detect any change.

• Be alert for restlessness, confusion, unresponsiveness, or decreased LOC. But remember that subtle changes in the patient's condition, rather than the abrupt development of any one sign or symptom, commonly signal increasing ICP.

Also known as decerebrate rigidity or abnormal extensor reflex, decerebrate posture usually heralds neurologic deterioration. It's characterized by adduction and extension of the arms, pronated wrists, and flexed fingers. The legs are stiffly extended, with plantar flexion of the feet. This sign indicates upper brain stem damage, which may result from primary lesions, such as infarction, hemorrhage, or tumor; metabolic encephalopathy; head injury; or brain stem compression and increased intracranial pressure (ICP).

Unilateral or bilateral decerebrate posture may follow noxious stimuli or may occur spontaneously. In concurrent brain stem and cerebral damage, decerebrate posture may affect only the arms, while the legs remain flaccid. Or decerebrate posture may affect one side of the body and decorticate posture the other. Or the two postures may alternate. The duration of each posturing episode correlates with the severity of brain stem damage.

▶ **Emergency interventions**
Notify the doctor of decerebrate posture immediately. Ensure a patent airway: Insert an artificial airway, elevate the head of the bed, and turn the patient's head to the side to prevent aspiration (don't disrupt spinal alignment if you suspect spinal cord injury). Give supplemental oxygen and ventilate the patient with a manual resuscitation bag, if necessary. Or prepare to assist with intubation and mechanical ventilation. Keep emergency resuscitation equipment handy. Check the patient's chart for a no-code order.

**History**
If you can't obtain history information, look for clues to the causative disorder, such as hepatomegaly, cyanosis, diabetic skin changes, needle tracks, or obvious trauma. If a family member is available, find out when the patient's level of consciousness (LOC) began deteriorating. Did it occur abruptly? What did the patient complain of before he lost consciousness? Does he have a history of diabetes, liver disease, cancer, blood clots, or aneurysm? Ask about any accident or trauma.

**Physical exam**
After taking vital signs, assess the patient's LOC using the Glasgow Coma Scale. Evaluate the pupils for size, equality, and response to light. Test deep tendon reflexes, cranial nerve reflexes, and for doll's eye sign.

**Causes**
*Cerebral lesion.* Any cerebral lesion that increases ICP may also produce decerebrate posture, typically as a late sign. Associated findings vary with the lesion's site and extent but commonly include coma, abnormal pupil size and response to light, and signs of increased ICP.

*Hypoxic encephalopathy.* Severe hypoxia may produce decerebrate posture — the result of brain stem compression associated with anaerobic metabolism and increased ICP. Other findings include coma, a positive Babinski's reflex, absence of doll's eye sign, hypoactive deep tendon reflexes and, possibly, fixed pupils and respiratory arrest.

*Pontine hemorrhage.* This life-threatening disorder usually leads rapidly to decerebrate posture with coma. Accompanying signs include total paralysis, absence of doll's eye sign, a positive Babinski's reflex, and small reactive pupils.

*Posterior fossa hemorrhage.* This subtentorial lesion causes decerebrate posture. Earlier effects include vomiting, vertigo, ataxia, stiff neck, drowsiness, and cranial nerve palsies. The patient eventually slips into a coma and may suffer respiratory arrest.

*Other causes.* Brain stem infarct; brain stem tumor; hepatic encephalopathy; and hypoglycemic encephalopathy.

**Nursing considerations**
• Monitor neurologic status and vital signs every 30 minutes or hourly. Be alert for signs of increased ICP and neurologic deterioration. Report subtle changes in the patient's condition.

**D**

# Pulse pressure, narrowed

Pulse pressure—the difference between systolic and diastolic blood pressures—is measured by sphygmomanometry or intra-arterial monitoring. Normally, systolic pressure exceeds diastolic by about 40 mm Hg.

Narrowed pressure—a difference of less than 30 mm Hg—occurs when peripheral vascular resistance increases, cardiac output declines, or intravascular volume markedly decreases. In conditions that cause mechanical obstruction, such as aortic stenosis, pulse pressure is directly related to the severity of the underlying condition. Usually a late sign, narrowed pulse pressure alone doesn't signal an emergency, even though it commonly occurs in shock and other life-threatening disorders.

## Physical exam

After you detect a narrowed pulse pressure, check for other signs of heart failure, such as hypotension, tachycardia, dyspnea, distended neck veins, and decreased urine output. Also check for changes in skin temperature or color, strength of peripheral pulses, and level of consciousness (LOC). Auscultate the heart for murmurs, and ask about a history of chest pain, dizziness, or syncope. Inform the doctor of your findings.

## Causes

*Aortic stenosis.* Narrowed pulse pressure occurs late in significant stenosis. Other findings include an atrial or ventricular gallop, chest pain, a harsh systolic ejection murmur, dyspnea, and syncope.

*Cardiac tamponade.* In this life-threatening disorder, pulse pressure narrows approximately 10 to 20 mm Hg. Pulsus paradoxus, neck vein distention, hypotension, and muffled heart sounds are classic. The patient may be anxious and cyanotic, with clammy skin and chest pain. He may exhibit dyspnea, tachypnea, decreased LOC, and a weak, rapid pulse. Pericardial friction rub and hepatomegaly may also occur.

*Congestive heart failure.* Narrowed pulse pressure occurs relatively late. It may accompany tachypnea, palpitations, dependent edema, steady weight gain despite nausea and anorexia, chest tightness, slowed mental response, hypotension, diaphoresis, pallor, and oliguria. Assessment reveals a ventricular gallop, inspiratory crackles, and possibly a tender, palpable liver. Later, dullness develops over the lung bases, and hemoptysis, cyanosis, marked hepatomegaly, and marked pitting edema may occur.

*Shock.* In *anaphylactic shock,* narrowed pulse pressure occurs late, preceded by a rapid, weak pulse that soon becomes uniformly absent. Within seconds or minutes after exposure to an allergen, the patient experiences hypotension, restlessness, and feelings of doom, along with intense itching and a pounding headache.

In *cardiogenic shock,* narrowed pulse pressure occurs relatively late. Typically, peripheral pulses are absent and central pulses are weak. A drop in systolic pressure to 30 mm Hg below baseline, or a sustained reading below 80 mm Hg not attributable to medication, produces poor tissue perfusion, which causes tachycardia; tachypnea; pale, clammy skin; cyanosis; oliguria; restlessness; and obtundation.

In *hypovolemic shock,* narrowed pulse pressure occurs as a late sign. All peripheral pulses become weak, then uniformly absent. Deepening shock leads to hypotension, decreased urine output, confusion, and decreased LOC.

In *septic shock,* narrowed pulse pressure is a relatively late sign. All of the patient's peripheral pulses become weak, then uniformly absent. As shock progresses, the patient experiences oliguria, thirst, anxiety, confusion, and hypotension. His extremities become cool and cyanotic, and eventually his skin becomes cold and clammy.

## Nursing considerations

• Monitor the patient closely for changes in pulse rate or quality and for hypotension. Prepare him for diagnostic studies, as necessary.

Also called decorticate rigidity or abnormal flexor response, decorticate posture is a sign of corticospinal damage characterized by adduction and flexion of the arms, with the wrists and fingers flexed on the chest. The legs are extended and internally rotated, with plantar flexion of the feet.

This posture may occur unilaterally or bilaterally. Most often, it results from cerebrovascular accident (CVA) or head injury. It may be elicited by noxious stimuli or may occur spontaneously. The intensity of the required stimulus, the duration of the posture, and the frequency of spontaneous episodes vary with the severity of cerebral injury.

Although a serious sign, decorticate posture carries a more favorable prognosis than decerebrate posture. However, if the causative disorder extends lower in the brain stem, decorticate posture may progress to decerebrate posture.

▶ **Emergency interventions**
When the patient displays decorticate posture, notify the doctor and begin a neurologic assessment. First evaluate level of consciousness (LOC). If consciousness is impaired, insert an oropharyngeal airway, elevate the head of the bed 30 degrees, and turn the patient's head to the side to prevent aspiration (unless spinal cord injury is suspected). Assess respiratory rate, rhythm, and depth. Prepare to assist respirations with a manual resuscitation bag or intubation and mechanical ventilation, if necessary. Also, institute seizure precautions. Then record other vital signs.

**History**
Ask a family member if the patient complained of headache, dizziness, nausea, abnormal vision, or numbness and tingling. When did he first notice these symptoms? Did he exhibit any behavior changes? Also ask about a history of cerebrovascular disease, cancer, meningitis, encephalitis, upper respiratory tract infection, and recent trauma.

**Physical exam**
Test the patient's motor and sensory functions. Evaluate pupil size, equality, and response to light. Test cranial nerve and deep tendon reflexes.

**Causes**
*Brain abscess.* Decorticate posture may occur. Related findings vary, depending on the size and location of the abscess, but may include aphasia, hemiparesis, headache, dizziness, seizures, nausea, and vomiting. Behavior changes, altered vital signs, and decreased LOC may also occur.

*Brain tumor.* Decorticate posture is usually bilateral—the result of increased ICP associated with tumor growth. Related signs and symptoms include headache, behavior changes, memory loss, diplopia, blurred vision or vision loss, seizures, ataxia, dizziness, apraxia, aphasia, paresis, sensory loss, paresthesia, vomiting, papilledema, and signs of hormonal imbalance.

*Cerebrovascular accident.* Typically, a CVA involving the cerebral cortex produces unilateral decorticate posture, also called spastic hemiplegia. Other clinical features are hemiplegia (contralateral to the lesion), dysarthria, dysphagia, unilateral sensory loss, apraxia, agnosia, aphasia, memory loss, decreased LOC, urine retention, urinary incontinence, and constipation. Ocular effects include homonymous hemianopia, diplopia, and blurred vision.

*Head injury.* Decorticate posture may be among the variable features of this disorder, depending on the site and severity of head injury. Associated signs and symptoms may include headache, nausea and vomiting, dizziness, irritability, decreased LOC, aphasia, hemiparesis, unilateral numbness, seizures, and pupil dilation.

**Nursing considerations**
• Assess the patient frequently to detect subtle signs of neurologic deterioration. Also monitor neurologic status and vital signs every 30 minutes to 2 hours. Be alert for signs of increased ICP, including bradycardia, increasing systolic blood pressure, and widening pulse pressure.

**D**

Produced by large waves of pressure as blood ejects from the left ventricle with each contraction, a bounding pulse is strong and easily palpable and may be visible over superficial peripheral arteries. It's characterized by regular, recurrent expansion and contraction of the arterial walls and isn't obliterated by the pressure of palpation.

A healthy person develops a bounding pulse during exercise, pregnancy, or periods of anxiety. However, this sign also results from fever and certain endocrine, hematologic, and cardiovascular disorders that increase the basal metabolic rate.

## History
Ask the patient if he has noticed any weakness, fatigue, shortness of breath, or other changes in his health. Review his medical history for hyperthyroidism, anemia, or cardiovascular disorders, and ask about his use of alcohol.

## Physical exam
After you detect a bounding pulse, check other vital signs, then auscultate the heart and lungs for any abnormal sounds, rates, or rhythms.

## Causes
*Alcoholism (acute).* Vasodilation of acute alcoholism produces a rapid, bounding pulse and flushed face. An odor of alcohol on the patient's breath and an ataxic gait are common. Other findings may include hypothermia, bradypnea, stertorous respirations, nausea, vomiting, diuresis, decreased level of consciousness, and seizures.

*Anemia.* In this disorder, a bounding pulse may be accompanied by capillary pulsations, a systolic ejection murmur, tachycardia, an atrial gallop ($S_4$), and a systolic bruit over the carotid artery. Associated findings include fatigue, pallor, dyspnea, and possibly bleeding tendencies.

*Aortic insufficiency.* Sometimes called a waterhammer pulse, the bounding pulse associated with this condition is characterized by a rapid, forceful expansion of the arterial pulse followed by rapid contraction. Widened pulse pressure also occurs. Acute aortic insufficiency may produce signs and symptoms of left ventricular failure and cardiovascular collapse, such as weakness, severe dyspnea, hypotension, a ventricular gallop ($S_3$), and tachycardia.

Additional findings may include pallor, chest pain, palpitations, or strong, abrupt carotid pulsations. The patient may also have pulsus bisferiens, an early systolic murmur, a murmur heard over the femoral artery during systole and diastole (Duroziez's sign), and a high-pitched diastolic murmur that starts with the second heart sound. An apical diastolic rumble (Austin Flint murmur) may also occur, especially with heart failure.

Most patients with chronic aortic insufficiency remain asymptomatic until the age of 40 or 50, when exertional dyspnea, increased fatigue, orthopnea and, eventually, paroxysmal nocturnal dyspnea may develop.

*Febrile disorder.* Fever can cause a bounding pulse. Accompanying findings reflect the specific disorder.

*Thyrotoxicosis.* This disorder produces a rapid, full, bounding pulse. Associated findings may include tachycardia, palpitations, an $S_3$ or $S_4$ gallop, and weight loss despite increased appetite. In addition, the patient may have diarrhea, an enlarged thyroid, dyspnea, tremors, nervousness, and exophthalmos. His skin will be warm, moist, and diaphoretic, and he may be hypersensitive to heat.

## Nursing considerations
• Prepare the patient for diagnostic laboratory and radiographic studies. If a bounding pulse is accompanied by a rapid or irregular heartbeat, you may need to connect the patient to a cardiac monitor for further evaluation.

A hyperactive deep tendon reflex (DTR) is an abnormally brisk muscle contraction in response to a sudden stretch induced by sharply tapping the muscle's tendon of insertion. This elicited sign may be graded as brisk (+ + +) or hyperactive (+ + + +).

The corticospinal tract governs the reflex arc—the relay cycle that produces any reflex response. A corticospinal lesion above the level of the reflex arc being tested may result in a hyperactive DTR. Abnormal neuromuscular transmission at the end of the reflex arc from a deficiency of calcium or magnesium may also cause a hyperactive DTR. Hyperactive DTRs often accompany other neurologic findings but usually lack specific diagnostic value. An exception is hypocalcemia, in which hyperactive DTRs are an early, cardinal sign.

## History

After eliciting hyperactive DTRs, ask about possible pregnancy, spinal cord injury or other trauma, and prolonged exposure to cold, wind, or water. A positive response to any of these questions requires prompt assessment to rule out life-threatening autonomic hyperreflexia, tetanus, preeclampsia, or hypothermia. Ask about the onset and progression of related signs and symptoms, paresthesia, vomiting, and altered bladder habits.

## Physical exam

Evaluate the patient's level of consciousness. Test motor and sensory function in the limbs. Check for ataxia, tremors, or speech and visual deficits. Test for Chvostek's and Trousseau's signs and for carpopedal spasm. Finally, take vital signs.

## Causes

*Autonomic hyperreflexia.* Associated signs include hypertension, bradycardia, piloerection, diaphoresis, and intestinal cramps.

*Hypocalcemia.* Generalized hyperactive DTRs may appear suddenly or gradually, with paresthesia, muscle twitching and cramping, positive Chvostek's and Trousseau's signs, carpopedal spasm, and tetany.

*Hypomagnesemia.* This disorder causes gradual onset of generalized hyperactive DTRs accompanied by muscle cramps, hypotension, ataxia, tachycardia, paresthesia, tetany, and possibly seizures.

*Hypothermia.* Mild hypothermia (90° to 94° F [32.2° to 34.4° C]) causes generalized hyperactive DTRs, shivering, weakness, lethargy, slurred speech, ataxia, muscle stiffness, tachycardia, bradypnea, hypotension, and cold, pale skin.

*Preeclampsia.* Occurring in pregnancy of at least 20 weeks' duration, preeclampsia may cause gradual onset of generalized hyperactive DTRs. Other findings include increased blood pressure; abnor-

mal weight gain; edema of the face, fingers, and abdomen after bed rest; oliguria; headache; blurred or double vision; nausea and vomiting; irritability; shortness of breath; and crackles.

*Spinal cord lesion.* Incomplete spinal cord lesions cause hyperactive DTRs below the level of the lesion. In a traumatic lesion, hyperactive DTRs follow resolution of spinal shock. In a neoplastic lesion, hyperactive DTRs gradually replace normal DTRs. Other signs and symptoms include paralysis and sensory loss below the level of the lesion, urine retention and overflow incontinence, and alternating constipation and diarrhea.

*Tetanus.* Sudden onset of generalized hyperactive DTRs accompanies tachycardia, diaphoresis, low-grade fever, painful and involuntary muscle contractions, trismus, and risus sardonicus.

*Other causes.* Amyotrophic lateral sclerosis, brain tumor, cerebrovascular accident, hepatic encephalopathy, and multiple sclerosis.

## Nursing considerations

• If motor weakness accompanies hyperactive DTRs, perform or encourage range-of-motion exercises to preserve muscle integrity. Also, reposition the patient frequently, provide a special mattress, and massage his back.

# Pulse, absent or weak

An absent or weak pulse may be generalized, as in shock, or affect only one extremity, as in arterial occlusion. Palpation may also temporarily diminish or obliterate superficial pulses, such as the posterior tibial or dorsal pedal. Thus, bilateral weakness or absence of these pulses doesn't necessarily indicate an underlying disorder.

## History
If the patient is unconscious, obtain a brief history from family members.

## Physical exam
After detecting an absent or weak pulse, quickly palpate the remaining pulses to distinguish between localized or generalized loss or weakness. Quickly check other vital signs and assess cardiopulmonary status. Based on your findings, proceed with emergency interventions.

## Causes
*Aortic aneurysm (dissecting).* When circulation to the innominate, left common carotid, subclavian, or femoral arteries is affected, it causes weak or absent pulses distal to the affected area in 75% of cases. Other findings include tearing pain in the chest and neck that may radiate to the back and abdomen, lower blood pressure in the legs than in the arms, syncope, diastolic murmur, hypoten-sion, and mottled skin below the waist.

*Arterial occlusion.* In acute occlusion, arterial pulses distal to the obstruction are weak and then absent. The affected limb is cool, pale, and cyanotic, with prolonged capillary refill time. The patient complains of pain, paresthesia and, possibly, paralysis. A line of color and temperature demarcation develops at the level of obstruction. In chronic occlusion, pulses weaken gradually.

*Cardiac tamponade.* Life-threatening cardiac tamponade causes a weak, rapid pulse with pulsus paradoxus, jugular vein distention, hypotension, and muffled heart sounds. Narrowed pulse pressure, pericardial friction rub, and hepatomegaly may occur. Other findings include anxiety, cyanosis, chest pain, clammy skin, dyspnea, and tachypnea.

*Peripheral vascular disease.* Peripheral pulses gradually weaken and disappear. The patient complains of aching pain distal to the occlusion that worsens with exercise and abates with rest. The skin is cool, with decreased hair growth.

*Pulmonary embolism.* This disorder causes generalized weak, rapid pulse. It also may cause abrupt onset of chest pain, tachycardia, apprehension, syncope, diaphoresis, and cyanosis. Respiratory effects may include tachypnea, dyspnea, decreased breath sounds, crackles, and a cough, possibly with blood-tinged sputum.

*Shock.* In *anaphylactic shock,* the patient experiences hypotension, feelings of doom, intense itching, and a pounding headache. Pulses become rapid and weak, then uniformly absent within seconds or minutes after exposure to an allergen.

In *cardiogenic shock,* peripheral pulses are absent and central pulses are weak. A drop in blood pressure produces poor tissue perfusion and causes tachycardia; rapid, shallow respirations; oliguria; obtundation; and pale, clammy skin.

In *hypovolemic shock,* all peripheral pulses become weak and then, depending on the degree of shock, absent. Later, remaining pulses become thready and more rapid.

In *septic shock,* all peripheral pulses become weak and then, possibly, uniformly absent. Shock is heralded by chills, sudden fever, tachycardia, tachypnea, and flushed, dry skin. Later, hypotension, anxiety, and confusion develop.

*Other causes.* Aortic arch syndrome; aortic bifurcation occlusion (acute); aortic stenosis; arrhythmias; thoracic outlet syndrome; and certain treatments, such as arteriovenous fistulas or shunts for dialysis.

## Nursing considerations
• Monitor the patient's vital signs, measure daily weight, monitor hourly or daily intake and output, and assess central venous pressure.

A hypoactive deep tendon reflex (DTR) is an abnormally diminished muscle contraction in response to a sudden stretch induced by sharply tapping the muscle's tendon of insertion. It may be graded as minimal ( + ) or absent (0).

Normally, a DTR operates via the reflex arc, which is governed by the corticospinal tract. A hypoactive DTR may result from damage to the reflex arc involving the specific muscle, the peripheral nerve, the nerve roots, or the spinal cord at that level. Hypoactive DTRs are an important sign of many disorders, especially when they appear with other neurologic signs and symptoms.

## History
After eliciting hypoactive DTRs, obtain a thorough history from the patient or a family member. Ask for a detailed description of current signs and symptoms. Then take a family and drug history.

## Physical exam
First assess the patient's level of consciousness. Test motor function in his limbs, and palpate for muscle atrophy or increased mass. Test sensory function, including pain, touch, temperature, and vibration sense. Ask about paresthesia. Have the patient take several steps so that you can observe his gait and coordination. To check for Romberg's sign, ask him to stand with feet together and eyes closed. During conversation, assess the patient's speech. Also observe for signs of vision or hearing loss. Assess for autonomic nervous system effects by taking vital signs. Also inspect the patient's skin for pallor, dryness, flushing, or diaphoresis. Auscultate for hypoactive bowel sounds. Ask about nausea, vomiting, constipation, and incontinence. Palpate for bladder distention.

## Causes
*Botulism.* In this disorder, generalized hypoactive DTRs accompany progressive descending muscle weakness. Initially, the patient usually complains of blurred and double vision and, occasionally, of anorexia, nausea, and vomiting. Other early bulbar signs and symptoms include vertigo, hearing loss, dysarthria, and dysphagia. The patient may have signs of respiratory distress and severe constipation marked by hypoactive bowel sounds.

*Guillain-Barré syndrome.* Bilateral hypoactive DTRs progress rapidly from hypotonia to areflexia in several days; muscle weakness typically begins in the legs, extends to the arms and perhaps to the trunk and neck muscles, possibly causing total paralysis. Other features include cranial nerve palsies, pain, paresthesia, and signs of brief autonomic dysfunction. Symptoms usually peak in 10 to 14 days, then begin to clear.

*Spinal cord lesions.* Spinal cord injury or transection produces spinal shock, resulting in hypoactive DTRs below the level of the lesion. Other findings may include quadriplegia or paraplegia, flaccidity, loss of sensation below the level of the lesion, urine retention with overflow incontinence, hypoactive bowel sounds, constipation, genital reflex loss, and dry, pale skin.

*Syringomyelia.* Permanent bilateral hypoactive DTRs occur early in this progressive disorder. Other findings include muscle weakness and atrophy; loss of sensation, usually extending in a capelike fashion over the arms, shoulders, neck, back, and occasionally the legs; deep, boring pain in the limbs; and signs of brain stem involvement.

*Other causes.* Drugs, such as barbiturates and paralyzing drugs (pancuronium and curare); Eaton-Lambert syndrome; peripheral neuropathy; polymyositis; and tabes dorsalis.

## Nursing considerations
• Promote independence while ensuring patient safety. In sensory deficits, protect the patient from injury caused by heat or pressure. Perform or encourage range-of-motion exercises. Also encourage a balanced diet with increased protein intake.

Ptosis is the excessive drooping of the upper eyelid. If severe, the patient may not be able to raise his eyelids. Ptosis can be constant, progressive, or intermittent, and unilateral or bilateral. Unilateral ptosis is detected easily by comparing the eyelids' relative positions. Bilateral or mild ptosis is difficult to detect; the eyelids may cover the upper part of the iris or pupil. Because ptosis can resemble enophthalmos, exophthalmometry may be required.

Congenital ptosis results from levator muscle underdevelopment or disorders of the third cranial nerve. Acquired ptosis may result from trauma to or inflammation of these muscles and nerves, or from certain drugs, systemic diseases, intracranial lesions, and life-threatening aneurysms. The most common cause is age, which reduces muscle elasticity and produces senile ptosis.

### History
Ask your patient when his ptosis began and if it has worsened or improved. Determine if he's had recent eye trauma. If so, avoid manipulating the eye. Ask about eye pain or headache, and determine its location and severity. Has the patient experienced any vision changes? If so, have him describe them. Obtain a drug history, noting especially use of any chemotherapeutic agents.

### Physical exam
Assess the degree of ptosis and check for eyelid edema, exophthalmos, deviation, or conjunctival injection. Evaluate extraocular muscle function by testing the six cardinal fields of gaze. Carefully examine the pupils' size, color, shape, and reaction to light, and test visual acuity.

Keep in mind that ptosis infrequently indicates a life-threatening condition. For example, sudden unilateral ptosis can herald a cerebral aneurysm.

### Causes
*Botulism.* Acute cranial nerve dysfunction causes the hallmark signs of ptosis, dysarthria, dysphagia, and diplopia. Other findings include dry mouth, sore throat, weakness, vomiting, diarrhea, hyporeflexia, and dyspnea.

*Cerebral aneurysm.* An aneurysm that compresses the oculomotor nerve can cause sudden ptosis, along with diplopia, a dilated pupil, and inability to rotate the eye. These may be the first signs of this life-threatening disorder. With rupture, an aneurysm typically produces sudden severe headache, nausea, vomiting, and decreased level of consciousness (LOC).

*Lacrimal gland tumor.* This disorder may cause mild to severe ptosis, depending on the tumor's size and location. It may also cause brow elevation, exophthalmos, eye deviation, and eye pain.

*Myasthenia gravis.* Gradual bilateral ptosis is often the first sign of this disorder. Mild to severe, it may be accompanied by weak eye closure and diplopia. Other characteristics include muscle weakness and fatigue leading to paralysis. Depending on the muscles affected, other findings may include masklike facies, difficulty chewing or swallowing, dyspnea, and cyanosis.

*Ocular trauma.* Trauma to the nerve or muscles that control the eyelids can cause mild to severe ptosis. Eye pain, lid swelling, ecchymosis, and decreased visual acuity may also occur.

*Subdural hematoma (chronic).* Ptosis may be a late sign, along with unilateral pupillary dilation and sluggishness. Headache, behavioral changes, and decreased LOC commonly occur.

*Other causes.* Alcoholism; dacryoadenitis; drugs, such as vinca alkaloids; hemangioma; Horner's syndrome; lead poisoning; myotonic dystrophy; ocular muscle dystrophy; Parinaud's syndrome; and Parry-Romberg syndrome.

### Nursing considerations
• Prepare the patient for diagnostic studies, such as the tensilon test and slit-lamp examination, and for surgery if indicated.
• If the patient has decreased visual acuity, orient him to his surroundings.

Depression defies easy definition, commonly eluding diagnosis and treatment. Its character, intensity, and duration vary from periodic bouts of "the blues" to persistent thoughts of suicide. Mild depression is transient and characterized by downheartedness, sadness, and dejection.

Moderate depression is marked by noticeably disturbed thought processes, impaired communication and socialization, and sensory dysfunction.

In severe depression, the patient may appear withdrawn, expressionless, or unaffected by his surroundings, and may exhibit delusional thinking, dramatic sensory dysfunction, and limited or agitated motor activity.

Depression is more common in women than men and is especially prevalent among adolescents.

## History

Try to determine how the patient feels about himself, his family, and his environment, exploring the nature of his depression, how other factors affect it, and his coping mechanisms. Ask the patient what's bothering him. Then ask him to describe the way he feels about himself. What are his plans and dreams? How realistic are they? Is he generally satisfied with what he has accomplished in his work, relationships, and other interests? Ask about any changes in his social interactions, sleep patterns, ability to make decisions or concentrate, or normal activities. Explore drug and alcohol use.

Ask about his family. What part does he feel he plays in his family life? Find out if other family members have been depressed and whether anyone important to the patient has been sick or has died in the past year. Finally, ask the patient about his environment. Has his life-style changed in the past month? Six months? Year? When he's feeling blue, where does he go and what does he do to feel better? Find out how he feels about his role in the community and the resources available to him. Try to determine if the patient has an adequate support network to help him cope with his depression.

## Causes

*Drugs.* Various drugs cause depression as an adverse effect. Among the more common are barbiturates; antineoplastic agents, such as asparaginase; anticonvulsants, such as diazepam; and antiarrhythmics, such as disopyramide. Other depression-inducing drugs include centrally acting antihypertensives, such as reserpine, methyldopa, and clonidine; beta-adrenergic blockers, such as propranolol; levodopa; indomethacin; cycloserine; corticosteroids; and oral contraceptives.

*Organic disorders.* Various organic disorders produce mild, moderate, or severe depression. Among these are metabolic and endocrine disorders, such as hypothyroidism, hyperthyroidism, and diabetes; infectious diseases, such as influenza, hepatitis, and encephalitis; degenerative diseases, such as Alzheimer's disease, multiple sclerosis, and multi-infarct dementia; and neoplastic disorders, such as cancer of the pancreas.

*Psychiatric disorders.* Affective disorders are commonly characterized by abrupt mood swings from depression to elation (mania) or by prolonged episodes of either mood. Severe depression may last for weeks. Moderate depression occurs in cyclothymic disorders and usually alternates with moderate mania. Moderate depression that is more or less constant over a 2-year period often results from dysthymic disorders. Chronic anxiety disorders, characterized by obsessive-compulsive behavior, may cause depression.

*Other causes.* Alcohol abuse.

## Nursing considerations

• Help the patient set realistic goals. Encourage him to promote feelings of self-worth by asserting his opinions and making decisions. Encourage him to talk about his emotions and feelings.

• Try to determine his suicide potential, and take steps to help ensure his safety.

• Make sure the patient receives adequate nourishment and rest, and keep his environment free from stress and excessive stimulation.

**D**

# Psychotic behavior

Psychotic behavior reflects an inability or unwillingness to recognize and acknowledge reality and to relate with others. It may begin suddenly or insidiously, progressing from vague complaints of fatigue, insomnia, or headache to withdrawal, social isolation, and preoccupation.

Various behaviors together or separately can constitute psychotic behavior. Delusions are persistent beliefs with no basis in reality or in the patient's knowledge or experience, such as delusions of grandeur. Illusions are misinterpretations of external sensory stimuli, such as a mirage in the desert. Hallucinations are sensory perceptions that do not result from external stimuli.

Bizarre language reflects a communication disruption. It can range from echolalia (purposeless repetition of a word or phrase) and clang association (repetition of words or phrases that sound similar) to neologisms (creation and use of words whose meaning only the patient knows).

Perseveration, a persistent verbal or motor response, may indicate organic brain disease. Motor changes include inactivity, excessive activity, and repetitive movements.

## History

Because the patient's behavior can make it difficult or dangerous to obtain information, conduct the interview in a calm, safe, and well-lit room. Provide personal space to avoid threatening or agitating the patient. Ask him to describe his problem and any circumstances that may have precipitated it. Explore his use of alcohol or drugs, noting duration of use and amount. Ask if he has had any illnesses or accidents in the last year.

Interview the patient's family. Which family members does the patient seem closest to? How does the family describe the patient's relationships, communication patterns, and role? Find out if anyone in his family has been hospitalized previously for psychiatric or emotional illness.

Evaluate the patient's environment. Ask about his educational and employment history. What is his (or his family's) socioeconomic status? Are community services available to them? How does the patient spend his leisure time? Does he have friends? Has he ever had a close emotional relationship?

## Physical exam

Watch for cognitive, linguistic, or perceptual abnormalities. Look for unusual gestures, posture, gait, tone, or mannerisms.

## Causes

*Organic disorders.* Various disorders, including alcohol withdrawal syndrome, cerebral hypoxia, and nutritional disorders, may produce psychotic behavior, as can endocrine disorders and severe infections. Neurologic causes include Alzheimer's disease and other dementias.

*Psychiatric disorders.* Psychotic behavior usually occurs with bipolar disorders, personality disorders, schizophrenia, and traumatic stress disorders.

*Other causes.* Many drugs, including albuterol, bromocriptine, corticosteroids, diazepam, thyroid hormones, and others (almost any drug can provoke psychotic behavior as a rare, severe adverse or idiosyncratic reaction); and postoperative delirium and depression.

## Nursing considerations

- Evaluate the patient's orientation to reality. Help him build a conception of reality by calling him by his preferred name, telling him your name, and using clocks and calendars.
- Encourage the patient's involvement in structured activities. If he's nonverbal or incoherent, spend time with him by sitting, walking, or talking about concrete topics.
- Refer the patient for psychological evaluation. Administer antipsychotics or other drugs, as ordered, and prepare him for transfer to a mental health center, if necessary.
- Check the patient's eating habits and monitor his elimination patterns.

# Diaphoresis

Diaphoresis is profuse sweating, possibly more than 1 liter per hour. This sign represents an autonomic nervous system response to physical or psychogenic stress, fever, or high environmental temperature. Usually diaphoresis begins abruptly; other autonomic system signs, such as tachycardia and increased blood pressure, may also occur.

Intermittent diaphoresis may accompany chronic disorders characterized by recurrent fever. Isolated diaphoresis may mark an episode of acute pain or fever. When caused by excessive external temperature, diaphoresis is a normal response.

## History

If the patient is diaphoretic, quickly rule out a life-threatening cause. Then ask about the chief complaint and explore associated signs and symptoms. Note general fatigue and weakness. Ask about insomnia, headache, changes in vision or hearing, and dizziness. Ask about pleuritic pain, cough, sputum, difficulty breathing, palpitations, nausea, vomiting, altered bowel or bladder habits, and abdominal pain. Ask the female patient about amenorrhea. Is she menopausal? Note weight loss or gain. Ask about paresthesia, muscle cramps or stiffness, and joint pain. Ask about travel to tropical countries, recent exposure to high environmental temperatures or pesticides, and a recent snake bite. Check for a history of partial gastrectomy or drug or alcohol abuse. Obtain a drug history.

## Physical exam

Inspect the trunk, extremities, palms, soles, and forehead for diaphoresis. Note whether diaphoresis occurs during the day or at night. Observe for flushing, abnormal skin texture or lesions, increased coarse body hair, poor skin turgor, dry mucous membranes, and splinter hemorrhages. Evaluate the patient's mental status and take his vital signs. Observe for fasciculations and flaccid paralysis. Note the patient's facial expression, and examine the eyes for pupillary dilation or constriction, exophthalmos, and excessive tearing. Test visual fields. Check for hearing loss and tooth or gum disease. Auscultate and percuss the lungs. Look for decreased respiratory excursion. Palpate for lymphadenopathy and hepatosplenomegaly.

## Causes

*Autonomic hyperreflexia.* Occurring after resolution of spinal shock in spinal cord injury above T6, hyperreflexia causes profuse diaphoresis, pounding headache, blurred vision, and dramatically elevated blood pressure. Diaphoresis occurs above the level of the injury along with flushing.

*Heat exhaustion.* Initially, profuse diaphoresis, fatigue, weakness, and anxiety occur, possibly leading to circulatory collapse and shock. Other findings include an ashen-gray appearance, dilated pupils, and normal or subnormal temperature.

*Hypoglycemia.* Rapidly induced hypoglycemia may cause diaphoresis accompanied by irritability, tremors, hypotension, blurred vision, tachycardia, hunger, and loss of consciousness.

*Myocardial infarction.* Usually, diaphoresis accompanies acute, substernal, radiating chest pain. Other findings include anxiety, dyspnea, nausea, tachycardia, a blood pressure change, fine crackles, pallor, and clammy skin.

*Other causes.* Acquired immunodeficiency syndrome; acromegaly; anxiety disorders; congestive heart failure; drug and alcohol withdrawal; drugs, such as sympathomimetics, some antipsychotics, thyroid hormone, and antipyretics; dumping syndrome; empyema; envenomization; Hodgkin's disease; immunoblastic lymphadenopathy; infective endocarditis (subacute); liver abscess; lung abscess; malaria; Ménière's disease; pesticide poisoning; pheochromocytoma; pneumonia; relapsing fever; tetanus; thyrotoxicosis; and tuberculosis.

## Nursing considerations

• Replace fluids and electrolytes. Regulate infusions of I.V. solutions; monitor urine output; and encourage oral fluids high in electrolytes.

A positive psoas sign—increased abdominal pain when the patient moves his leg against resistance—indicates direct or reflexive irritation of the psoas muscles. This sign, which can be elicited on the right or left side, usually indicates appendicitis but may also occur with localized abscesses. It's elicited in a patient with abdominal or lower back pain after completion of the abdominal examination to prevent spurious assessment findings.

## ▶ Emergency interventions
If you elicit a positive psoas sign in a patient with abdominal pain, suspect appendicitis. Quickly check the patient's vital signs and have another nurse notify the doctor. Prepare the patient for surgery: Explain the procedure, restrict food and fluids, and withhold analgesics, which can mask symptoms. Administer I.V. fluids to prevent dehydration, but don't give cathartics or enemas, which can cause a ruptured appendix and lead to peritonitis.

## Physical exam
Check for Rovsing's sign by deeply palpating the patient's left lower quadrant. If he reports right lower quadrant pain, the sign is positive, indicating peritoneal irritation.

## Causes
*Appendicitis.* An inflamed retrocecal appendix can cause a positive right psoas sign. Early epigastric and periumbilical pain disappear, only to worsen and localize in the right lower quadrant. This pain also worsens with walking or coughing. Related findings include nausea and vomiting, abdominal rigidity and rebound tenderness, and constipation or diarrhea. Fever, tachycardia, retractive respirations, anorexia, and malaise may also occur. If the appendix ruptures, additional findings may include sudden, severe pain, followed by signs of peritonitis, such as hypoactive or absent bowel sounds, high fever, and boardlike abdominal rigidity.

*Retroperitoneal abscess.* After a lower retroperitoneal infection, an iliac or lumbar abscess can produce a positive right or left psoas sign and fever. An iliac abscess causes iliac or inguinal pain that may radiate to the hip, thigh, or knee; a tender mass in the lower abdomen or groin may be palpable. A lumbar abscess usually produces back tenderness and spasms on the affected side with a palpable lumbar mass; a tender abdominal mass without back pain may occur instead.

## Nursing considerations
• Monitor vital signs to detect complications, such as peritonitis.

• Promote patient comfort by position changes. For example, have the patient lie down and flex his right leg. Then have him sit upright.
• Prepare the patient for diagnostic tests, such as electrolyte studies and abdominal X-rays.

Usually a chief sign of intestinal disorders, diarrhea is an increase in the frequency and fluidity of bowel movements. Acute diarrhea may result from acute infection, stress, fecal impaction, or the effects of drugs. Chronic diarrhea may result from chronic infection, obstructive and inflammatory bowel disease, malabsorption syndrome, certain endocrine disorders, and the effects of GI surgery. Periodic diarrhea may result from food allergy or from ingestion of spicy or high-fiber foods or caffeine. The fluid and electrolyte imbalances caused by diarrhea may precipitate life-threatening arrhythmias or hypovolemic shock.

▶ **Emergency interventions**

If the patient's diarrhea is profuse, check for signs of shock. Help the patient to a supine position and elevate his legs 20 degrees. Insert an I.V. line for fluid replacement. Also, assess for electrolyte imbalance; in hypokalemia, look for an irregular pulse, muscle weakness, anorexia, and nausea and vomiting. Report these signs and symptoms at once. Keep emergency resuscitation equipment handy.

## History

Ask the patient if he has abdominal pain and cramps, difficulty breathing, weakness, or fatigue. Find out his drug history. Has he had GI surgery

or radiation therapy? Ask him to briefly describe his diet. Does he have any food allergies? Is he under unusual stress?

## Physical exam

Assess hydration. Check skin turgor and take blood pressure with the patient lying down, sitting, and standing. Inspect the abdomen for distention and palpate for tenderness. Auscultate bowel sounds. Take the patient's temperature and note any chills.

## Causes

*Infections.* Acute viral, bacterial, and protozoal infections cause sudden, watery diarrhea along with abdominal pain, cramps, nausea, vomiting, and fever. Fluid and electrolyte loss can cause signs of dehydration and shock. Chronic tuberculosis and fungal and parasitic infections cause less severe but more persistent diarrhea accompanied by epigastric distress, vomiting, weight loss, and possibly passage of blood and mucus.

*Intestinal obstruction.* Partial intestinal obstruction increases intestinal motility, resulting in diarrhea, abdominal pain with tenderness and guarding, nausea, and possibly distention.

*Ischemic bowel disease.* In this life-threatening disorder, bloody diarrhea occurs with abdominal pain. If severe, signs of shock may be present.

*Large-bowel neoplasms.* Bloody diarrhea alter-

nates with pencil-thin stools. Other findings include abdominal pain, anorexia, weakness, and depression.

*Pseudomembranous enterocolitis.* This life-threatening disorder produces copious watery or bloody diarrhea that rapidly precipitates shock. Other features include abdominal pain and distention, fever, vomiting, and disorientation.

*Ulcerative colitis.* The hallmark of this disorder is recurrent bloody diarrhea with pus or mucus. Other findings include tenesmus, hyperactive bowel sounds, lower abdominal pain, low-grade fever, anorexia and, at times, nausea and vomiting.

*Other causes.* Carcinoid syndrome; Crohn's disease; drugs, such as antibiotics, magnesium-containing antacids, colchicine, guanethidine, lactulose, dantrolene, ethacrynic acid, mefenamic acid, methotrexate, metyrosine, and, in high doses, digitalis and quinidine; GI surgery; high-dose radiation therapy; irritable bowel syndrome; lactose intolerance; laxative abuse; lead poisoning; malabsorption syndrome; and thyrotoxicosis.

## Nursing considerations

• Measure liquid stools and weigh the patient daily. Encourage oral fluids, and administer I.V. fluid replacements.

• Advise the patient to avoid spicy and high-fiber foods, caffeine, and milk.

# Pruritus

Pruritus—itching—is an unpleasant sensation that affects the skin, certain mucous membranes, and the eyes. Most severe at night, pruritus may worsen with increased skin temperature, poor skin turgor, local vasodilation, dermatoses, and stress.

The most common symptom of dermatologic disease, pruritus may also result from local and systemic disorders and drug use. Physiologic pruritus may occur in primigravidas late in the third trimester. It can also stem from emotional upsets or contact with skin irritants.

## History

If the patient reports pruritus, have him describe its onset, frequency, and intensity. If it occurs at night, ask him whether it prevents him from falling asleep or if it awakens him. Does exercise, stress, fear, depression, or illness seem to aggravate the itching? Ask about contact with skin irritants, previous skin disorders, and related symptoms. Then obtain a complete drug history.

## Physical exam

Look for signs of scratching, such as excoriation, purpura, scabs, scars, or lichenification. Look for primary lesions to help confirm dermatoses.

## Causes

*Conjunctivitis.* All types cause eye itching, burning, and pain along with photophobia, conjunctival injection, a foreign body sensation, excessive tearing, and a feeling of fullness around the eye.

*Dermatitis.* Atopic dermatitis begins with intense, severe pruritus and an erythematous rash on dry skin at flexion points. Scratching may produce edema, scaling, and pustules. Mild irritants and allergies can cause contact dermatitis, with itchy small vesicles that may ooze and scale and are surrounded by redness. Dermatitis herpetiformis, most common in men between ages 20 and 50, initially causes intense pruritus and stinging. Eight to twelve hours later, symmetrically distributed lesions form on the buttocks, shoulders, elbows, and knees.

*Herpes zoster.* Pruritus may precede eruption of lesions and may be accompanied by malaise, fever, erythema, and sharp, shooting, or burning pain. Macular lesions erupt later, usually spreading over the thorax or the arms and legs. If nodules appear, they evolve into fluid- or pus-filled vesicles that dry and form scabs. Localized paresthesia or hyperesthesia may occur.

*Hodgkin's disease.* Most common in young adults, this disorder initially causes mild pruritus on the lower part of the body. Later, the pruritus may become severe and unresponsive to treatment. Early nonspecific findings include persistent fever, night sweats, fatigue, weight loss, and painless swelling of a cervical lymph node. Other nodes may enlarge rapidly or slowly and may or may not cause pain. Later findings may include retroperitoneal node enlargement, hepatosplenomegaly, dyspnea, dysphagia, cough, hyperpigmentation, and jaundice.

*Psoriasis.* Pruritus and pain are common. Psoriasis begins with small, erythematous papules that enlarge or coalesce to form red elevated plaques with silver scales on the scalp, chest, elbows, knees, back, buttocks, and genitals.

*Other causes.* Anemia (iron-deficiency), *Cimex lectularius* (bedbugs), drug hypersensitivity, hemorrhoids, leukemia (chronic lymphocytic), lichen planus, lichen simplex chronicus, multiple myeloma, mycosis fungoides, myringitis, pediculosis (lice), pityriasis rosea, polycythemia vera, psychogenic causes, renal failure (chronic), scabies, thyrotoxicosis, tinea pedis, urticaria, and vaginitis.

## Nursing considerations

• Administer topical corticosteroids, antihistamines, or tranquilizers, as ordered.
• If the patient doesn't have a localized infection or skin lesions, suspect a systemic disease and prepare him for a complete blood count and differential, erythrocyte sedimentation rate, protein electrophoresis, and radiologic studies.

Diplopia, or double vision, occurs when extraocular muscles fail to work together, causing images to fall on noncorresponding parts of the retinas. Diplopia can result from orbital lesions, the effects of surgery, or impaired function of cranial nerves that supply extraocular muscles.

Classified as monocular or binocular, diplopia usually begins intermittently or affects near or far vision exclusively. More common binocular diplopia may result from ocular deviation or displacement, extraocular muscle palsies, psychoneurosis, or retinal surgery. Monocular diplopia may result from an early cataract, retinal edema or scarring, iridodialysis, a subluxated lens, poorly fitting contact lenses, or an uncorrected refractive error. Diplopia may also occur in hysteria or malingering.

## ▶ Emergency interventions

If the patient complains of double vision, first check his neurologic status. Evaluate his level of consciousness (LOC), pupil size and response to light, and motor and sensory functions. Then take his vital signs. Briefly ask about associated neurologic symptoms, especially severe headache.

## History

Find out when the patient first noticed diplopia. Are the images side-by-side (horizontal), one above the other (vertical), or a combination? Does diplopia affect near or far vision? Does it affect certain directions of gaze? Has it worsened, remained the same, or subsided? Does its severity change throughout the day? Find out if the patient can correct diplopia by tilting his head. If so, ask him to show you and note the direction of the tilt. Also ask about eye pain and explore his medical history. Note a history of extraocular muscle disorders, trauma, or eye surgery.

## Physical exam

Observe the patient for ocular deviation, ptosis, exophthalmos, lid edema, and conjunctival injection. Have him occlude one eye at a time; if he sees double with either one, he has monocular diplopia. Test visual acuity and extraocular muscles.

## Causes

*Botulism.* Hallmark signs are diplopia, dysarthria, dysphagia, and ptosis. Early findings include dry mouth, sore throat, vomiting, and diarrhea. Later, descending weakness or paralysis of extremity and trunk muscles causes hyporeflexia and dyspnea.

*Brain tumor.* Diplopia may be an early symptom. Accompanying features vary with the tumor's size and location, and include eye deviation, emotional lability, headache, vomiting, and seizures.

*Cerebrovascular accident.* Diplopia characterizes this life-threatening disorder when it affects the vertebrobasilar artery. Other features may include unilateral motor weakness or paralysis, decreased LOC, dizziness, and aphasia.

*Intracranial aneurysm.* This life-threatening disorder initially produces diplopia and eye deviation, perhaps accompanied by ptosis and a dilated pupil on the affected side. Other findings include severe, unilateral, frontal headache, which becomes violent after rupture of the aneurysm; neck and spinal pain and rigidity; decreased LOC; tinnitus; dizziness; vomiting; and unilateral muscle weakness or paralysis.

*Myasthenia gravis.* Initially, diplopia and ptosis occur, worsening throughout the course of the day. Later findings include a blank facial expression; difficulty chewing, swallowing, and making fine hand movements; and possibly life-threatening respiratory muscle weakness.

*Other causes.* Alcohol intoxication, cavernous sinus thrombosis, diabetes mellitus, encephalitis, eye surgery, head injury, multiple sclerosis, ophthalmoplegic migraine, orbital blowout fracture, orbital cellulitis, orbital tumors, and thyrotoxicosis.

## Nursing considerations

• Continue to monitor vital signs and neurologic status if an acute neurologic disorder is suspected.
• Provide a safe environment.

A urologic emergency, priapism is a persistent, painful erection unrelated to sexual excitement. This relatively rare sign may begin during sleep and appear to be a normal erection, but it may last for hours or days. It's usually accompanied by a severe, constant, dull aching in the penis. Despite this, the patient may avoid medical help and try to achieve detumescence through sexual activity.

Priapism occurs when the veins of the corpora cavernosa fail to drain correctly, resulting in persistent engorgement. Without prompt treatment, penile ischemia and thrombosis occur. About half of all cases develop without apparent predisposing factors. Secondary priapism results from blood disorders, neoplasms, trauma, and certain drugs.

▶ **Emergency interventions**
If your patient has priapism, notify the doctor immediately. Apply an ice pack to the patient's penis, administer analgesics, and insert an indwelling urinary catheter to relieve urine retention, as ordered. If ordered, assist with procedures to remove blood from the corpora cavernosa, such as irrigation and surgery.

**History**
As appropriate, ask the patient when the priapism began. Is it continuous or intermittent? Has he had a prolonged erection before? If so, what did he do

to relieve it? How long did he remain detumescent? Does he have pain or tenderness when he urinates? Has he noticed any changes in sexual function? If the patient reports sickle cell anemia, find out about any factors that could precipitate a crisis. Ask if he has recently suffered genital trauma, and obtain a thorough drug history.

**Physical exam**
Examine the patient's penis, noting its color and temperature. Check for any loss of sensation, and look for signs of infection. Take his vital signs, particularly noting fever.

**Causes**
*Cerebrovascular accident (CVA).* A CVA may cause priapism, but sensory loss and aphasia may prevent the patient from noticing or describing it. Other findings depend on the CVA's location and extent but may include hemiplegia, seizures, headache, dysarthria, dysphagia, ataxia, apraxia, agnosia, and visual deficits.

*Penile carcinoma.* Carcinoma that exerts pressure on the corpora cavernosa can cause priapism. Usually, the first sign is a painless ulcerative lesion or an enlarging warty growth on the glans or foreskin, which may be accompanied by localized pain, a foul-smelling discharge from the prepuce, a firm lump near the glans, and lymphade-

nopathy. Later findings may include bleeding, dysuria, urine retention, and bladder distention.

*Penile trauma.* Priapism can occur with bruising, abrasions, swelling, pain, and hematuria.

*Sickle cell anemia.* Painful priapism can occur without warning, usually on awakening. The patient may have a history of priapism, impaired growth and development, and increased susceptibility to infection. Related findings include tachycardia, pallor, weakness, hepatomegaly, dyspnea, joint swelling and pain, chest pain, murmurs, leg ulcers and, possibly, jaundice and gross hematuria.

*Spinal cord injury.* The patient may be unaware of the onset of priapism. Related effects depend on the extent and level of the injury and may include autonomic signs such as bradycardia.

*Other causes.* Drugs, such as phenothiazines, thioridazine, trazodone, androgenic steroids, and some antihypertensives; genitourinary infection; granulocytic leukemia (chronic); and thrombocytopenia.

**Nursing considerations**
• As ordered, prepare the patient for blood tests. If he requires surgery, keep his penis flaccid postoperatively by applying a pressure dressing.
• At least every 30 minutes, inspect the glans for signs of vascular compromise.

A common symptom, dizziness is a sensation of imbalance or faintness sometimes associated with weakness, confusion, and blurred or double vision. Usually, episodes are brief; they may be mild or severe with abrupt or gradual onset. Dizziness may be aggravated by standing up quickly and alleviated by lying down. Dizziness typically results from inadequate blood flow and oxygen supply to the cerebrum and spinal cord. It may occur in anxiety, in respiratory and cardiovascular disorders, and in postconcussion syndrome. It's a key symptom in certain serious disorders, such as hypertension and vertebrobasilar insufficiency.

## ▶ Emergency interventions

First, assess the severity of the patient's dizziness. When did it begin? Is it associated with headache or blurred vision? Take the patient's vital signs and ask about a history of high blood pressure. If his diastolic pressure exceeds 100 mm Hg, notify the doctor immediately. Tell the patient to lie down, and recheck his vital signs every 15 minutes until the doctor arrives. Start an I.V. line, and prepare to administer an antihypertensive.

## History

Ask about a history of diabetes, cardiovascular disease, myocardial infarction, congestive heart failure, atherosclerosis, anemia, chronic obstruc-tive pulmonary disease, anxiety disorders, or head injury. Obtain a complete drug history. Ask how often dizziness occurs. How long does each episode last? Does the dizziness abate spontaneously? Is it triggered by sitting up suddenly or stooping over? Has the patient been irritable or anxious? Ask about palpitations, chest pain, diaphoresis, shortness of breath, and chronic cough.

## Physical exam

Assess level of consciousness, motor and sensory functions, and reflexes. Inspect for poor skin turgor, dry mucous membranes, barrel chest, clubbing, cyanosis, and accessory muscle use. Auscultate heart rate and rhythm and breath sounds. Take the patient's blood pressure while he's lying down, sitting, and standing; test capillary refill in the extremities; and palpate for edema.

## Causes

*Cardiac arrhythmias.* Dizziness lasts for several minutes or longer and may precede fainting. The patient may experience palpitations; irregular, rapid, or thready pulse; hypotension; weakness; blurred vision; paresthesia; and confusion.

*Carotid sinus hypersensitivity.* Brief episodes of dizziness that usually terminate in fainting are characteristic. These episodes are precipitated by stimulation of one or both carotid arteries by wearing a tight collar, moving the patient's head, or other seemingly minor actions.

*Hypertension.* Dizziness may precede fainting but may be relieved by rest. Other findings may include elevated blood pressure, headache, blurred vision, retinal hemorrhage and exudate, and papilledema.

*Transient ischemic attack (TIA).* Lasting from a few seconds to 24 hours, an attack commonly signals impending stroke and may be triggered by turning the head to the side. Dizziness of varying severity, diplopia, blindness or visual field deficits, ptosis, tinnitus, hearing loss, paresis, and numbness may occur during an attack.

*Other causes.* Anemia; drugs, such as antianxiety drugs, central nervous system depressants, narcotics, decongestants, antihistamines, antihypertensives, and vasodilators; emphysema; generalized anxiety disorder; hyperventilation syndrome; orthostatic hypotension; panic disorder; and postconcussion syndrome.

## Nursing considerations

• If the patient is hyperventilating, have him breathe and rebreathe into cupped hands or a paper bag. Instruct the patient who risks a TIA from vertebrobasilar insufficiency to turn his body instead of just turning his head to one side.

**D**

# Postnasal drip

A sinus or nasal discharge that flows behind the nose and into the throat, a postnasal drip usually results from infection, suggested by a thick, tenacious, and purulent discharge, or allergies, suggested by a watery discharge. Postnasal drip may also result from environmental irritants.

## History
Ask the patient when his postnasal drip began and if it's continuous or intermittent. Does it occur during a certain season? What relieves the postnasal drip? What aggravates it? Ask about related signs and symptoms, such as a cough, sinus pain, headache, and nasal congestion. Next, take an allergy history and find out about occupational exposure to environmental irritants, such as chemical fumes or dust.

## Physical exam
If the patient has mucosal swelling, use a vasoconstricting nasal spray before beginning the nasal examination. Then use a nasal speculum to assess the mucous membranes, which are normally pink to dull red. Observe the size and shape of the turbinates and septum, noting any abnormal structures and characterizing the secretions. If the patient wears dentures, ask him to remove them before you examine his throat. Use a warmed, size 0 postnasal mirror and a tongue blade to examine the oropharynx and nasopharynx for drainage. Finally, palpate the sinus areas for swelling and tenderness.

## Causes
*Environmental irritants.* Exposure to environmental irritants, such as fumes, smoke, or dust, may cause postnasal drip. Other findings depend on the type of irritant and the duration of exposure but may include a cough and itching or burning eyes, nose, and throat.

*Rhinitis.* Two types of rhinitis — allergic and vasomotor — can produce postnasal drip. In allergic rhinitis, symptoms can occur seasonally, as with hay fever, or year-round, as with chronic rhinitis. Nasal obstruction and edematous, pale nasal mucosa may be apparent. The mucosal surface appears smooth and shiny, and the turbinates fill the air space and press against the nasal septum. The patient has swollen, red eyelids and conjunctivae and excessive tearing. He also has paroxysmal sneezing, a thin nasal discharge, a diminished sense of smell, frontal or temporal headache, and eye, nose, and possibly throat itching.

A recurrent postnasal drip occurs with vasomotor rhinitis, which can be aggravated by dry air. Related effects may include engorged inferior turbinates, nasal obstruction, sneezing, watery or sticky rhinorrhea, a pink nasal septum, and bluish mucosa.

*Sinusitis.* This disorder commonly produces postnasal drip. It may also cause headache, sinus pain, purulent rhinorrhea, halitosis, fever, sore throat, cough, malaise, and red, swollen nasal mucosa and turbinates.

## Nursing considerations
• Teach the patient with postnasal drip how to use medications safely. Remind him not to use decongestants for more than a month at a time. If he has hypertension, instruct him to avoid systemic decongestants. Caution him against overuse of nose drops, which can produce rebound rhinitis. If he has allergic rhinitis, recommend antihistamines.
• If sinus pain accompanies postnasal drip, apply wet hot packs to the sinuses. Instruct the patient to avoid nasal irritants, such as tobacco smoke.
• As ordered, prepare the patient for diagnostic tests, such as sinus X-rays and culture and sensitivity studies.

Also known as a negative oculocephalic reflex, the absence of the doll's eye sign is an ominous indicator of brain stem dysfunction detected by the rapid but gentle turning of the patient's head from side to side. The eyes remain fixed in mid-position instead of moving laterally away from the direction of the head turn. Usually, this sign can't be elicited in the conscious patient because he voluntarily controls eye movements.

Absent doll's eye sign indicates injury to the midbrain, pons, and cranial nerves III, VI, and VIII. Typically, it accompanies coma caused by lesions of the cerebellum and brain stem. When it's detected in deep coma, absent doll's eye sign is a mark of brain death.

A variant of absent doll's eye sign that develops gradually is known as abnormal doll's eye sign: One eye may move laterally while the other remains fixed or moves in the opposite direction. Usually, an abnormal doll's eye sign accompanies metabolic coma or increased intracranial pressure (ICP). The associated brain stem dysfunction may be reversible or may progress to deeper coma with absent doll's eye sign.

## Physical exam

After detecting an absent doll's eye sign, assess the patient's level of consciousness using the Glasgow Coma Scale. Look for lightening or deepening coma, and note decerebrate or decorticate posture. Examine the pupils for size, equality, and response to light. Check for signs of increased ICP: increased blood pressure, increasing pulse pressure, and bradycardia.

## Causes

*Brain stem infarction.* This infarction causes absent doll's eye sign with coma. It also causes limb paralysis, cranial nerve palsies (facial weakness, diplopia, blindness or visual field deficits, nystagmus), bilateral cerebellar ataxia, and variable sensory loss. Late signs include a positive Babinski's reflex, decerebrate posture, and flaccidity.

*Brain stem tumor.* Absent doll's eye sign accompanies coma in this disorder. This sign may be preceded by hemiparesis, nystagmus, extraocular nerve palsies, facial pain or sensory loss, facial paralysis, diminished corneal reflex, tinnitus, hearing loss, dysphagia, drooling, vertigo, dizziness, ataxia, and vomiting.

*Central midbrain infarction.* Accompanying absent doll's eye sign are coma, Weber's syndrome (oculomotor palsy with contralateral hemiplegia), contralateral ataxic tremor, nystagmus, and pupillary abnormalities.

*Cerebellar lesion.* Whether associated with abscess, hemorrhage, or tumor, a cerebellar lesion that progresses to coma may cause an absent doll's eye sign. Coma may be preceded by headache, nystagmus, ocular deviation to the side of the lesion, unequal pupils, dysarthria, dysphagia, ipsilateral facial paresis, and cerebellar ataxia. Characteristic signs of increased ICP may also occur.

*Pontine hemorrhage.* Absent doll's eye sign and coma develop within minutes in this life-threatening disorder. Other ominous signs, such as complete paralysis, decerebrate posture, a positive Babinski's reflex, and small reactive pupils, may then rapidly progress to death.

*Posterior fossa hematoma.* A subdural hematoma at this location typically causes absent doll's eye sign and coma. These signs may be preceded by headache, vomiting, drowsiness, confusion, unequal pupils, dysphagia, cranial nerve palsies, stiff neck, and cerebellar ataxia.

*Other causes.* Drugs, such as barbiturates.

## Nursing considerations

● Do not attempt to elicit doll's eye sign in the comatose patient with suspected cervical spine injury. Instead, use the caloric test.
● Continue to monitor vital signs and neurologic status in the patient with an absent doll's eye sign.

The daily excretion of more than 2,500 ml (2.5 liters) of urine, polyuria is a relatively common sign usually reported by the patient as increased voidings, especially when it occurs at night. Aggravated by overhydration, caffeine or alcohol consumption, and excessive ingestion of salt, glucose, or other hyperosmolar substances, polyuria usually results from the use of certain drugs, such as diuretics, and from psychological, neurologic, and renal disorders. It can reflect renal impairment or central nervous system dysfunction that diminishes or suppresses secretion of antidiuretic hormone. In both cases, the renal tubules fail to reabsorb sufficient water, causing polyuria.

## History

If the patient doesn't display signs of hypovolemia, explore the frequency and pattern of the polyuria. When did it begin? How long has it lasted? Was it precipitated by a certain event? Ask the patient to describe the pattern and amount of his daily fluid intake. Find out about any current or past psychiatric disorders and chronic hypokalemia or hypercalcemia. Check for a history of visual deficits, headaches, or head trauma. Also check for a history of urinary tract obstruction, diabetes mellitus, and renal disorders. Find out the dosage of any drugs the patient is taking.

## Physical exam

Evaluate fluid status first. Take vital signs, noting increased body temperature, tachycardia, and orthostatic hypotension. Inspect for dry skin and mucous membranes, decreased skin turgor and elasticity, and reduced perspiration. Is the patient unusually tired or thirsty? Has he recently lost more than 5% of his body weight? If you detect these effects of hypovolemia, notify the doctor and infuse replacement fluids, as ordered.

Perform a neurologic examination, noting any change in the patient's level of consciousness. Then palpate the bladder and inspect the urethral meatus. Obtain a urine specimen and check its specific gravity.

## Causes

*Acute tubular necrosis.* During the diuretic phase, polyuria of less than 8 liters/day gradually subsides after 8 to 10 days. Urine specific gravity (1.010 or less) increases as polyuria subsides. Related findings include weight loss, decreasing edema, and nocturia.

*Diabetes insipidus.* Polyuria of about 5 liters/day with a specific gravity of 1.005 or less usually occurs. Other findings include polydipsia, nocturia, fatigue, and signs of dehydration.

*Diabetes mellitus.* Polyuria seldom exceeds 5 liters/day, and urine specific gravity exceeds 1.020. The patient has polydipsia, polyphagia, weight loss, weakness, fatigue, and nocturia. He may also display signs of dehydration.

*Glomerulonephritis (chronic).* Polyuria gradually progresses to oliguria. Urine output is usually less than 4 liters/day; specific gravity is about 1.010. Related effects include nausea and vomiting, fatigue, edema, and elevated blood pressure.

*Hypokalemia.* Prolonged potassium depletion may lead to nephropathy, producing polyuria of less than 5 liters/day with a specific gravity of about 1.010. Associated findings include polydipsia, muscle weakness or paralysis, hypoactive deep tendon reflexes, fatigue, and arrhythmias.

*Postobstructive uropathy.* After resolution of a urinary tract obstruction, polyuria of more than 5 liters/day with a specific gravity of less than 1.010 occurs for several days, then subsides.

*Other causes.* Diagnostic tests using contrast media; drugs, such as diuretics, cardiotonics, vitamin D, demeclocycline, phenytoin, lithium, methoxyflurane, and propoxyphene; hypercalcemia; psychogenic polydipsia; pyelonephritis; Sheehan's syndrome; and sickle cell anemia.

## Nursing considerations

• Record fluid intake and output accurately, and weigh the patient daily. Closely monitor vital signs, and encourage him to drink adequate fluids.

The flow of saliva from the mouth, drooling may stem from facial muscle paralysis or weakness that prevents mouth closure, from neuromuscular disorders or local pain that causes dysphagia, or from the effects of drugs or toxins that induce salivation. Drooling may be scant or copious (up to 1 liter daily) and may cause circumoral irritation.

## History
Ask the patient when his drooling began. Ask about sore throat and difficulty in swallowing, chewing, speaking, or breathing. Have the patient describe any pain or stiffness in the face and neck, and any muscle weakness in the face and extremities. Has he noticed unusual drowsiness or agitation? Ask about changes in vision, hearing, and sense of taste. Ask about anorexia, weight loss, fatigue, nausea, vomiting, and altered bowel or bladder habits. Has he recently had a cold or infection, been bitten by an animal, or been exposed to pesticides? Finally, obtain a complete drug history.

## Physical exam
Observe whether drooling is scant or copious. Inspect for circumoral irritation. Take vital signs. Inspect for signs of facial paralysis or abnormal expression. Examine the mouth and neck for swelling, the throat for edema and redness, and the tonsils for exudate. Note foul breath odor. Examine the tongue for bilateral furrowing. Look for pallor and skin lesions and for frontal baldness. Carefully assess any bite or puncture marks. Assess cranial nerves II through VII, IX, and X. Check pupil size and response to light. Assess the patient's speech. Evaluate muscle strength, and palpate for tenderness or atrophy. Also palpate for lymphadenopathy, especially in the cervical area. Test for poor balance, hyperreflexia, and positive Babinski's reflex. Assess sensory function.

## Causes
*Acoustic neuroma.* When this malignant tumor involves the facial nerve, it produces facial weakness or paralysis with constant scant to copious drooling, along with tinnitus, unilateral hearing loss, and vertigo. Other symptoms include dysphagia, poor balance, and ear or eye pain.

*Bell's palsy.* Constant drooling accompanies sudden onset of facial hemiplegia. The affected side of the face sags and is expressionless, the nasolabial fold flattens, and the palpebral fissure widens. The patient usually complains of pain in or behind the ear. Other findings include unilateral diminished or absent corneal reflex, decreased lacrimation, upward deviation of the eye with attempt at lid closure, and altered sense of taste.

*Esophageal tumor.* Copious and persistent drooling is preceded by weight loss and progressively severe dysphagia. Other findings include substernal, back, or neck pain, and blood-flecked regurgitation.

*Peritonsillar abscess.* Severe sore throat causes dysphagia with moderate to copious drooling. It's accompanied by high fever, rancid breath, and enlarged, reddened, edematous tonsils that may be covered by a soft gray exudate.

*Retropharyngeal abscess.* This disorder causes painful swallowing, resulting in moderate to copious drooling. The patient complains of a lump in his throat and dyspnea when he's sitting, which disappears when he lies down. Other findings include coughing, snoring, choking, noisy breathing, and a "cry of a duck" voice tone.

*Other causes.* Achalasia; amyotrophic lateral sclerosis; cerebrovascular accident; diphtheria; drugs, such as clonazepam, ethionamide, and haloperidol; glossopharyngeal neuralgia; Guillain-Barré syndrome; hypocalcemia; Ludwig's angina; myasthenia gravis; myotonic dystrophy; paralytic poliomyelitis; Parkinson's disease; pesticide poisoning; rabies; seizures (generalized); and tetanus.

## Nursing considerations
● Be alert for aspiration. Position the patient upright or on his side. Provide frequent mouth care and suction, as necessary, to control drooling.

**D**

Also called hyperphagia, polyphagia refers to voracious eating before satiety. A common symptom that can be persistent or intermittent, it results primarily from endocrine and psychological disorders, as well as from use of certain drugs. Depending on the underlying cause, polyphagia may or may not cause weight gain.

## History
Ask the patient what he has eaten and drunk within the last 24 hours and, if he can recall, within the last 48 hours. Note the frequency of his meals and the amount and types of food eaten. Find out if the patient's eating habits have changed recently or if he has always had a large appetite. Does his overeating alternate with periods of anorexia? Ask about conditions that may trigger overeating, such as stress, depression, or menstruation. Does the patient actually feel hungry, or does he eat simply because food is available? Does he ever vomit or have a headache after overeating?

Explore related signs and symptoms. Has the patient recently gained or lost weight? Does he feel tired, nervous, or excitable? Has he experienced heat intolerance, dizziness, or palpitations? Diarrhea or increased thirst or urination? Obtain a complete drug history, including his use of laxatives or enemas.

## Physical exam
Weigh the patient. Tell him his current weight and watch for any expression of disbelief or anger. Inspect the skin to detect dryness or poor turgor. Palpate the thyroid for enlargement.

## Causes
*Anxiety.* Mild to moderate anxiety or stress may produce polyphagia. Typically, mild anxiety produces restlessness, sleeplessness, irritability, repetitive questioning, and constant seeking of attention and reassurance. With moderate anxiety, selective inattention and difficulty concentrating may occur. Other effects may include muscle tension, diaphoresis, GI distress, palpitations, tachycardia, and urinary and sexual dysfunction.

*Bulimia.* Most common in women ages 18 to 29, bulimia causes polyphagia that alternates with self-induced vomiting, fasting, or diarrhea. The patient typically weighs less than normal but has a morbid fear of obesity. She appears depressed, has low self-esteem, and conceals her overeating.

*Diabetes mellitus.* Polyphagia occurs with weight loss, polydipsia, and polyuria. It's accompanied by nocturia, weakness, fatigue, and signs of dehydration, such as dry mucous membranes and poor skin turgor.

*Migraine headache.* Polyphagia sometimes precedes a migraine headache. Other prodromal signs and symptoms may include fatigue, nausea, vomiting, and a visual aura. Light and noise sensitivity may also occur.

*Premenstrual syndrome.* Food cravings and binges are common. Abdominal bloating may occur with behavioral changes, such as depression and insomnia. Headache, paresthesia, and other neurologic symptoms may also occur. Related findings include diarrhea or constipation, edema and temporary weight gain, palpitations, back pain, breast swelling and tenderness, oliguria, and easy bruising.

*Thyrotoxicosis.* This disorder can produce weight loss despite constant polyphagia. Other characteristics include weakness, nervousness, diarrhea, tremors, diaphoresis, and dyspnea. The patient's hair and nails are thin and brittle; his thyroid is enlarged. He may have palpitations, tachycardia, heat intolerance, and possibly exophthalmos and an atrial or ventricular gallop.

*Other causes.* Drugs, such as corticosteroids and cyproheptadine.

## Nursing considerations
• Offer the patient emotional support, and help him understand the underlying cause of his polyphagia. As needed, refer the patient and his family for psychological counseling.

Dysarthia is poorly articulated speech, characterized by slurring and a labored, irregular rhythm. It may be accompanied by a nasal voice tone caused by palate weakness. Dysarthria is occasionally confused with aphasia—loss of the ability to produce or comprehend speech. Dysarthria is commonly caused by degenerative neurologic disorders but may also result from ill-fitting dentures.

## ▶ Emergency interventions
If the patient displays dysarthria, ask him about difficulty swallowing. Then assess respiratory rate and depth, and measure vital capacity. Next, obtain blood pressure and heart rate. Usually, tachycardia and slightly increased blood pressure are early signs of respiratory muscle weakness. Notify the doctor immediately if these signs accompany shortness of breath.

Ensure a patent airway. Place the patient in Fowler's position and suction him, if necessary. Administer oxygen and keep resuscitation equipment nearby. Expect to provide intubation and mechanical ventilation in progressive respiratory muscle weakness. Withhold oral fluids in the patient with associated dysphagia.

## History
If the patient isn't in distress, ask him when his dysarthria began and if it has improved. (Speech improves with resolution of a transient ischemic attack, but not in a completed stroke.) Ask if dysarthria worsens during the day. Obtain a drug and alcohol history, and note a history of seizures.

## Physical exam
If the patient's dysarthria is not accompanied by respiratory muscle weakness and dysphagia, continue to assess for other neurologic deficits. Compare muscle strength and tone in the limbs. Then evaluate tactile sensation. Ask the patient about numbness or tingling. Test deep tendon reflexes. Also, note gait ataxia. Next, test visual fields and ask about double vision. Check for signs of facial weakness, such as ptosis. Finally, assess level of consciousness and mental status.

## Causes
*Alcoholic cerebellar degeneration.* Chronic, progressive dysarthria is common along with ataxia, diplopia, ophthalmoplegia, hypotension, and altered mental status.

*Amyotrophic lateral sclerosis.* Dysarthria occurs when this disorder affects the brain stem nuclei. It may worsen as the disease progresses.

*Botulism.* This is marked by acute cranial nerve dysfunction, causing dysarthria, dysphagia, diplopia, and ptosis. Early findings include dry mouth, sore throat, weakness, vomiting, and diarrhea.

*Brain stem cerebrovascular accident (CVA).* This CVA is marked by bulbar palsy, resulting in the triad of dysarthria, dysphonia, and dysphagia. The dysarthria is most severe at the onset of stroke; it may lessen or disappear with rehabilitation.

*Multiple sclerosis.* Dysarthria is accompanied by nystagmus, blurred or double vision, dysphagia, ataxia, and intention tremor. These effects wax and wane along with the disorder.

*Myasthenia gravis.* Dysarthria typically worsens during the day. Other findings include nasal voice tone, dysphagia, facial weakness, diplopia, dyspnea, and skeletal muscle weakness.

*Olivopontocerebellar degeneration.* Dysarthria, a major sign, accompanies cerebellar ataxia and spasticity.

*Parkinson's disease.* Dysarthria accompanies low-pitched monotonic speech. Other findings: muscle rigidity, bradykinesia, involuntary tremor (usually in the fingers), and difficulty walking.

*Other causes.* Basilar artery insufficiency; cerebral CVA; chronic mercury or manganese poisoning; drugs, such as anticonvulsants and barbiturates; and Shy-Drager syndrome.

## Nursing considerations
• Encourage the patient with dysarthria to speak slowly so that he can be understood. Encourage him to use gestures.

Polydipsia is excessive thirst—a common symptom associated with endocrine disorders and use of certain drugs. It may reflect reduced fluid intake, increased urine output (as in diabetes mellitus), or excessive loss of water and salt (as in profuse sweating).

## History

Find out how much fluid the patient drinks each day. How often does he urinate? How much does he typically urinate? Does the need to urinate awaken him at night? Ask about any recent weight loss or change in appetite. Determine if he or anyone in his family has diabetes or kidney disease. Ask about medications he uses and recent lifestyle changes that may have upset him.

## Physical exam

Take the patient's blood pressure and pulse rate in the supine and standing positions. A decrease of 10 mm Hg in systolic pressure and a pulse rate increase of 10 beats/minute from the supine to the standing position may indicate hypovolemia. If these changes occur, notify the doctor and ask the patient about recent weight loss. Check for signs of dehydration, such as dry mucous membranes and decreased skin turgor.

## Causes

*Diabetes insipidus.* Characteristically causing polydipsia, diabetes insipidus may also cause excessive voiding of dilute urine and mild to moderate nocturia. If severe, it causes fatigue and signs of dehydration.

*Diabetes mellitus.* Polydipsia is a classic finding. Other effects include polyuria, polyphagia, nocturia, weakness, fatigue, and weight loss. Signs of dehydration may occur.

*Hypercalcemia.* As this disorder progresses, the patient develops polydipsia, polyuria, nocturia, constipation, paresthesia and, occasionally, hematuria and pyuria. Severe hypercalcemia can progress quickly to vomiting, decreased level of consciousness, and renal failure.

*Hypokalemia.* This disorder can cause nephropathy, resulting in polydipsia, polyuria, and nocturia. Related hypokalemic effects include muscle weakness or paralysis, fatigue, decreased bowel sounds, hypoactive deep tendon reflexes, and arrhythmias.

*Renal disorders (chronic).* Chronic renal disorders, such as glomerulonephritis and pyelonephritis, damage the kidneys, causing polydipsia and polyuria. Associated signs and symptoms may include nocturia, weakness, elevated blood pressure, pallor and, in later stages, oliguria.

*Sheehan's syndrome.* Polydipsia, polyuria, and nocturia occur in this syndrome of postpartum pituitary necrosis. Other features include fatigue, failure to lactate, amenorrhea, decreased pubic and axillary hair growth, and reduced libido.

*Sickle cell anemia.* As nephropathy develops, polydipsia and polyuria occur. They may be accompanied by abdominal pain and cramps, arthralgia and, occasionally, lower extremity skin ulcers and bone deformities, such as kyphosis and scoliosis.

*Other causes.* Drugs, such as diuretics, demeclocycline, phenothiazines, and anticholinergics; psychogenic polydipsia; and thyrotoxicosis.

## Nursing considerations

- If ordered, infuse I.V. replacement fluids.
- Carefully monitor the patient's fluid balance by recording his total intake and output. Weigh the patient at the same time each day, in the same clothing, and using the same scale.
- Regularly check blood pressure and pulse in the supine and standing positions to detect orthostatic hypotension, which may indicate hypovolemia. Because thirst is usually the body's way of compensating for water loss, give the patient ample liquids.

# Dysmenorrhea

Painful menstruation, dysmenorrhea affects over 50% of menstruating women, causing sharp, intermittent pain or dull, aching pain. Usually, it's characterized by mild to severe cramping or colicky pain in the pelvis or lower abdomen that may radiate to the thighs and lower sacrum. This pain may precede menstruation by several days or may accompany it. The pain gradually subsides as bleeding tapers off.

Dysmenorrhea may be idiopathic or may result from endometriosis or other pelvic disorders or from structural abnormalities, such as an imperforate hymen. Stress and poor health may aggravate dysmenorrhea, whereas rest and mild exercise may relieve it.

## History

Ask whether dysmenorrhea is intermittent or continuous. Is the pain sharp, cramping, or aching? Where is the pain located? Is it bilateral? How long has the patient been experiencing it? Find out when the pain begins and ends, and when it's severe. Does it radiate to the back? Explore associated symptoms, such as nausea, vomiting, altered bowel habits, bloating, pelvic or rectal pressure, and unusual fatigue, irritability, or depression.

Ask the patient if her menstrual flow is heavy or scant. Have her describe any vaginal discharge between menses. Does she experience dyspareunia with menses? Find out what relieves her cramps. Does she take pain medication? Does it relieve cramping? Note her method of contraception, and check for a history of pelvic infection or signs and symptoms of urinary obstruction. Determine how the patient copes with stress.

## Physical exam

Take vital signs, noting fever and any accompanying chills. Inspect the abdomen for distention and palpate for tenderness and masses. Note costovertebral angle tenderness.

## Causes

*Adenomyosis.* Endometrial tissue invades the myometrium, resulting in severe dysmenorrhea with pain radiating to the back or rectum, menorrhagia, and an enlarged, globular uterus.

*Endometriosis.* Typically, this disorder produces steady, aching pain that begins before menses and peaks at the height of menstrual flow. The pain may also occur between menstrual periods. Other findings include menorrhagia, irregular menses, dyspareunia, infertility, nausea and vomiting, painful defecation, and rectal bleeding and hematuria with menses.

*Pelvic inflammatory disease.* Chronic infection produces dysmenorrhea accompanied by fever; malaise; menorrhagia; foul-smelling, purulent vaginal discharge; dyspareunia; soft, enlarged uterus; severe abdominal pain; vomiting; and diarrhea.

*Premenstrual syndrome (PMS).* Usually, PMS follows an ovulatory cycle. As a result, it's rare during the first 12 months after menarche. The cramping pain usually begins with menstrual flow and persists for hours or days, diminishing with decreasing flow. Common effects precede menses by several days to 2 weeks and include abdominal bloating, breast tenderness, palpitations, diaphoresis, flushing, depression, and irritability.

*Primary (idiopathic) dysmenorrhea.* Increased prostaglandin secretion intensifies uterine contractions, apparently causing mild to severe spasmodic cramping pain in the lower abdomen, which radiates to the sacrum and inner thighs. Cramping abdominal pain peaks a few hours before menses.

*Other causes.* Cervical stenosis, intrauterine devices, uterine leiomyomas; and uterine prolapse.

## Nursing considerations

• If dysmenorrhea is idiopathic, advise the patient to place a heating pad on her abdomen to relieve pain. A light circular massage with the fingertips may also provide relief, as may warm beverages, warm showers, waist-bending and pelvic-rocking exercises, and walking.

## 89

A common result of pulmonary disorders or trauma, a pleural friction rub is a loud, coarse, grating, creaking, or squeaking sound that may be auscultated during late inspiration or early expiration. It's heard best over the low axilla or the anterior, lateral, or posterior bases of the lungs with the patient sitting upright. Sometimes intermittent, it may resemble crackles or a pericardial friction rub.

A pleural friction rub indicates inflammation of the visceral and parietal pleural lining. Resultant fibrinous exudate covers both pleural surfaces, displacing the fluid that's normally between them and causing the surfaces to rub together.

## ▶ Emergency interventions

When you detect a pleural friction rub, quickly assess for signs of respiratory distress: shallow or decreased respirations; crowing, wheezing, or stridor; dyspnea; increased accessory muscle use; intercostal or suprasternal retractions; cyanosis; and nasal flaring. Also check for hypotension, tachycardia, and a decreased level of consciousness. If you detect signs of distress, have another nurse notify the doctor while you maintain an airway. Elevate the patient's head 30 degrees, and monitor his cardiac status constantly.

## History

Ask the patient if he has had chest pain and, if so, its location, severity, and duration. Does it radiate to his shoulder, neck, or upper abdomen? Does it worsen with breathing, movement, or coughing? Does it abate if he splints his chest, holds his breath, or exerts pressure on the affected side? Ask about a history of rheumatoid arthritis, respiratory or cardiovascular disorders, recent trauma, and exposure to asbestos or radiation. If he smokes, obtain a history in pack years.

## Physical exam

Auscultate the patient's lungs with the patient sitting upright and breathing deeply and slowly through his mouth. Is the friction rub unilateral or bilateral? Listen for absent or diminished breath sounds, noting their location and timing in the respiratory cycle. Do abnormal breath sounds clear with coughing? Observe for clubbing and pedal edema. Then palpate for decreased chest motion, and percuss for flatness or dullness.

## Causes

*Asbestosis.* Besides a pleural friction rub, this disorder may cause dyspnea on exertion, a cough, chest pain, and crackles. Clubbing is a late sign.

*Lung cancer.* A pleural friction rub may be heard in the affected area. Other findings may include a cough, dyspnea, chest pain, weight loss, anorexia, fatigue, clubbing, fever, and wheezing.

*Pleurisy.* A pleural friction rub occurs early, along with sudden, intense unilateral chest pain in the lower lateral chest. Deep breathing, coughing, or thoracic movement aggravates the pain. Decreased breath sounds and inspiratory crackles may be heard over the painful area.

*Pneumonia (bacterial).* A pleural friction rub occurs along with a dry, painful, hacking cough that rapidly becomes productive. Related effects develop suddenly: chills, high fever, headache, dyspnea, pleuritic chest pain, and tachypnea.

*Pulmonary embolism.* A pleural friction rub can occur over the affected area. Usually, the first symptom is sudden dyspnea, possibly accompanied by anginal or pleuritic chest pain. Other features include a nonproductive cough or a cough that produces blood-tinged sputum, tachycardia, tachypnea, low-grade fever, and restlessness.

*Other causes.* Radiation therapy, rheumatoid arthritis, systemic lupus erythematosus, thoracic surgery, and tuberculosis.

## Nursing considerations

• Monitor the patient's respiratory status and vital signs.
• Teach your patient splinting maneuvers, apply a heating pad over the affected area and, as ordered, administer analgesics for pain relief.
• Instruct the patient not to suppress coughing.

# Dyspepsia

## 90

Usually described as an uncomfortable fullness after meals, dyspepsia is associated with nausea, belching, heartburn, and possibly cramping and abdominal distention. It's aggravated by spicy, fatty, or high-fiber foods and excessive caffeine consumption, and indicates impaired digestive function. Dyspepsia apparently results when altered gastric secretions lead to excess stomach acidity. It can be caused by GI disorders and, less often, from cardiac, respiratory, and renal disorders and the effects of drugs. It may also result from emotional upset and overly rapid eating or improper chewing.

## History
Ask the patient to describe his dyspepsia. How often and when does it occur? Do any drugs or activities relieve or aggravate it? Has he had nausea, vomiting, melena, hematemesis, a cough, or chest pain? Has he noticed any change in the amount or color of his urine? Also ask about recent surgery and a history of renal, cardiovascular, or respiratory disease.

## Physical exam
Inspect the abdomen for distention, ascites, scars, jaundice, uremic frost, and bruising. Then auscultate for bowel sounds and characterize their motility. Palpate and percuss the abdomen, noting any tenderness, pain, organ enlargement, or tympany. Finally, assess other body systems. Ask about behavioral changes and evaluate level of consciousness. Auscultate for gallops and crackles, and percuss the lungs to detect consolidation. Note peripheral edema.

## Causes
***Cholelithiasis.*** Heavy or greasy meals can precipitate dyspepsia with bloating, flatulence, nausea, vomiting, belching, and biliary colic. Acute pain in the right upper quadrant may radiate to the back, shoulders, and chest.

***Cirrhosis.*** Dyspepsia varies in intensity and duration and is relieved by antacids. Other GI effects include anorexia, nausea, flatulence, diarrhea, constipation, abdominal distention, and epigastric or right upper quadrant pain.

***Congestive heart failure.*** Common in right ventricular failure, transient dyspepsia may be accompanied by chest tightness and a constant ache or sharp pain in the right upper quadrant.

***Duodenal ulcer.*** Dyspepsia is a primary sign, ranging from a vague feeling of fullness or pressure to a boring or aching sensation in the middle or right epigastrium. It usually occurs 1½ to 3 hours after eating and is relieved by food or antacids.

***Gastric ulcer.*** Dyspepsia after eating occurs early in this disorder. The primary symptom is epigastric pain that may be relieved by food. Other findings include vomiting, distention, weight loss, and GI bleeding.

***Gastritis (chronic).*** Dyspepsia is relieved by antacids and aggravated by spicy foods or excessive caffeine intake. It occurs with anorexia, a feeling of fullness, vague epigastric pain, belching, nausea, and vomiting.

***GI neoplasms.*** These neoplasms usually produce chronic dyspepsia. Other features include fatigue, anorexia, jaundice, melena, hematemesis, constipation, and abdominal pain.

***Uremia.*** Dyspepsia may be the earliest and most important symptom. Others include anorexia, nausea, vomiting, abdominal cramps, bloating, diarrhea, epigastric pain, and weight gain.

***Other causes.*** Chronic pancreatitis; drugs, such as antibiotics, antihypertensives, diuretics, and nonsteroidal anti-inflammatory agents; hepatitis; postoperative gastritis; pulmonary embolus; and pulmonary tuberculosis.

## Nursing considerations
• Food or antacids may relieve dyspepsia, so have both available at all times. Give antacids, as ordered, 30 minutes before a meal or 1 hour after it. Give drugs after meals, if possible. Make sure the patient gets plenty of rest.
• If ordered, prepare the patient for endoscopy.

Pica refers to the craving and ingestion of normally inedible substances, such as plaster, charcoal, clay, wool, ashes, paint, or dirt. In children, the most commonly affected group, pica typically results from nutritional deficiencies. In adults, however, it may reflect a psychological disturbance. Depending on the substance ingested, pica can lead to poisoning and GI disorders.

## History
Determine what substances the patient has been eating. If he has eaten toxic substances, such as lead, notify the doctor and the poison control center. Ask the parents to describe their child's eating habits and nutritional history. Ask them when he first displayed pica, if he always craves the same substance, and whether he's listless or irritable.

## Physical exam
Check the patient's vital signs, noting especially bradycardia, tachycardia, or hypotension. Then inspect the abdomen for visible peristaltic waves or other abnormalities. Also observe the hair, skin, and mucous membranes for changes, such as dryness or pallor.

## Causes
*Anemia (iron-deficiency).* Chronic, severe iron-deficiency anemia may cause pica for dirt, paint, cornstarch, nails, or clay. It may also cause fatigue, irritability, listlessness, and anorexia. The patient may complain of light-headedness, headache, an inability to concentrate, dysphagia, and dyspnea on exertion. His muscle tone is poor and his extremities may have paresthesia. His nails are brittle and spoon-shaped, his tongue is smooth, and his skin and mucous membranes are pale.

*Malnutrition.* Severe malnutrition and starvation may cause pica for any substance, including dirt. Besides marked weight loss, the patient may have muscle wasting and paresthesia in the extremities. He appears lethargic and apathetic. His skin is dry, thin, and flaky. His sparse, dull hair falls out easily. His nails are brittle, his cheeks dark and swollen, his lips red and swollen. The patient may have nausea, vomiting, hepatomegaly, bradycardia, hypotension, slow and shallow respirations, and amenorrhea or gonadal atrophy.

*Psychological disorders.* Profound psychological impairments, such as schizophrenia and autism, can lead to pica.

## Nursing considerations
• Explain to the child's parents the effects of poisoning.
• Provide them with the telephone number of the local poison control center. Refer them to a dietitian for nutritional counseling.
• As ordered, prepare the patient for blood tests, a toxicology screen, and stool examination for ova and parasites. If these tests fail to reveal an organic disorder, refer the patient for psychological evaluation.

Dysphagia — difficulty swallowing — usually results from esophageal disorders. It may also be caused by oropharyngeal, respiratory, neurologic, and collagen disorders; toxins; and treatments.

## ▶ Emergency interventions

If the patient suddenly complains of difficulty swallowing and is in respiratory distress, suspect an airway obstruction and perform abdominal thrusts. Have another nurse call the doctor if this maneuver fails. Prepare to administer oxygen and to assist with endotracheal intubation.

## History

If the patient is stable, ask him if it's painful to swallow. If so, is the pain constant or intermittent? Have him point to where the problem is. Ask if eating alleviates or aggravates the symptom. Is it harder to swallow solids or liquids? Does the symptom disappear after he tries to swallow a few times? Is swallowing easier if he changes position?

## Physical exam

Evaluate the patient's swallowing, cough, and gag reflexes. Evaluate speech for signs of muscle weakness. Does he have aphasia or dysarthria? Is his voice nasal or hoarse? Check his mouth for dry mucous membranes and thick secretions. Observe for tongue and facial weakness.

## Causes

*Achalasia.* Dysphagia in the form of regurgitation of undigested food may cause wheezing, coughing, or choking as well as halitosis.

*Airway obstruction.* Life-threatening upper airway obstruction is marked by respiratory distress. Dysphagia occurs with gagging and dysphonia.

*Amyotrophic lateral sclerosis (ALS).* Besides dysphagia, ALS causes muscle weakness and atrophy, fasciculations, and shallow respirations.

*Esophageal carcinoma.* Typically, painless dysphagia accompanies rapid weight loss. As carcinoma advances, painful dysphagia, chest pain, and cough with hemoptysis occur.

*Esophageal spasm.* Distinctive symptoms of this disorder are dysphagia for solids and liquids and dull or squeezing substernal chest pain.

*Esophagitis.* Dysphagia accompanied by excessive salivation, hematemesis, tachypnea, fever, and intense pain in the mouth and anterior chest is characteristic of *corrosive esophagitis. Monilial esophagitis* causes dysphagia and sore throat. In *reflux esophagitis,* dysphagia is a late symptom that usually accompanies strictures.

*Gastric carcinoma.* Dysphagia is accompanied by nausea, vomiting, and pain that may radiate to the neck, back, or retrosternum.

*Hiatal hernia.* This causes dysphagia with retrosternal or substernal chest pain. Other signs include dyspepsia, and heartburn and regurgitation aggravated by lying down or stooping over.

*Mediastinitis.* Dysphagia may be insidious or rapid in onset. Other findings include chills, fever, and retrosternal chest pain that may radiate.

*Myasthenia gravis.* Progressive muscle weakness, causing painless dysphagia and choking, characterizes this disorder, along with fatigue.

*Other causes.* Botulism; bulbar paralysis; chronic pharyngitis; dysphagia lusoria; esophageal diverticulum, leiomyoma, or obstruction; external esophageal compression; extrinsic laryngeal carcinoma; hypocalcemia; laryngeal nerve damage; lead poisoning; oral cavity tumor; Parkinson's disease; Plummer-Vinson syndrome; progressive systemic sclerosis; rabies; radiation therapy; syphilis; systemic lupus erythematosus; tetanus; and tracheostomy.

## Nursing considerations

• At mealtime, position the patient upright and have him flex his neck forward slightly and keep his chin at midline. Provide mouth care before and after meals. Give an anticholinergic or antiemetic to control excess salivation.

• If the patient has a weak or absent cough reflex, consider giving tube feedings.

# Photophobia

An abnormal sensitivity to light, photophobia usually indicates increased eye sensitivity without an underlying disorder. In some patients, however, it can indicate excessive wearing of—or poorly fitted—contact lenses. Photophobia may also indicate systemic or ocular disorders, trauma, or the use of certain drugs.

## History
Ask the patient about the onset and severity of photophobia and whether it followed eye trauma, a chemical splash, or exposure to a sun lamp. If it resulted from trauma, avoid eye manipulation. Ask the patient to describe any eye pain, along with its location, duration, and intensity. Does he have a sensation of a foreign body in his eye, tearing, vision changes, or other symptoms?

## Physical exam
Take the patient's vital signs and assess his neurologic status. Next, carefully inspect the eyes' external structures. Examine the conjunctiva and sclera, noting especially their color. Characterize the amount and consistency of any discharge. Check pupillary reaction to light. Test the six cardinal fields of gaze and visual acuity in both eyes.

Keep in mind that photophobia can accompany life-threatening meningitis, although it's not a cardinal sign of meningeal irritation.

## Causes
*Burns.* In chemical burns, photophobia and eye pain may accompany erythema and blistering on the face and lids, miosis, diffuse conjunctival injection, and corneal changes. The patient may be unable to keep his eye(s) open, and his vision will be blurred. In ultraviolet radiation burns, photophobia occurs with moderate to severe eye pain about 12 hours after exposure.

*Conjunctivitis.* When conjunctivitis affects the cornea, it causes photophobia. Other findings include conjunctival injection, increased tearing, a foreign body sensation, a feeling of fullness around the eyes, and eye pain, burning, and itching. *Allergic conjunctivitis* produces a stringy eye discharge and milky red injection. *Bacterial conjunctivitis* causes a copious, mucopurulent, flaky eye discharge and a brilliant red conjunctiva. *Fungal conjunctivitis* produces a thick, purulent discharge, extreme redness, and crusting, sticky eyelids. *Viral conjunctivitis* causes copious tearing with little discharge as well as enlargement of the preauricular lymph nodes.

*Corneal abrasion.* Photophobia accompanies excessive tearing, conjunctival injection, visible corneal damage, and a foreign body sensation. Blurred vision and eye pain may occur.

*Corneal ulcer.* This vision-threatening disorder causes severe photophobia and eye pain that is aggravated by blinking. Impaired visual acuity may accompany blurring, eye discharge, and sticky eyelids. Conjunctival injection may occur.

*Iritis (acute).* Severe photophobia may accompany conjunctival injection, moderate to severe eye pain, and blurred vision. The pupil may be constricted and may respond poorly to light.

*Meningitis (acute bacterial).* Photophobia occurs with nuchal rigidity, hyperreflexia, opisthotonos, and positive Brudzinski's and Kernig's signs. Other findings include early fever, headache, vomiting, ocular palsies, facial weakness, pupillary abnormalities, and hearing loss. In severe meningitis, seizures, stupor, or coma may occur.

*Migraine headache.* Photophobia and noise sensitivity are prominent. Other findings include fatigue, blurred vision, nausea, and vomiting.

*Other causes.* Corneal foreign body; drugs, including mydriatics, amphetamines, cocaine, and ophthalmic antifungal agents; dry eye syndrome; keratitis (interstitial); scleritis; sclerokeratitis; trachoma; and uveitis.

## Nursing considerations
• Darken the patient's room, and tell him to close both eyes. If photophobia persists at home, suggest that he wear dark glasses.

The patient usually reports this sensation of difficult or uncomfortable breathing as shortness of breath. Pathologic causes of dyspnea include respiratory, cardiac, neuromuscular, and allergic disorders. It may also be caused by anxiety.

## ▶ Emergency interventions

If the patient shows signs of respiratory distress, notify the doctor immediately. Prepare to administer oxygen. Start an I.V. infusion and begin cardiac monitoring to detect arrhythmias.

## History

If the patient is stable, ask if dyspnea began suddenly or gradually, if it's constant or intermittent, and if it occurs with activity or while at rest. Does he have a productive or nonproductive cough or chest pain? Ask about recent trauma and a history of upper respiratory tract infections or phlebitis.

## Physical exam

Look for accessory muscle hypertrophy as well as pursed-lip exhalation, clubbing, peripheral edema, barrel chest, diaphoresis, and distended neck veins. Check blood pressure, and auscultate for heart and breath sounds.

## Causes

*Adult respiratory distress syndrome.* Dyspnea is followed by progressive respiratory distress, anxiety, tachycardia, crackles, and rhonchi.

*Aspiration of a foreign body.* Acute dyspnea, inspiratory stridor, and decreased or absent breath sounds mark this life-threatening condition.

*Asthma.* Acute dyspneic attacks occur along with audible wheezing, a dry cough, and accessory muscle use.

*Congestive heart failure (CHF).* Chronic paroxysmal nocturnal dyspnea, orthopnea, tachypnea, tachycardia, ventricular gallop, dependent peripheral edema, and weight gain may occur. With acute onset, CHF may produce distended neck veins.

*Emphysema.* Progressive exertional dyspnea may accompany barrel chest, accessory muscle hypertrophy, diminished breath sounds, peripheral cyanosis, tachypnea, and pursed-lip breathing.

*Flail chest.* Sudden dyspnea usually results from multiple rib fractures. Other findings include paradoxical chest movement, chest pain, tachypnea, and tachycardia.

*Myocardial infarction.* Sudden dyspnea occurs with crushing substernal chest pain that may radiate to the back, neck, jaw, and arms.

*Pneumonia.* Dyspnea occurs suddenly, usually accompanied by fever, chills, pleuritic chest pain, and a productive cough.

*Pneumothorax.* This causes dyspnea and sudden, stabbing chest pain. Other signs include a dry cough and decreased or absent breath sounds.

*Pulmonary edema.* Commonly preceded by signs of CHF, this life-threatening disorder causes acute dyspnea, crackles in both lung fields, and a ventricular gallop.

*Pulmonary embolism.* Acute dyspnea, usually accompanied by sudden pleuritic chest pain, marks this life-threatening disorder. Related findings include cough with hemoptysis, pleural friction rub, crackles, and wheezing.

*Shock.* Dyspnea arises suddenly and worsens progressively in this life-threatening disorder. Related findings include severe hypotension and cool, clammy skin.

*Tuberculosis.* Dyspnea commonly occurs with chest pain, crackles, and a productive cough. Other findings: night sweats, fever, and weight loss.

*Other causes.* Acute epiglottitis, amyotrophic lateral sclerosis, anemia, anxiety, cardiac arrhythmias, cor pulmonale, Guillain-Barré syndrome, inhalation injury, interstitial fibrosis, laryngotracheobronchitis (croup), lung cancer, myasthenia gravis, pleural effusion, poliomyelitis, and sepsis.

## Nursing considerations

• Reassure the patient and help him into a high Fowler or forward-leaning position. Give oxygen, as ordered.

In intestinal obstruction, peristalsis temporarily increases in strength and frequency as the intestine tries to force its contents past the obstruction. Peristaltic waves may visibly roll across the abdomen. Typically, these waves appear suddenly and vanish quickly because increased peristalsis overcomes the obstruction or the GI tract becomes atonic. Peristaltic waves are best detected by stooping at the supine patient's side and inspecting the abdominal contour.

Visible peristaltic waves may also reflect normal stomach and intestinal contractions in thin patients or in malnourished patients with abdominal muscle atrophy.

## History

After observing peristaltic waves, ask about a history of pyloric ulcer, stomach cancer, or chronic gastritis, which can lead to pyloric obstruction. Also ask about conditions leading to intestinal obstruction, such as intestinal tumors or polyps, gallstones, chronic constipation, and a hernia. Has the patient recently had abdominal surgery?

Determine if the patient has related symptoms. Spasmodic abdominal pain, for example, accompanies small-bowel obstruction, whereas colicky pain accompanies pyloric obstruction. Is the patient nauseated? Has he vomited? If he has vomited, ask about the consistency and color of the vomitus. Lumpy vomitus may contain undigested food particles. Green or brown vomitus may contain bile or fecal matter.

## Physical exam

With the patient supine, inspect the abdomen for distention, surgical scars and adhesions, or visible loops of bowel. Auscultate for bowel sounds, noting high-pitched, tinkling sounds. Next, jar the patient's bed (or roll the patient from side to side) and auscultate for a succussion splash — a splashing sound in the stomach that indicates pyloric obstruction. Palpate the abdomen for rigidity and tenderness, and percuss for tympany. Check the skin and mucous membranes for dryness and poor skin turgor, indicating dehydration. Take the patient's vital signs, noting especially tachycardia and hypotension, which indicate hypovolemia.

## Causes

*Large-bowel obstruction.* Visible peristaltic waves in the upper abdomen and obstipation are early signs of this obstruction. Other signs and symptoms develop more slowly than in a small-bowel obstruction; they may include nausea, colicky abdominal pain (milder than in small-bowel obstruction), gradual and eventually marked abdominal distention, and hyperactive bowel sounds.

*Pyloric obstruction.* Peristaltic waves may be detected in a swollen epigastrium or in the left upper quadrant, usually beginning near the left rib margin and rolling from left to right. Related findings include vague epigastric discomfort or colicky pain after eating, nausea, vomiting, anorexia, and weight loss. Auscultation reveals a loud succussion splash.

*Small-bowel obstruction.* Early signs include peristaltic waves rolling across the upper abdomen and intermittent, cramping periumbilical pain. Other findings include nausea, vomiting of bilious or fecal material, and constipation. In partial obstruction, diarrhea may be present. Hyperactive bowel sounds and slight abdominal distention also occur early.

## Nursing considerations

• Monitor the patient's status and prepare him for diagnostic evaluation and treatment. Be sure to withhold food and fluids, and explain the purpose and procedure of any diagnostic tests.

• If tests confirm obstruction, nasogastric suctioning may be used to decompress the stomach and small bowel. Provide frequent oral hygiene, and watch for a thick, swollen tongue and dry mucous membranes, indicating dehydration. Monitor vital signs and intake and output frequently.

Characterized by slow, involuntary movements of large muscle groups of the limbs, trunk, and neck, dystonia is an extrapyramidal sign that may involve flexion of the foot, hyperextension of the legs, extension and pronation of the arms, arching of the back, and extension and rotation of the neck (spasmodic torticollis). It's typically aggravated by walking and emotional stress and relieved by sleep. It may be intermittent—lasting just a few minutes—or continuous and painful. Although dystonia may be hereditary or idiopathic, it results more often from extrapyramidal disorders or drugs.

## History
If possible, include the patient's family in history taking. Ask when dystonia occurs. Is it aggravated by emotional upset? Does it disappear during sleep? Ask about a family history of dystonia. Take a drug history, especially noting use of phenothiazines and antipsychotics. If you suspect dystonia is drug-induced, notify the doctor.

## Physical exam
Examine the patient's coordination and voluntary muscle movement. Observe his gait as he walks across the room. Have him squeeze your fingers to assess muscle strength. Check coordination by having him touch your fingertip and then his nose repeatedly. Then test gross motor movement of the leg: Have him place his heel on one knee, slide it down his shin, then return it to his knee. Finally, assess fine motor movement of the fingers.

## Causes
*Alzheimer's disease.* Dystonia is a late sign of this disorder. The patient typically displays decreased attention span, amnesia, agitation, an inability to carry out activities of daily living, dysarthria, and emotional lability.

*Drugs.* All three types of phenothiazines may cause dystonia, but piperazine phenothiazines such as acetophenazine produce it most frequently. Haloperidol and loxapine usually produce acute facial dystonia, as do antiemetic doses of metoclopramide, excessive doses of levodopa, and metyrosine.

*Dystonia musculorum deformans.* Prolonged, generalized dystonia is the hallmark of this disorder, which usually develops in childhood and worsens with age. Initially, it causes foot inversion followed by growth retardation and scoliosis. Late signs include dysarthria, limb contractures, and twisted, bizarre postures.

*Hallervorden-Spatz syndrome.* This degenerative disorder causes dystonic trunk movements accompanied by choreoathetosis, ataxia, myoclonus, and generalized rigidity. The patient also shows progressive intellectual decline and dysarthria.

*Huntington's chorea.* Dystonic movements mark the preterminal stage of Huntington's chorea, a disorder that leads to dementia and emotional lability. Other findings include choreoathetosis, dysarthria, dysphagia, facial grimacing, and wide-based prancing gait.

*Parkinson's disease.* Dystonic spasms are common. Classic features include uniform or jerky rigidity, "pill-rolling" tremors, bradykinesia, dysarthria, dysphagia, drooling, masklike facies, monotone voice, stooping, and propulsive gait.

*Wilson's disease.* Progressive dystonia and chorea of the arms and legs mark this disorder. Other features include hoarseness, bradykinesia, behavior changes, dysphagia, drooling, dysarthria, tremors, and Kayser-Fleischer rings (rusty-brown rings at the periphery of the cornea).

*Other causes.* Olivopontocerebellar atrophies, Pick's disease, and supranuclear ophthalmoplegia (Steele-Richardson-Olszewski syndrome).

## Nursing considerations
• Encourage the patient to obtain adequate sleep and avoid emotional upset. Avoid range-of-motion exercises, which can aggravate dystonia.
• If dystonia is severe, protect the patient from injury by raising and padding his bed rails. Provide an uncluttered environment if he's ambulatory.

Typically transient, a pericardial friction rub is a scratching, grating, or crunching sound that occurs when two inflamed layers of the pericardium slide over one another. Ranging from faint to loud, this abnormal sound is heard best along the lower left sternal border during deep inspiration.

A pericardial friction rub indicates pericarditis, which can result from acute infection, cardiac and renal disorders, postpericardiotomy syndrome, and certain drugs, such as procainamide and antineoplastic agents.

Occasionally, it can resemble a murmur or a pleural friction rub.

## History
Obtain a complete medical history, noting especially cardiac dysfunction. Has the patient recently had a myocardial infarction or cardiac surgery? Has he ever had pericarditis or rheumatic disorders, such as rheumatoid arthritis or systemic lupus erythematosus? Does he have chronic renal failure or an infection? If the patient complains of chest pain, ask him to describe its character and location. What relieves the pain? What worsens it?

## Physical exam
Take the patient's vital signs, noting especially hypotension, tachycardia, irregular pulse rate, tachypnea, and fever. Inspect for jugular vein distention, edema, ascites, and hepatomegaly. Auscultate the lungs for crackles.

## Causes
*Acute pericarditis.* A pericardial friction rub is the hallmark of this disorder, which also causes sharp precordial or retrosternal pain that usually radiates to the left shoulder and neck. The pain worsens when the patient breathes deeply, coughs, lies flat or, possibly, when he swallows. It abates when he sits up and leans forward. He may also have fever, dyspnea, tachycardia, and arrhythmias.

*Chronic constrictive pericarditis.* A pericardial friction rub develops gradually. It's accompanied by signs of decreased cardiac filling and output, such as peripheral edema, ascites, jugular vein distention on inspiration (Kussmaul's sign), and hepatomegaly. Dyspnea, orthopnea, pulsus paradoxus, and chest pain may also occur.

## Nursing considerations
• Continue to monitor the patient's cardiovascular status. If the pericardial friction rub disappears, be alert for signs of cardiac tamponade: pallor; cool, clammy skin; hypotension; tachycardia; tachypnea; pulsus paradoxus; and increased jugular vein distention. If these signs occur, prepare the patient for pericardiocentesis to prevent cardiovascular collapse.
• Ensure that the patient gets adequate rest. As ordered, give anti-inflammatory drugs, antiarrhythmics, diuretics, or antimicrobials to treat the underlying cause. If necessary, prepare him for a pericardiectomy to promote adequate cardiac filling and contraction.

Painful or difficult urination, dysuria is commonly accompanied by urinary frequency, urgency, or hesitancy. It usually reflects lower urinary tract infection—a common disorder, especially in women. Dysuria also results from lower urinary tract irritation or inflammation, which stimulates nerve endings in the bladder and urethra.

## History

Have the patient describe the severity and location of dysuria. Ask him when he first noticed it, what precipitates it, and if anything aggravates or alleviates it. Ask about previous urinary or genital tract infections; invasive procedures, such as cystoscopy or urethral dilatation; and a history of intestinal disease. Ask the female patient about menstrual disorders and the use of products that irritate the urinary tract, such as bath salts, feminine deodorants, contraceptive gels, and perineal lotions.

## Physical exam

During the physical examination, inspect the urethral meatus for discharge, irritation, and other abnormalities. Assist the doctor with a pelvic or rectal examination, as ordered.

## Causes

*Bladder cancer.* Dysuria is a late symptom in this mostly male disorder. Findings include urinary frequency and urgency, nocturia, hematuria, and perineal, back, or flank pain.

*Chemical irritants.* Dysuria may result from irritating substances, such as bubble bath salts and feminine deodorants. It's usually most intense at the end of voiding. Other features may include urinary frequency and urgency, diminished urine stream and, possibly, hematuria.

*Cystitis.* Dysuria throughout voiding is common in all types of cystitis, as are urinary urgency and frequency, flank pain, nocturia, straining to void, and hematuria.

*Paraurethral gland inflammation.* Dysuria throughout voiding occurs with urinary frequency and urgency, diminished urine stream, mild perineal pain and, occasionally, hematuria.

*Prostatitis.* Dysuria occurs throughout or toward the end of voiding, accompanied by diminished urine stream, urinary frequency and urgency, hematuria, perineal fullness, fever, chills, fatigue, myalgia, nausea, vomiting, and constipation.

*Pyelonephritis (acute).* Dysuria occurs throughout voiding. Other features include high fever with chills, costovertebral angle tenderness, flank pain, weakness, urinary urgency and frequency, nocturia, and hematuria.

*Reiter's syndrome.* In this male disorder, dysuria occurs 1 to 2 weeks after sexual contact. Other findings include mucopurulent discharge, urinary urgency and frequency, meatal swelling and redness, suprapubic pain, anorexia, weight loss, and low-grade fever.

*Urethral syndrome.* This syndrome occurs in women and mimics urethritis. Dysuria throughout voiding may occur with urinary frequency, diminished urine stream, suprapubic aching and cramping, tenesmus, low back and unilateral flank pain.

*Urethritis.* This primarily male infection causes dysuria throughout voiding. It's accompanied by a reddened meatus and a yellow, purulent discharge (gonorrheal infection) or a white or clear mucoid discharge (nongonorrheal infection).

*Urinary obstruction.* Outflow obstruction by urethral strictures or calculi produces dysuria throughout voiding.

*Vaginitis.* Dysuria occurs throughout voiding as urine touches inflamed or ulcerated labia. Other findings include urinary frequency and urgency, nocturia, hematuria, perineal pain, and vaginal discharge.

*Other causes.* Appendicitis, diverticulitis, monoamine oxidase inhibitors, and metyrosine.

## Nursing considerations

• Monitor vital signs, intake, and output. Administer drugs, as ordered, and prepare the patient for such tests as urinalysis and cystoscopy.

Also called "orange-peel" skin, peau d'orange refers to the edematous thickening and pitting of skin on the breasts. Usually a late sign of breast cancer, peau d'orange develops slowly and can also occur with breast or axillary lymph node infection. Its striking orange-peel appearance stems from development of lymphatic edema around deepened hair follicles.

## History
Ask the patient when she first detected peau d'orange and whether she has noticed any lumps, pain, or other breast changes. Does she have related symptoms, such as malaise and achiness? Is she lactating or has she recently weaned her infant?

## Physical exam
Examine the patient's breasts. Estimate the extent of the peau d'orange and check for erythema. Assess the nipples for discharge, deviation, retraction, dimpling, and cracking. Then gently palpate the area of peau d'orange, noting warmth or induration. Next, palpate the entire breast, noting any fixed or mobile lumps, and the axillary lymph nodes, noting enlargement. Finally, take the patient's temperature.

## Causes
*Breast abscess.* Usually affecting lactating women with milk stasis, this infection causes peau d'orange, malaise, breast tenderness and erythema, and a sudden fever that may be accompanied by shaking chills. A cracked nipple may exude pus, and an indurated or palpable soft mass may be present.

*Breast cancer.* Advanced breast cancer is the most likely cause of peau d'orange, which usually begins in the dependent part of the breast or the areola. Palpation typically reveals a firm, immobile mass that adheres to the skin above the area of peau d'orange. Inspection of the breasts may reveal changes in contour, size, or symmetry. Inspection of the nipples may reveal deviation, erosion, or retraction. The nipples may exude a thin and watery, bloody, or purulent discharge. The patient may report a burning and itching sensation in the nipples; she also may feel a sensation of warmth or heat in the breast. Although the patient may complain of breast pain, this sign is not a reliable indicator of cancer.

*Tuberculosis of the axillary lymph nodes.* Rarely, peau d'orange occurs as one or more axillary lymph nodes enlarge. Nodal enlargement is usually painless but may be accompanied by mild fever, fatigue, and weight loss.

## Nursing considerations
• Because peau d'orange usually signals advanced breast cancer, you'll need to provide emotional support for the patient. Encourage her to express her fears and concerns.
• Clearly explain expected diagnostic tests, such as mammography and breast biopsy.

Also called otalgia, earache usually results from disorders of the external and middle ear associated with infection, obstruction, or trauma. Its severity ranges from a feeling of fullness or blockage to deep, boring pain. At times, it may be difficult to localize precisely. This common symptom may be intermittent or continuous and may develop suddenly or gradually.

## History
Ask the patient how long he has had an earache. Is it intermittent or continuous? Painful or slightly annoying? Can he localize the site of ear pain? Does he have pain in other areas, such as the jaw?

Ask about recent illnesses or ear injury. Does swimming or showering trigger ear pain? Does the ear itch? If so, find out where itching is most intense and when it began. Ask about ear drainage and, if present, have the patient characterize it. Does he have ringing or noise in his ears? Dizziness or vertigo? Difficulty swallowing, hoarseness, neck pain, or pain from opening the mouth?

## Physical exam
Inspect the external ear for redness, drainage, swelling, or deformity. Apply pressure to the mastoid process and tragus to elicit tenderness. Using an otoscope, check the external auditory canal for lesions, bleeding or discharge, impacted cerumen, foreign bodies, tenderness, or swelling. Examine the tympanic membrane and look for landmarks: cone of light, umbo, pars tensa, and malleus's handle and short process. Perform watch tick, Rinne, and Weber's tests to detect hearing loss.

## Causes
*Ear canal obstruction.* An obstruction by a foreign body (such as an insect) may cause severe pain.

*Mastoiditis (acute).* This bacterial infection causes a dull ache behind the ear, low-grade fever, and thick, purulent discharge. The eardrum appears dull and edematous and may be perforated.

*Otitis externa.* Acute otitis externa begins with mild to moderate ear pain that occurs with tragus manipulation. The pain may occur with low-grade fever, sticky yellow or purulent ear discharge, partial hearing loss, and a feeling of blockage. Later, ear pain intensifies and fever may reach 104° F (40° C). Examination reveals swelling of the tragus, external meatus, and external canal; eardrum erythema; and lymphadenopathy. The patient also complains of dizziness and malaise.

*Malignant otitis externa* abruptly causes ear pain that's aggravated by moving the auricle or tragus. The pain occurs with intense itching, purulent ear discharge, fever, parotid gland swelling, and trismus. Examination reveals a swollen external canal with exposed cartilage and temporal bone.

*Otitis media (acute).* Acute serous otitis media may cause a feeling of fullness in the ear, hearing loss, and a vague sensation of top-heaviness. The eardrum may be slightly retracted, amber-colored, and marked by air bubbles and a meniscus, or it may be blue-black from hemorrhage.

Severe, deep, throbbing ear pain and fever that may reach 102° F (38.9° C) characterize *acute suppurative otitis media.* The pain increases steadily over several hours or days and may be aggravated by pressure on the mastoid antrum. Typically, the patient experiences mild hearing loss, slight dizziness, nausea, and vomiting. Rupture causes purulent drainage and relieves the pain.

*Temporomandibular joint infection.* Typically unilateral, this infection produces ear pain that's referred from the jaw joint. The pain is aggravated by jaw movement and commonly radiates.

*Other causes.* Acute barotrauma, cerumen impaction, chondrodermatitis nodularis chronica helicis, extradural abscess, frostbite, furunculosis, herpes zoster oticus, keratosis obturans, Ménière's disease, middle ear tumor, myringitis bullosa, perichondritis, and petrositis.

## Nursing considerations
Give analgesics and apply heat to relieve pain. Instill eardrops, if necessary. Teach the patient how to instill drops if prescribed for home use.

An early sign of left ventricular failure, paroxysmal nocturnal dyspnea is an attack of dyspnea that abruptly awakens the patient and commonly causes diaphoresis, coughing, and wheezing. Dramatic and terrifying, it usually abates after the patient sits up or stands for several minutes but may recur every 2 to 3 hours.

Paroxysmal nocturnal dyspnea can reflect decreased respiratory drive, impaired left ventricular function, enhanced reabsorption of interstitial fluid, and increased thoracic blood volume. All of these pathophysiologic mechanisms cause dyspnea to worsen when the patient lies down.

## History

Begin by exploring the patient's complaint of dyspnea. Does he have a dyspneic attack at other times, such as after exertion or while sitting down? If so, what type of activity triggers the attack? Does he experience coughing, wheezing, fatigue, or weakness during an attack? Find out if the patient sleeps with his head elevated and, if so, on how many pillows. Obtain a cardiopulmonary history. Does the patient or a family member have a history of myocardial infarction, coronary artery disease, or hypertension? Chronic bronchitis, emphysema, or asthma? Has the patient had cardiac surgery?

## Physical exam

Take the patient's vital signs and form an overall impression of his appearance. Is he noticeably cyanotic or edematous? Auscultate the lungs for crackles and wheezing. Auscultate the heart for gallops and arrhythmias.

## Cause

*Left ventricular failure.* Dyspnea upon exertion, during sleep, and even at rest is an early sign of left ventricular failure. It's characteristically accompanied by Cheyne-Stokes respirations, diaphoresis, weakness, wheezing, and a persistent, nonproductive cough or a cough that produces clear or blood-tinged sputum.

As the patient's condition worsens, he develops tachycardia, tachypnea, pulsus alternans (typically initiated by a premature beat), a ventricular gallop, and crackles.

In advanced left ventricular failure, the patient may also have severe orthopnea, cyanosis, clubbing, hemoptysis, and cardiac arrhythmias. He may also develop signs and symptoms of shock, such as hypotension, weak pulse, and cold, clammy skin.

## Nursing considerations

• Prepare the patient for diagnostic tests, such as chest X-ray, echocardiography, exercise electrocardiography, and cardiac blood pool imaging.
• If the hospitalized patient experiences paroxysmal nocturnal dyspnea, help him into a sitting position or assist him in walking around the room.
• If necessary, provide low-flow supplemental oxygen. Try to keep the patient calm because anxiety can exacerbate dyspnea.

A common sign in severely ill patients, generalized edema is the excessive accumulation of interstitial fluid throughout the body. Its severity varies widely; slight edema may be difficult to detect, especially if the patient is obese, whereas massive edema is immediately apparent.

Typically, generalized edema is chronic and progressive. It may stem from cardiac, renal, endocrine, or hepatic disorders; severe burns; or drug effects. Common causes are hypoalbuminemia and excess sodium ingestion or retention — both of which influence plasma osmotic pressure.

▶ **Emergency interventions**

Assess edema's severity, including degree of pitting. If the patient has severe edema, take vital signs and check for distended neck veins and cyanotic lips. Auscultate lungs and heart. If you hear signs of pulmonary congestion or heart failure, such as crackles or ventricular gallop, notify the doctor. Put the patient in Fowler's position to promote lung expansion, unless he's hypotensive. Prepare to give oxygen and I.V. diuretics. Have resuscitation equipment nearby.

## History

When the patient's condition permits, obtain a full history. Note when edema began. Is it affected by position changes? Accompanied by dyspnea or arm or leg pain? Find out how much weight the patient has gained. Has his urine output changed?

Next, ask about previous burns or cardiac, renal, hepatic, endocrine, or GI disorders. Explore his drug history and note recent I.V. therapy.

## Physical exam

Compare arms and legs for symmetrical edema. Note ecchymoses and cyanosis. Assess the bedridden patient's back, sacrum, and hips for dependent edema. Palpate peripheral pulses, noting if his hands and feet feel cold. Perform a complete cardiopulmonary assessment.

## Causes

*Angioneurotic edema.* Recurrent attacks of acute, painless, pitting edema affect skin and mucous membranes (especially of the respiratory tract).

*Burns.* Edema and associated tissue damage vary with burn severity. Severe generalized edema (4 +) may occur within 2 days of a major burn.

*Congestive heart failure.* Severe, pitting, generalized edema — occasionally anasarca — may follow leg edema late in this disorder. The edema may improve with exercise or limb elevation. Other classic late findings: hemoptysis, cyanosis, marked hepatomegaly, crackles, and ventricular gallop.

*Drugs.* Any drug that causes sodium retention may aggravate or produce generalized edema. Some examples: antihypertensives, corticosteroids, androgenic and anabolic steroids, estrogens, and nonsteroidal anti-inflammatory drugs.

*Myxedema.* In this severe form of hypothyroidism, nonpitting generalized edema occurs with dry, waxy, pale skin. Other findings: masklike facies, hair loss or coarsening, hoarseness, weight gain, fatigue, cold intolerance, bradycardia, constipation, impotence, and infertility.

*Nephrotic syndrome.* Pitting generalized edema is characteristic. In severe cases, anasarca develops. Other common features: ascites, anorexia, fatigue, malaise, depression, and pallor.

*Other causes.* Cirrhosis, I.V. infusions and feedings, malnutrition, pericardial effusion, pericarditis (chronic constrictive), protein-wasting enteropathy, renal failure, and septic shock.

## Nursing considerations

• Position the patient with his limbs above heart level to promote drainage. If he develops dyspnea, lower his limbs, elevate the head of the bed, and give oxygen. Massage reddened areas. Prevent skin breakdown by placing a pressure mattress or lamb's wool pad on the patient's bed.
• Restrict fluids and sodium, and give diuretics or I.V. albumin, as ordered. Monitor intake, output, daily weight, and serum electrolyte (especially sodium) and albumin levels.

Commonly described as numbness, prickling, or tingling, paresthesia is an abnormal sensation felt along peripheral nerve pathways. Generally painless, this sensation commonly occurs in many neurologic disorders and may also result from certain systemic disorders and the effects of drugs.

## History
Ask the patient when the paresthesia began and have him describe its character and distribution. Take a medical history, including neurologic, cardiovascular, metabolic, renal, and chronic inflammatory disorders, such as arthritis or lupus. Also find out if the patient sustained trauma or had recent surgery or invasive procedures that may have injured peripheral nerves.

## Physical exam
Assess the patient's level of consciousness and cranial nerve function. Test muscle strength and deep tendon reflexes in limbs. Evaluate touch, pain, temperature, vibration, and position sensation. Note skin color and temperature. Palpate pulses.

## Causes
*Arterial occlusion (acute).* Sudden paresthesia and coldness may develop in one or both legs with a saddle embolus. Other findings may include intermittent claudication and aching pain at rest.

*Arteriosclerosis obliterans.* This disorder produces paresthesia, intermittent claudication, diminished or absent popliteal and pedal pulses, pallor, paresis, and coldness in the affected leg.

*Brain tumor.* Tumors affecting the parietal lobe may cause progressive contralateral paresthesia accompanied by agnosia, apraxia, agraphia, homonymous hemianopia, and loss of proprioception.

*Buerger's disease.* Exposure to cold makes the feet cold, cyanotic, and numb; later, they redden, become hot, and tingle. Intermittent claudication, which is aggravated by exercise, is also common.

*Guillain-Barré syndrome.* Transient paresthesia may precede muscle weakness, which usually begins in the legs and ascends to the arms and facial nerves.

*Herpes zoster.* Paresthesia occurs early in the dermatome supplied by the affected spinal nerve. Other findings include pruritic, erythematous rash and sharp, shooting pain.

*Rabies.* Prodromal signs include paresthesia, coldness, and itching at the site of an animal bite.

*Raynaud's disease.* Rewarming of pale, cold fingers causes paresthesia and redness.

*Seizure disorders.* Seizures originating in the parietal lobe usually cause paresthesia of the lips, fingers, and toes. Paresthesia may also be an aura that warns of tonic-clonic seizures.

*Spinal cord injury.* Paresthesia may occur in partial spinal cord transection after spinal shock resolves. It may be unilateral or bilateral, occurring at or below the level of the lesion.

*Spinal cord tumors.* Typically, these tumors produce paresthesia, paresis, pain, and variable sensory loss along the nerve distribution pathway served by the affected cord segment.

*Thoracic outlet syndrome.* Paresthesia occurs suddenly in this syndrome when the affected arm is raised and abducted. The arm also becomes pale and cool with diminished pulses.

*Transient ischemic attack.* Typically, paresthesia occurs abruptly in an attack and is limited to one arm or another isolated part of the body.

*Other causes.* Arthritis, cerebrovascular accident; drugs, such as phenytoin, chemotherapeutic agents, D-penicillamine, isoniazid, nitrofurantoin, chloroquine, and parenteral gold therapy; heavy metal or solvent poisoning; herniated disk; hyperventilation syndrome; hypocalcemia; long-term radiation therapy; migraine headache; multiple sclerosis; peripheral nerve trauma; peripheral neuropathy; systemic lupus erythematosus; tabes dorsalis; and vitamin $B_{12}$ deficiency.

## Nursing considerations
• Teach the patient how to avoid injuries from sensory loss.

The result of excess interstitial fluid in the arm, this edema may be unilateral or bilateral and may develop gradually or abruptly. It may be aggravated by immobility and alleviated by arm elevation and exercise. Arm edema signals localized fluid imbalance between vascular and interstitial spaces. Commonly, it results from trauma, venous disorders, toxins, and treatments.

## History
When taking the patient's history, one of the first questions to ask is, "How long has your arm been swollen?" Then find out if the patient also has arm pain, numbness, or tingling. Does exercise or arm elevation decrease the edema? Ask about recent arm injury, such as burns or insect stings. Also note recent I.V. therapy or breast surgery.

## Physical exam
Assess the edema's severity by comparing the size and symmetry of both arms. Use a tape measure to determine the exact girth. Note whether the edema is unilateral or bilateral, and test for pitting. Next, assess and compare the color and temperature of both arms. Look for erythema and for ecchymoses or wounds that suggest injury. Palpate and compare radial and brachial pulses. Finally, assess for arm tenderness and decreased mobility. If you detect signs of neurovascular compromise, elevate the arm and notify the doctor immediately.

## Causes
*Angioneurotic edema.* This common reaction is characterized by sudden onset of painless, nonpruritic edema affecting the hands, feet, eyelids, lips, face, neck, genitalia, or viscera. Although these swellings usually don't itch, they may burn and tingle.

*Arm trauma.* Shortly after a crush injury, severe edema may affect the entire arm. Ecchymoses or superficial bleeding, pain or numbness, and paralysis may occur.

*Burns.* Two days or less after injury, arm burns may cause mild to severe edema, pain, and tissue damage.

*Envenomization.* Initially, envenomization by snakes, aquatic animals, or insects may cause edema around the bite or sting that quickly spreads to the entire arm. Pain at the site is common, as are erythema, pruritus, and, occasionally, paresthesia. Later, generalized signs and symptoms may develop, such as nausea, vomiting, weakness, muscle cramps, fever, chills, hypotension, headache and, in severe cases, dyspnea, seizures, and paralysis.

*Superior vena cava syndrome.* Usually, bilateral arm edema progresses slowly and is accompanied by facial and neck edema. Dilated veins mark these edematous areas. The patient also complains of headache, vertigo, and visual disturbances.

*Thrombophlebitis.* This disorder may cause arm edema, pain, and warmth. *Deep vein thrombophlebitis* can also produce cyanosis, fever, chills, and malaise, whereas *superficial thrombophlebitis* also causes redness, tenderness, and induration along the vein.

*Treatments.* Localized arm edema may result from infiltration of I.V. fluid into the interstitial tissue. A radical or modified radical mastectomy that disrupts lymphatic drainage may cause edema of the entire arm. Also, radiation therapy for breast cancer may produce arm edema immediately after treatment or months later.

## Nursing considerations
• Treatment reflects the underlying cause. However, general measures include arm elevation, frequent repositioning, and appropriate use of bandages and dressings to promote drainage and circulation.
• Provide meticulous skin care to prevent breakdown and pressure sores.
• Give prescribed drugs, such as analgesics and anticoagulants.

Total loss of voluntary motor function, paralysis results from severe cortical or pyramidal tract damage. It occurs in cerebrovascular disorders, degenerative neuromuscular disease, trauma, tumors, or central nervous system infection.

## ▶ Emergency interventions

If sudden paralysis occurs, suspect trauma or an acute vascular insult. After immobilizing the patient's spine, assess his level of consciousness (LOC) and take vital signs. Elevated systolic blood pressure, widening pulse pressure, and bradycardia may signal increasing intracranial pressure; notify the doctor immediately. Assess the patient's respiratory status; be prepared to administer oxygen, insert an artificial airway, or assist with intubation and mechanical ventilation, as needed.

## History

Ask the patient about the onset, duration, and intensity of paralysis, and the events preceding its development. Note any fever, headache, visual disturbances, dysphagia, bowel or bladder dysfunction, muscle pain or weakness, or fatigue.

## Physical exam

Perform a complete neurologic examination, testing cranial nerve, motor, and sensory function, and deep tendon reflexes. Assess strength in all major muscle groups, and note any muscle atrophy.

## Causes

*Amyotrophic lateral sclerosis.* Spastic or flaccid paralysis in the body's major muscle groups eventually progresses to total paralysis. Other findings include muscle atrophy, dyspnea, and possibly respiratory distress.

*Brain abscess.* Hemiplegia — along with ocular disturbances, unequal pupils, and decreased LOC — suggests frontal or temporal lobe abscess.

*Brain tumor.* A tumor affecting the frontal lobe may cause contralateral hemiparesis that progresses to hemiplegia. Early findings may include frontal headache and behavioral changes.

*Cerebrovascular accident.* Paralysis may occur along with headache, vomiting, seizures, decreased LOC, dysarthria, dysphagia, visual disturbances, and bowel and bladder dysfunction.

*Guillain-Barré syndrome.* Reversible ascending paralysis develops rapidly. Leg muscle weakness leads to dysphagia, nasal speech, and dysarthria.

*Multiple sclerosis.* Paralysis commonly waxes and wanes but may later become permanent.

*Myasthenia gravis.* Paralysis is usually transient in early stages but becomes more persistent as the disease progresses.

*Poliomyelitis.* This disorder can cause insidious, permanent flaccid paralysis and hyporeflexia.

*Rabies.* Progressive flaccid paralysis, vascular collapse, coma, and death occur within 2 weeks of initial infection. Prodromal findings include fever, headache, paresthesia, photophobia, and excessive salivation, lacrimation, and perspiration.

*Spinal cord injury.* Spinal cord transection results in permanent spastic paralysis below the level of injury. Partial transection causes variable paralysis and paresthesia.

*Subarachnoid hemorrhage.* Sudden paralysis occurs, along with severe headache, mydriasis, photophobia, aphasia, sharply decreased LOC, and nuchal rigidity.

*Other causes.* Bell's palsy, botulism, conversion disorder, electroconvulsive therapy, encephalitis, head trauma, migraine headache, neuromuscular blocking agents, neurosyphilis, Parkinson's disease, peripheral nerve trauma, peripheral neuropathy, seizure disorders, spinal cord tumor, syringomyelia, thoracic aortic aneurysm, and transient ischemic attacks.

## Nursing considerations

• Provide frequent position changes, meticulous skin care, and frequent chest physiotherapy.
• If the patient has difficulty chewing and swallowing, provide a liquid or soft diet, and keep suction equipment on hand. Consider using feeding tubes or total parenteral nutrition.

Facial edema refers to a generalized swelling encompassing the face and possibly extending to the neck and upper arms. Occasionally painful, this sign may develop gradually or abruptly. At times, it precedes onset of peripheral or generalized edema. Mild edema may be difficult to detect.

Facial edema stems from disruption of the hydrostatic and osmotic pressures that govern fluid movement between the arteries, veins, and lymphatics. It may result from venous, inflammatory, and certain systemic disorders; trauma; allergy; or the effects of drugs, tests, and treatments.

▶ **Emergency interventions**
If the patient has facial edema caused by burns or if he reports recent allergen exposure, quickly assess his respiratory status: Edema may also affect his upper airway, causing life-threatening obstruction. If you detect wheezes, inspiratory stridor, or other signs of distress, notify the doctor and give epinephrine, as ordered. In severe distress — with absent breath sounds and cyanosis — assist with endotracheal intubation, cricothyroidotomy, or tracheotomy. Give oxygen, as ordered.

## History
If the patient isn't in severe distress, take his history. Ask if facial edema developed suddenly or gradually. Has he gained weight? If so, how much and over what duration? Has his urine color or output changed? Has his appetite? Take a drug history and ask about recent facial trauma.

## Physical exam
Characterize the edema. Does it affect the whole face? Part of it? Other body areas? Determine if it's pitting or nonpitting and grade its severity. Take vital signs and assess neurologic status.

## Causes
*Allergic reaction.* Facial edema may characterize local allergic reactions and anaphylaxis. In life-threatening anaphylaxis, angioneurotic facial edema may occur with urticaria and flushing. Airway edema causes hoarseness, stridor, and bronchospasm with dyspnea and tachypnea. Signs of shock may also occur. A localized reaction produces facial edema, erythema, and urticaria.

*Drugs.* Long-term use of glucocorticoids may produce facial edema. Any drug that causes an allergic reaction (such as aspirin, penicillin, and sulfa preparations) may have the same effect.

*Facial burns.* These may cause extensive edema that impairs respiration. Additional findings may include singed nasal hairs, red mucosa, sooty sputum, and signs of respiratory distress.

*Facial trauma.* In this disorder, edema depends on the type of injury. For example, contusion may cause localized edema, whereas nasal or maxillary fracture causes more generalized edema. Associated features also depend on the injury.

*Myxedema.* This disorder eventually causes generalized facial edema, waxy dry skin, hair loss or coarsening, and other signs of hypothyroidism.

*Nephrotic syndrome.* Often the first sign of this syndrome, periorbital edema precedes dependent and abdominal edema. Associated findings: weight gain, nausea, anorexia, lethargy, and pallor.

*Pregnancy-induced hypertension.* Edema of the face, hands, and ankles is an early sign of this disorder. Other characteristics include excessive weight gain, severe headache, blurred vision, hypertension, and midepigastric pain.

*Other causes.* Chalazion, conjunctivitis, contrast media for diagnostic tests, corneal ulcers (fungal), dacryoadenitis, dacryocystitis, herpes zoster ophthalmicus, malnutrition, osteomyelitis, peritonsillar abscess, rhinitis, sinusitis, stye, superior vena cava syndrome, surgery, and trachoma.

## Nursing considerations
• Give analgesics for facial edema and apply creams to reduce itching, as ordered.
• Unless contraindicated, apply cold compresses to the patient's eyes to decrease edema. Elevate the head of his bed to help drain the accumulated fluid.
• Prepare the patient for urine and blood tests.

# Papular rash

This rash consists of small, raised, circumscribed, and possibly discolored lesions known as papules. Acute or chronic, a papular rash may erupt anywhere on the body in various configurations. It is characteristic in many cutaneous disorders and may also result from allergies or from infectious, neoplastic, or systemic disorders.

## History
Find out when the rash erupted and if it has changed since then. Is it itchy or burning? Painful or tender? Have the patient describe associated signs and symptoms, such as fever, headache, and GI distress. Ask about allergies, previous skin disorders, infections, childhood diseases, sexually transmitted diseases, and neoplasms. Has the patient recently been bitten by an insect or rodent or been exposed to anyone with an infectious disease?

## Physical exam
Note the rash's color, configuration, and location.

## Causes
*Acne vulgaris.* Rupture of enlarged comedones produces inflamed and possibly painful and pruritic papules, pustules, nodules, or cysts on the face and occasionally on the shoulders, chest, and back.

*Insect bites.* Venom from insect bites—especially from ticks, lice, flies, and mosquitoes—may produce an allergic reaction associated with a papular, macular, or petechial rash. Other findings include fever, myalgia, headache, lymphadenopathy, nausea, and vomiting.

*Kaposi's sarcoma.* This neoplastic disorder produces purple or blue papules or macules on the extremities, ears, and nose. Firm pressure reduces lesion size; lesions return to original size in 10 to 15 seconds. Two variants—classic and acute generalized—affect elderly patients and those with acquired immunodeficiency syndrome.

*Psoriasis.* This disorder begins with small, erythematous papules on the scalp, chest, elbows, knees, back, buttocks, and genitalia. Papules are pruritic and may be painful. They enlarge and coalesce, forming elevated, red, scaly plaques covered by silver scales, except in moist areas such as the genitalia. The scales may flake off easily or thicken, covering the plaque. Other findings include pitted fingernails and arthralgia.

*Syphilis.* A discrete, reddish brown, mucocutaneous rash and general lymphadenopathy signal secondary syphilis. The rash may be papular, macular, pustular, or nodular. It erupts between rolls of fat on the trunk and on the arms, palms, soles, face, and scalp. Lesions in warm, moist areas enlarge and erode, producing highly contagious, pink or grayish white condylomata lata.

*Systemic lupus erythematosus.* A "butterfly rash" of erythematous maculopapules or discoid plaques appears in a malar distribution across the nose and cheeks. Similar rashes may appear on exposed body areas. Other features include photosensitivity and nondeforming arthritis in the hands, feet, and large joints.

*Other causes.* Dermatomyositis; drugs, including antibiotics, sulfonamides, benzodiazepines, lithium, phenylbutazone, gold salts, allopurinol, isoniazid, and salicylates; erythema chronicum migrans; follicular mucinosis; Fox-Fordyce disease; gonococcemia; granuloma annulare; infectious mononucleosis; leprosy; lichen amyloidosis; lichen planus; mycosis fungoides; necrotizing vasculitis; parapsoriasis; perioral dermatitis; pityriasis rosea; pityriasis rubra pilaris; polymorphic light eruption; rat-bite fever; rosacea; sarcoidosis; seborrheic keratosis; and syringoma.

## Nursing considerations
• Advise the patient to keep his skin clean and dry; to wear loose-fitting, nonirritating clothing; and to avoid scratching his rash. Instruct him to report promptly any change in its color, size, or configuration and the onset of itching or bleeding. Have him avoid excessive direct sunlight and apply a protective sunscreen before going outdoors.

**P-Q**

This edema results when excess interstitial fluid accumulates in one or both legs. It may affect just the foot and ankle or extend to the thigh. This common sign may be slight or dramatic, pitting or nonpitting. It may result from venous disorders, trauma, and certain bone and cardiac disorders that disturb normal fluid balance. However, nonpathologic mechanisms may also cause it. Prolonged sitting, standing, or immobility may cause bilateral orthostatic edema. Usually, this pitting edema affects the foot and vanishes with rest and leg elevation. Increased venous pressure late in pregnancy may also cause ankle edema.

## History
Ask when leg edema began. Did it develop suddenly or gradually? Does it decrease if the patient raises his legs? Is it painful when touched? When he walks? Ask about recent surgery or illness that may have caused immobilization. Does he have a history of cardiovascular disease? Also ask about recent leg injury. Obtain a drug history.

## Physical exam
Assess each leg for pitting edema. Because leg edema may compromise arterial flow, palpate peripheral pulses to detect any insufficiency. Observe leg color and look for unusual vein patterns. Palpate for warmth, tenderness, or cords, and gently squeeze the calf muscle against the tibia to check for deep pain. If leg edema is unilateral, dorsiflex the foot to assess for Homans' sign. Note skin thickening or ulceration in the edematous areas.

## Causes
*Burns.* Within 2 days, leg burns may cause mild to severe edema, pain, and tissue damage.

*Congestive heart failure.* Bilateral leg edema is an early sign of right ventricular failure. Other findings: weight gain despite anorexia, nausea, hypotension, pallor, tachypnea, palpitations, ventricular gallop, and inspiratory crackles. Pitting ankle edema signals more advanced heart failure, as do hepatomegaly, hemoptysis, and cyanosis.

*Envenomization.* Mild to severe localized edema may develop suddenly at the site of a bite or sting, along with erythema, pain, urticaria, pruritus, and a burning sensation.

*Leg trauma.* Mild to severe localized edema may form around the trauma site.

*Osteomyelitis.* When this bone infection affects the lower leg, it usually produces localized, mild to moderate edema, which may spread to the adjacent joint. Typically, edema follows fever, local tenderness, and pain that worsens with leg movement.

*Thrombophlebitis.* Both deep and superficial vein thrombosis may cause sudden onset of unilateral mild to moderate edema. *Deep vein thrombophlebitis* may be asymptomatic or may cause mild to severe pain, warmth, and cyanosis in the affected leg as well as fever, chills, and malaise. *Superficial thrombophlebitis* typically causes pain, warmth, redness, tenderness, and induration along the affected vein.

*Venous insufficiency (chronic).* Unilateral or bilateral leg edema is moderate to severe. Initially, the edema is soft and pitting; later, it becomes hard as tissues thicken. Other signs include darkened skin and painless, easily infected stasis ulcers that develop around the ankle.

*Other causes.* Infiltration of the I.V. site and phlegmasia cerulea dolens.

## Nursing considerations
- Show the patient how to apply antiembolism stockings or bandages to promote venous return.
- Encourage leg exercises and provide analgesics as necessary.
- If ordered, apply a zinc-gelatin compression boot (Unna boot) to help reduce the edema.
- Have the patient avoid prolonged sitting or standing, and elevate his legs as necessary.
- Monitor intake and output, and check weight and leg circumference daily to detect change in edema.
- Prepare the patient for diagnostic tests, such as blood and urine studies and X-rays.

Normally unaware of his own heartbeat, a patient with palpitations may say that his heart is pounding, jumping, fluttering, or missing beats. Palpitations may be regular or irregular, fast or slow, paroxysmal or sustained. Usually, the patient feels them over the precordium or in the throat or neck.

Although usually insignificant, palpitations may result from cardiac and metabolic disorders and certain drugs. Nonpathologic palpitations may occur with a newly implanted prosthetic valve. Transient palpitations may accompany emotional or physical stress, or the use of stimulants, such as tobacco and caffeine.

## ▶ Emergency interventions

If the patient complains of palpitations, ask about dizziness and shortness of breath, then inspect for pale, cool, clammy skin. Take his vital signs, noting hypotension and irregular or abnormal pulse. If these signs are present, suspect cardiac arrhythmias and notify the doctor immediately. Prepare to begin cardiac monitoring, and start an I.V. line to administer antiarrhythmic drugs.

## History

Ask about cardiovascular or pulmonary disorders. Does the patient have a history of hypertension or hypoglycemia? Obtain a drug history. Has the patient recently started digitalis therapy? Also ask about caffeine, tobacco, and alcohol consumption. Then explore associated symptoms, such as weakness, fatigue, and anginal pain.

## Physical exam

Ask the patient to simulate the palpitations by tapping his finger. An irregular rhythm points to premature ventricular contractions; episodic racing suggests paroxysmal atrial tachycardia.

Auscultate for gallops, murmurs, and abnormal breath sounds.

## Causes

*Acute anxiety attack.* Palpitations may be accompanied by diaphoresis, facial flushing, and trembling. The patient usually hyperventilates, which may lead to dizziness, weakness, and syncope.

*Aortic insufficiency.* May produce sustained or paroxysmal palpitations, with anginal pain, pallor, and dyspnea. Strong, abrupt carotid pulsations may occur. Auscultatory findings may include Duroziez's sign; a large, diffuse apical heave; a decrescendo, high-pitched, and blowing diastolic murmur along the lower left sternal border; an early systolic murmur; and a ventricular gallop.

*Cardiac arrhythmias.* Paroxysmal or sustained palpitations may occur with dizziness, weakness, and fatigue. Other findings may include irregular, rapid, or slow pulse; decreased blood pressure; confusion; pallor; oliguria; and diaphoresis.

*Hypertension.* The patient may be asymptomatic or may complain of sustained palpitations alone or with headache, dizziness, tinnitus, and fatigue.

*Hypoglycemia.* In hypoglycemia, the sympathetic nervous system triggers epinephrine production, which may cause palpitations along with fatigue, irritability, hunger, cold sweats, tremors, tachycardia, anxiety, and headache.

*Mitral stenosis.* Early features include sustained palpitations with dyspnea and fatigue on exertion. Auscultation reveals a loud $S_1$ and a rumbling diastolic murmur at the apex. Related effects may include an atrial gallop and, later, orthopnea, dyspnea at rest, and paroxysmal nocturnal dyspnea.

*Thyrotoxicosis.* Sustained palpitations may accompany tachycardia, dyspnea, weight loss despite increased appetite, diarrhea, tremors, nervousness, diaphoresis, heat intolerance and, possibly, exophthalmos and an enlarged thyroid.

*Other causes.* Anemia; drugs, such as cardiac glycosides, sympathomimetics, ganglionic blockers, and atropine; hypocalcemia; mitral prolapse; and pheochromocytoma.

## Nursing considerations

• Prepare the patient for diagnostic tests, such as an ECG and chest X-ray.

Enophthalmos is the backward displacement of the eye into the orbit. This sign may develop suddenly or gradually. It may be severe or mild enough to go unnoticed by the patient. Most often, enophthalmos results from trauma. It may also result from severe dehydration and eye disorders. In the elderly patient, senile atrophy of orbital fat may produce physiologic enophthalmos.

Because enophthalmos allows the upper lid to droop over the sunken eye, it may be mistaken for ptosis. However, exophthalmometry can differentiate between these signs.

## History
Begin by asking the patient how long he's had enophthalmos. Is it accompanied by headache or eye pain? If so, ask him to describe its severity and location. Next, ask about a history of trauma, cancer, or other eye disorders.

## Physical exam
If you suspect an orbital fracture, do not open the patient's eye or place any pressure on the eyeball; this risks ocular laceration. Apply a metal (Fox) or plastic eye shield until the ophthalmologist can perform a complete exam.

Otherwise, perform a visual acuity test, with and without correction. Then evaluate extraocular muscle movements and assess intraocular pressure. Using a direct ophthalmoscope, check for papilledema and other abnormalities. Next, check pupil response to light. Also note eyelid drooping.

## Causes
*Dehydration.* Mild to severe enophthalmos may accompany severe dehydration. Typically, the patient also displays poor skin turgor, dry mucous membranes, extreme thirst, weight loss, fatigue, tachycardia, hypotension, nausea, vomiting, and diarrhea.

*Duane's syndrome.* In this congenital syndrome, transient enophthalmos occurs when the patient looks to the side. Visual acuity is usually normal, but horizontal eye movement is impaired.

*Greig's syndrome (craniofacial dystosis).* Typically, enophthalmos is accompanied by an abnormally wide distance between the pupils in this syndrome. Other common findings include mental deficiency, astigmatism, epicanthal folds, skull deformity and, occasionally, ocular deviation.

*Orbital fracture.* Here, enophthalmos may not be apparent until edema subsides. The affected eyeball is displaced down and in and is surrounded by ecchymosis. Other findings include diplopia in the affected eye, eye or head pain, subconjunctival hemorrhage, and a dilated or unreactive pupil.

*Parinaud's syndrome.* In this form of ophthalmoplegia, enophthalmos is accompanied by nystagmus when the patient tries to look up. Ocular muscles show absent voluntary movement but normal conjugate movement. Other signs include lid retraction, ptosis, dilated pupils with poor or absent light response, and papilledema.

*Parry-Romberg syndrome.* This syndrome produces enophthalmos and, possibly, irises that differ in color. The patient may have facial hemiatrophy, miotic pupils with a sluggish response to dim light, nystagmus, ocular muscle paralysis, and ptosis.

## Nursing considerations
• Regularly monitor vital signs and assess pupillary response to light.
• As ordered, prepare the trauma patient for skull X-rays and eye examination.

An abnormal paleness or loss of skin color, pallor may develop suddenly or gradually. Generalized pallor affects the entire body but is most apparent on the face, conjunctiva, oral mucosa, and nail beds. Localized pallor commonly affects a single limb. The detectability of pallor varies with skin color and the thickness and vascularity of underlying tissue. Pallor may result from anemia, its chief cause, or from reduced peripheral blood flow.

▶ **Emergency interventions**

If the patient suddenly develops generalized pallor, quickly assess for signs of shock. Notify the doctor immediately and prepare to infuse fluids or blood rapidly. Keep emergency resuscitation equipment nearby.

### History

Ask the patient if he or anyone in his family has a history of anemia or a chronic disorder, such as renal failure, congestive heart failure, or diabetes, that might lead to anemia. Ask about the patient's diet. Ask when the patient first noticed the pallor, whether it's constant or intermittent, and if it occurs when he's exposed to the cold. Determine if the patient is under emotional stress.

Explore other signs and symptoms, such as dizziness, fainting, weakness and fatigue on exertion, chest pain, palpitations, menstrual irregularities, or loss of libido. If the pallor is confined to one or both legs, ask if walking is painful, or if his legs feel cold or numb. If the pallor is confined to his fingers, ask about tingling and numbness.

### Physical exam

Take the patient's vital signs, checking for orthostatic hypotension. Auscultate the heart for gallops and murmurs. Auscultate the lungs for crackles. Check the patient's skin temperature; cold extremities commonly occur with vasoconstriction or arterial occlusion. Note skin ulceration, and palpate peripheral pulses.

### Causes

*Anemia.* Pallor usually develops gradually. The patient's skin may also appear sallow or grayish. Other effects may include fatigue, dyspnea, tachycardia, bounding pulse, atrial gallop, systolic bruit over the carotid arteries, crackles, and bleeding tendencies.

*Arterial occlusion (acute).* Pallor develops abruptly in the affected extremity and is usually the result of an embolus. A line of demarcation separates the cool, pale skin below the occlusion from the normal skin above it. Severe pain, intense intermittent claudication, paresthesia, and paresis in the affected extremity may also occur.

*Arterial occlusive disease (chronic).* Pallor is usually specific to an extremity. It develops gradually and is aggravated by elevating the extremity. Other findings include intermittent claudication, weakness, cool skin, diminished pulses, and possibly ulceration and gangrene.

*Frostbite.* Pallor is localized to the frostbitten area. Typically, the area feels cold, waxy and, in deep frostbite, hard. The skin doesn't blanch, and sensation may be absent. As it thaws, the skin turns purplish blue. If frostbite is severe, blistering and gangrene may follow.

*Raynaud's disease.* The fingers abruptly turn pale, then cyanotic with exposure to cold or stress; with rewarming, they become red and paresthetic. In chronic disease, ulceration may occur.

*Shock.* Initially, shock causes acute pallor and cool, clammy skin. In hypovolemic shock, other early signs include restlessness, thirst, slight tachycardia, and tachypnea. In cardiogenic shock, the signs and symptoms are more profound.

*Other causes.* Arrhythmias, orthostatic hypotension, and vasopressor syncope.

### Nursing considerations

• Prepare the patient with chronic generalized pallor for blood studies and, possibly, bone marrow biopsy. If the patient has localized pallor, he may require arteriography.

Usually, enuresis refers to nighttime urinary incontinence in a girl over age 5 or a boy over age 6. Rarely, this sign may continue into adulthood. It's most common in boys and may be classified as primary or secondary. *Primary enuresis* describes the child who has never achieved bladder control; *secondary enuresis* describes the child who achieved bladder control for at least 3 months but has since lost it.

Factors that may contribute to enuresis include delayed development of detrusor muscle control, unusually deep or sound sleep, organic disorders such as urinary tract infection or obstruction, and psychological stress. Probably the most important factor, psychological stress commonly results from the birth of a sibling, the death of a parent or loved one, or premature, rigorous toilet training. The child may be embarrassed or ashamed, which intensifies stress and makes enuresis more likely — thus creating a vicious cycle.

## History

When taking a history, consult the parents as well as the child. First, determine the number of nights each week or month that the child wets the bed. Is there a family history of enuresis? Ask about the child's daily fluid intake. Does he drink much after supper? What are his typical sleep and voiding patterns?

Find out if the child has ever had control of his bladder. If so, try to pinpoint what may have precipitated enuresis, such as an organic disorder or psychological stress. Does the bed-wetting occur at home and away from home?

Ask the parents how they have tried to manage the problem and have them describe the child's toilet training. Observe the child's and parents' attitudes toward bed-wetting. Finally, ask the child if it hurts when he urinates.

## Physical exam

Check for signs of neurologic or urinary tract disorders. Observe the child's gait to assess for motor dysfunction. Also test sensory function in the legs. Inspect the urethral meatus for erythema and obtain a urine specimen. Assist the doctor with a rectal examination to assess sphincter control.

## Causes

*Detrusor muscle hyperactivity.* Involuntary detrusor muscle contractions may cause primary or secondary enuresis associated with urinary urgency, frequency, and incontinence. Signs and symptoms of urinary tract infection are also common.

*Urinary tract infection.* In children, most urinary tract infections produce secondary enuresis. Associated features include urinary frequency and urgency, dysuria, straining to urinate, and hematuria. Lower back pain, fatigue, and suprapubic discomfort may also occur.

*Urinary tract obstruction.* Although daytime incontinence occurs more frequently, this disorder may produce primary or secondary enuresis. It may also cause flank and lower back pain; upper abdominal distention; urinary frequency, urgency, hesitancy, and dribbling; dysuria; diminished urine stream; hematuria; and variable urine output.

## Nursing considerations

• Provide emotional support for the child and his family. Encourage the parents to accept and support the child, and tell them how to manage enuresis at home.

• If the child has detrusor muscle hyperactivity, bladder training may help control enuresis. Another treatment uses a moisture-sensitive device that fits in the child's mattress and triggers an alarm when the mattress becomes wet. The alarm wakes the child immediately, conditioning him to avoid bed-wetting. This device is most useful for the child over age 8.

Drainage from the ear, otorrhea may be bloody, purulent, clear, or serosanguineous. Its onset, duration, and severity provide clues to the underlying cause. Otorrhea may result from disorders of the external ear canal or middle ear, including allergy, infection, neoplasms, trauma, and collagen diseases. It may occur alone or with other symptoms, such as ear pain.

## History

Ask the patient when the otorrhea began and how he recognized it. Did he clean the drainage from within the ear canal, or did he wipe it from the auricle? Is the drainage clear, purulent, or bloody? Does it occur in one or both ears? Is it continuous or intermittent? Ask about associated symptoms, such as pain, tenderness, vertigo, and tinnitus.

Check the patient's history for recent upper respiratory infection or head trauma, cancer, dermatitis, or immunosuppressive therapy. Ask how he cleans his ears and if he's an avid swimmer.

## Physical exam

Inspect the external ear, applying pressure on the tragus and mastoid area to elicit tenderness. Insert an otoscope and observe for edema, erythema, crusts, or polyps. Inspect the tympanic membrane for color, perforation, absence of a light reflex, and bulging.

To test hearing, stand behind the patient, have him occlude one ear, then whisper. Have the patient repeat what he heard. Use a tuning fork to perform the Weber and Rinne tests. Then palpate the patient's neck and preauricular, parotid, and mastoid areas for lymphadenopathy. Finally, test cranial nerves VII, IX, X, and XI.

## Causes

*Allergy.* When associated with tympanic membrane perforation, allergy may cause clear or cloudy otorrhea, rhinorrhea, and itchy, watery eyes.

*Basilar skull fracture.* Otorrhea may be clear and watery (from cerebrospinal fluid [CSF] leakage) or bloody (from hemorrhage). Other findings may include hearing loss, CSF or bloody rhinorrhea, periorbital or mastoid ecchymosis, cranial nerve palsies, decreased level of consciousness, and headache.

*Mastoiditis.* Otorrhea is thick, purulent, yellow, and profuse. Other findings are low-grade fever, aching in the mastoid area and, possibly, conductive hearing loss.

*Otitis externa.* Acute otitis externa, or swimmer's ear, causes purulent, yellow, sticky, foul-smelling otorrhea and white-green debris in the external ear canal. Other findings include edema, erythema, pain, and itching; tenderness and swelling of surrounding nodes; and partial conductive

hearing loss. Chronic otitis externa causes scanty, intermittent otorrhea and itching.

*Otitis media.* In acute otitis media, tympanic membrane rupture produces bloody, purulent otorrhea and relieves pain. A conductive hearing loss usually worsens over several hours. Acute suppurative otitis media resembles an upper respiratory infection. Chronic otitis media causes intermittent, foul-smelling otorrhea; perforation of the tympanic membrane; and gradual hearing loss.

*Tumor.* A benign tumor may cause bloody otorrhea, and squamous cell carcinoma of the external ear causes purulent otorrhea with itching, pain, hearing loss, and, later, facial paralysis. Squamous cell carcinoma of the middle ear causes blood-tinged otorrhea with hearing loss on the affected side. Later, facial paralysis occurs.

*Other causes.* Aural polyps, dermatitis of the external ear canal, epidural abscess, myringitis, perichondritis, trauma, tuberculosis, and Wegener's granulomatosis.

## Nursing considerations

• As ordered, apply warm, moist heat to the patient's ears. Keep ear drops at room temperature.
• The patient with ear problems should avoid forceful nose blowing and should clean his ears with a washcloth only. Swimmers should wear earplugs and wash and dry their ears after swimming.

A common sign, epistaxis can be spontaneous or induced from the front or back of the nose. Most nosebleeds occur in the anterior-inferior nasal septum, but they may also occur at the point where the inferior turbinates meet the nasopharynx.

Commonly unilateral, nosebleeds range from mild oozing to severe blood loss. They can result from trauma, certain disorders, and certain drugs and treatments.

## ▶ Emergency interventions

If your patient has severe epistaxis, take his vital signs. If you detect signs of hypovolemic shock, such as tachycardia, notify the doctor. Insert a large-gauge I.V. line for rapid fluid and blood replacement, and attempt to control bleeding by pinching the nares closed. However, if you suspect nasal fracture, don't pinch the nares. Instead, place gauze under the nose to absorb blood.

Have the hypovolemic patient lie down and turn his head to the side to prevent blood aspiration. If the patient isn't hypovolemic, have him sit upright and tilt his head forward. Constantly check airway patency.

## History

If the patient isn't in distress, ask if he has had a traumatic injury or surgery recently. Ask about the number, severity, and length of nosebleeds.

Obtain a medical and drug history, noting use of anti-inflammatories, such as aspirin, and anticoagulants, such as warfarin.

## Physical exam

Inspect the skin for signs of bleeding, such as ecchymoses and petechiae. Assess the trauma patient for associated injuries. Assist the doctor with nasal examination.

## Causes

*Coagulation disorders.* These can cause epistaxis, ecchymoses, petechiae, and mouth and gum bleeding. Menorrhagia and signs of GI bleeding, such as melena and hematemesis, can occur.

*Drugs.* Anticoagulants and anti-inflammatories can cause epistaxis.

*Fracture.* Nasal or skull fracture can cause epistaxis. In *nasal fracture,* bilateral epistaxis occurs with nasal swelling, edema, pain, and deformity. In *skull fracture,* blood may flow directly down the nares or through the eustachian tube into the nose.

*Hypertension.* If severe, hypertension can cause extreme epistaxis with pulsation above the middle turbinate. Other findings: dizziness, throbbing headache, anxiety, peripheral edema, nocturia, nausea, vomiting, and drowsiness.

*Leukemia.* In *acute leukemia,* sudden epistaxis is accompanied by high fever and other abnormal

bleeding. In *chronic leukemia,* epistaxis and other abnormal bleeding are late signs.

*Maxillofacial injury.* A pumping arterial bleed usually causes severe epistaxis, facial pain and edema, diplopia, and other signs.

*Polycythemia vera.* A common sign of this disorder, spontaneous epistaxis may be accompanied by bleeding gums, ecchymosis, ruddy facial cyanosis, and other signs.

*Other causes.* Aplastic anemia, barotrauma, biliary obstruction, chemical irritants, cirrhosis, facial and nasal surgery, glomerulonephritis (chronic), hepatitis, hereditary hemorrhagic telangiectasia, infectious mononucleosis, influenza, juvenile angiofibroma, nasal tumors, orbital floor fracture, renal failure, sarcoidosis, scleroma, scurvy, sinusitis, sinus procedures, syphilis, systemic lupus erythematosus, and typhoid fever.

## Nursing considerations

• Monitor vital signs until bleeding is controlled.
• If external pressure doesn't control bleeding, help the doctor insert vasoconstrictor-impregnated cotton or anterior or posterior nasal packing.
• If the patient has posterior nasal packing, give humidified oxygen by face mask.
• Prepare the patient for a complete blood count, clotting studies or, if trauma occurred recently, X-rays.

A rare but reliable sign of infective endocarditis, Osler's nodes are tender, raised, pea-sized, red or purple lesions that erupt on the palms, soles, and especially the pads of the fingers and toes. The nodes usually develop after other signs and symptoms and disappear spontaneously within several days.

How and why Osler's nodes develop is uncertain. They may result from emboli caught in peripheral capillaries or may reflect an immunologic reaction to the causative organism. Osler's nodes must be distinguished from the less common Janeway's spots — small, painless, erythematous lesions that erupt on the palms and soles.

## History

If you discover Osler's nodes, explore the patient's history for clues to the cause of infective endocarditis. Has the patient had recent surgery or dental work? Invasive procedures of the urinary or gynecologic tract? Does he have a prosthetic valve or an arteriovenous fistula for hemodialysis? Note any history of cardiac disorders and murmurs, or a recent upper respiratory tract, skin, or urinary tract infection. Find out if the patient has been using intravenous drugs, and explore associated complaints, such as chills, fatigue, anorexia, and night sweats.

## Physical exam

After taking the patient's vital signs, auscultate the heart for murmurs and gallops. Also auscultate the lungs for crackles. Inspect the skin and mucous membranes for petechiae and other lesions. If you suspect intravenous drug abuse, inspect the patient's arms and other areas for needle tracks.

## Causes

*Acute infective endocarditis.* Occasionally, Osler's nodes develop in this disorder. Classic features include acute onset of high, intermittent fever with chills, and signs of congestive heart failure, such as dyspnea, peripheral edema, and distended jugular veins. Janeway's and Roth's spots are common; petechiae may also occur.

Embolization may occur abruptly, causing organ infarction or peripheral vascular occlusion with hematuria, chest or limb pain, paralysis, blindness, and other diverse effects.

*Subacute infective endocarditis.* Osler's nodes are characteristic in this form of endocarditis. A suddenly changing murmur or a new murmur is another cardinal sign. Associated signs and symptoms include intermittent fever, pallor, weakness, fatigue, arthralgia, night sweats, tachycardia, anorexia and weight loss, splenomegaly, clubbing, and petechiae. Occasionally, Janeway's spots, sub-

ungual splinter hemorrhages, and Roth's spots also appear. Signs of congestive heart failure may occur with extensive valvular damage.

Embolization may develop, producing signs and symptoms that vary with the location of the emboli.

## Nursing considerations

• Monitor the patient's vital signs to evaluate the effectiveness of antibiotic therapy against infective endocarditis.

• Later, discuss measures to prevent reinfection, such as prophylactic antibiotic administration before dental or invasive procedures.

# Eructation

Commonly called belching, eructation occurs when gas or acidic fluid escapes from the stomach, producing a characteristic sound. Depending on the cause, it may vary in duration and intensity.

Occasionally, this sign results from GI disorders. More often, though, it results from aerophagia—the unconscious swallowing of air—or from ingestion of gas-producing food. Eructation may relieve associated symptoms, most notably nausea, heartburn, or dyspepsia.

## History
Focus your history to help decipher the cause of eructation. Ask if belching occurs after drinking carbonated beverages. Does it occur immediately after eating or several hours later? Is it relieved by vomiting or antacids? By changing position?

Find out if the patient has associated abdominal pain. If so, ask him to describe its location, duration, and intensity. Also ask about recent weight loss, lack of appetite, heartburn, nausea, or vomiting. Has the patient noticed a change in his bowel habits? Does he have trouble breathing when he's lying down?

## Physical exam
Take the patient's vital signs. As you do so, note his facial expression and posture. Does he appear to guard his abdomen? Is he sitting still or moving about? Check for foul-smelling breath.

Inspect the patient's abdomen for distention or visible peristalsis. Auscultate for bowel sounds and characterize their motility. Then palpate or percuss for abdominal tenderness, rigidity, distention, and masses.

## Causes
*Abdominal lymphadenopathy.* The result of infectious or neoplastic disorders, enlarged abdominal lymph nodes may cause belching and other digestive effects, such as abdominal discomfort and distention, constipation, and jaundice. Edema, backache, and fever may also occur.

*Gastric outlet obstruction.* This common complication of duodenal ulcer disease causes eructation, epigastric fullness and discomfort, anorexia, nausea, and vomiting.

*Hiatal hernia.* In this disorder, eructation occurs after eating and is accompanied by heartburn, regurgitation of sour-tasting fluid, and abdominal distention. The patient complains of dull substernal or epigastric pain that may radiate to the shoulder. Other features include dysphagia, nausea, weight loss, dyspnea, tachypnea, cough, and halitosis.

*Peptic ulcer.* This common disorder may cause eructation. Its classic symptoms, though, are heartburn and gnawing or burning stomach pain that's relieved by food or antacids. Associated signs and symptoms may include nausea, vomiting, abdominal distention, and epigastric tenderness.

*Superior mesenteric artery syndrome (acute).* Eructation and halitosis are late signs of this uncommon syndrome. Typically, the eructation occurs after eating and is accompanied by regurgitation.

## Nursing considerations
• Place the patient in a side-lying or knee-chest position to help relieve eructation.
• To prevent aerophagia, advise him not to chew gum or smoke. If he's sensitive to gas-producing food, such as onions and cucumbers, adjust his diet as necessary.

Orthopnea — difficulty breathing in the supine position — is a common symptom of cardiopulmonary disorders that produce dyspnea. It's commonly a subtle symptom; the patient may complain that he can't catch his breath when lying down or mention that he sleeps most comfortably in a reclining chair or propped up by pillows. Derived from this complaint is the common classification as two- or three-pillow orthopnea.

Orthopnea presumably results from increased hydrostatic pressure in the pulmonary vasculature associated with increased venous return in the supine position. It may be aggravated by obesity, which restricts diaphragmatic excursion. Sitting upright relieves orthopnea by impairing venous return, which reduces hydrostatic pressure, and by enhancing diaphragmatic excursion, which increases inspiratory volume.

## History

Begin your assessment by asking the patient if he has a history of cardiopulmonary disorders, such as myocardial infarction, rheumatic heart disease, valvular disease, emphysema, or chronic bronchitis. Does the patient smoke? If so, how much? Explore associated symptoms, noting especially any complaints of cough, nocturnal or exertional dyspnea, fatigue, weakness, loss of appetite, or chest pain.

## Physical exam

Check for other signs of increased respiratory effort, such as accessory muscle use, shallow respirations, and tachypnea. Also note barrel chest. Inspect the patient's skin for pallor or cyanosis, and the fingers for clubbing. Observe and palpate for dependent edema, and check for jugular vein distention. Auscultate the heart and lungs.

## Causes

*Chronic obstructive pulmonary disease (COPD).* This disorder typically produces orthopnea and other dyspneic complaints accompanied by accessory muscle use, tachypnea, tachycardia, and paradoxical pulse. Auscultation may reveal diminished breath sounds, rhonchi, crackles, and wheezing. The patient may also have a dry or productive cough with copious sputum. Other features include anorexia, weight loss, and edema. Barrel chest, cyanosis, and clubbing are usually late signs.

*Left ventricular failure.* Orthopnea occurs late in this disorder. If heart failure is acute, orthopnea may begin suddenly; if chronic, it may be constant. The earliest symptom of this disorder is progressively severe dyspnea. Other common early symptoms include Cheyne-Stokes respirations, paroxysmal nocturnal dyspnea, fatigue, weakness, and a cough that may occasionally produce clear or blood-tinged sputum. Tachycardia, tachy-

pnea, and crackles may also occur.

Other late findings may include cyanosis, clubbing, ventricular gallop, and hemoptysis. Left ventricular failure may also lead to signs of shock — hypotension, thready pulse, and cold, clammy skin.

*Mediastinal tumor.* Orthopnea is an early sign of this disorder, resulting from pressure of the tumor against the trachea, bronchus, or lung when the patient lies down. But many patients are asymptomatic until the tumor enlarges, producing retrosternal chest pain, dry cough, hoarseness, dysphagia, stertorous respirations, palpitations, and cyanosis. Examination reveals suprasternal retractions on inspiration, bulging of the chest wall, tracheal deviation, dilated jugular and superficial chest veins, and edema of the face, neck, and arms.

## Nursing considerations

• To relieve orthopnea, place the patient in semi-Fowler's or high Fowler's position; if this doesn't help, have him lean over a bedside table with his chest forward. If necessary, administer oxygen via nasal cannula. (Remember that patients with COPD require a low flow rate of 1 to 3 liters/minute.) If dyspnea persists when the patient's in the upright position, notify the doctor. He may order an ECG, a chest X-ray, and pulmonary function tests for further evaluation.

Erythema, or erythroderma, is a characteristic sign of skin inflammation, with changes in skin color ranging from bright red in acute conditions to pale violet or brown in chronic problems. To differentiate erythema from purpura, which causes redness from bleeding into the skin, apply pressure directly to the skin. Erythema blanches; purpura does not.

## ▶ Emergency interventions

Sudden progressive erythema (as urticaria) along with tachycardia, dyspnea, hoarseness, and agitation may be signs of anaphylactic shock. Take vital signs and have another nurse contact the doctor immediately. Provide emergency respiratory support and give epinephrine, as ordered.

## History

Ask the patient how long he's had the erythema and where it began. Has he had any associated pain or itching? Has he recently had a fever, an upper respiratory infection, or joint pain? Does he have a history of skin disease or other illness? Does he or anyone in his family have allergies, asthma, or eczema? Has he been exposed to someone who has had a similar rash?

Obtain a complete drug history, including recent immunizations. Ask about food intake and exposure to chemicals.

## Physical exam

Assess the extent, distribution, and intensity of erythema. Look for edema and skin lesions, such as urticaria. Also check for warmth and tenderness.

## Causes

*Allergic reactions.* Many kinds of allergens can cause a mild to severe allergic reaction and erythema. Anaphylaxis, a life-threatening condition, produces sudden urticaria as well as flushing, facial edema, diaphoresis, bronchospasm, and shock.

*Dermatitis.* In *atopic dermatitis,* erythema and pruritus precede the development of small papules that may redden, weep, scale, and become lichenified. In *contact dermatitis,* erythema, blisters, and vesicles quickly develop on exposed skin.

*Erythema multiforme. Erythema multiforme major* (Stevens-Johnson syndrome) produces sudden hivelike erythema with blisters and petechial or "iris" lesions on the face, hands, and feet. In *erythema multiforme minor,* erythematous macules and papules, purpura and, occasionally, blisters occur. Characteristic urticarial iris lesions may burn or itch.

*Erythema nodosum.* Sudden bilateral eruption of tender erythematous nodules characterizes this disorder. These firm, round nodules usually appear in crops on the shins, knees, and ankles.

*Rubella.* Flat solitary lesions join to form a blotchy pink erythematous rash that spreads to the trunk and extremities. The rash usually follows fever, headache, malaise, and sore throat.

*Toxic shock syndrome.* Sudden, diffuse erythema occurs as a macular rash. It's accompanied by a sudden high fever, myalgia, vomiting, severe diarrhea, and shock.

*Other causes.* Blood transfusion; chronic liver disease; dermatomyositis; drugs, such as anticoagulants, antimetabolites, barbiturates, cephalosporins, corticosteroids, nonsteroidal anti-inflammatory drugs, oral contraceptives, salicylates, sulfonamides, sulfonylureas, tetracyclines, and thiazides; erythema marginatum rheumaticum; erythema toxicum neonatorum; lupus erythematosus; polymorphous light eruption; psoriasis; radiation therapy; roseola; rubeola; scarlet fever; and toxic epidermal necrolysis.

## Nursing considerations

- Withhold all medications until after diagnosis. Then expect to administer antibiotics and topical or systemic corticosteroids.
- Advise a patient with leg erythema to keep his legs elevated above heart level.

A cardinal sign of meningeal irritation, opisthotonos is characterized by a severely arched, rigid back; a hyperextended neck; heels bent back; and arms and hands flexed at the joints. This posture usually occurs spontaneously and continuously, but it may be aggravated by movement.

Most commonly caused by meningitis, opisthotonos may also result from subarachnoid hemorrhage, Arnold-Chiari syndrome, and tetanus.

Opisthotonos is far more common in children—especially infants—than in adults. It's also more exaggerated in children because of nervous system immaturity.

### ▶ Emergency interventions

Report opisthotonos to the doctor at once. If the patient is stuporous or comatose, quickly assess his vital signs, and use appropriate resuscitative measures. Place the patient in a bed, with side rails raised and padded, or in a crib.

### History

When the patient's condition permits, obtain a history. If the patient is a young child or an infant, consult a family member. Ask about a history of cerebral aneurysm or arteriovenous malformation and about hypertension. Also note any recent infection that may have spread to the nervous system. Explore associated signs and symptoms, such as headache, chills, and vomiting.

### Physical exam

Focus the physical examination on the patient's neurologic status. Assess level of consciousness (LOC), and test sensorimotor and cranial nerve function. Then check for positive Brudzinski's and Kernig's signs and for nuchal rigidity.

### Causes

*Arnold-Chiari syndrome.* In this syndrome, opisthotonos is typically accompanied by hydrocephalus with its characteristic enlarged head; thin, shiny scalp with distended veins; and underdeveloped neck muscles. The infant usually also has a high-pitched, shrill cry; abnormal leg muscle tone; anorexia; vomiting; nuchal rigidity; irritability; noisy respirations; and a weak sucking reflex.

*Meningitis.* Opisthotonos accompanies other signs of meningeal irritation, including nuchal rigidity, positive Brudzinski's and Kernig's signs, and hyperreflexia. Meningitis also causes cardinal signs of infection—moderate to high fever with chills and malaise—and of increased intracranial pressure—headache, vomiting, and, rarely, papilledema. Additional findings include irritability; photophobia; diplopia, deafness, and other cranial nerve palsies; and decreased LOC, which may progress to seizures and coma.

*Subarachnoid hemorrhage.* This acute disorder may produce opisthotonos along with other signs of meningeal irritation, such as nuchal rigidity and positive Brudzinski's and Kernig's signs. Focal signs of hemorrhage—severe headache, hemiplegia or hemiparesis, aphasia, and photophobia—and other vision problems may also occur.

*Tetanus.* This life-threatening infection can cause opisthotonos. Initially, trismus occurs. Eventually, muscle spasms may affect the abdomen, producing boardlike rigidity; the back, resulting in opisthotonos; or the face, producing risus sardonicus.

*Other causes.* Drugs, such as phenothiazines and other antipsychotics.

### Nursing considerations

• Assess neurologic status and vital signs frequently. Make the patient as comfortable as possible; place him in a side-lying position with pillows for support.

• If meningitis is suspected, institute respiratory isolation. A lumbar puncture may be ordered to identify the causative microorganism and to analyze cerebrospinal fluid. If subarachnoid hemorrhage is suspected, prepare the patient for a computed tomography scan.

Also known as erythroderma, localized erythema is the most common sign of skin inflammation or irritation, with skin color ranging from bright red in acute conditions to pale violet or brown in chronic problems. To differentiate erythema from purpura, which causes redness from bleeding into the skin, apply pressure directly to the skin. Erythema blanches; purpura does not.

## History
Ask the patient how long he's had the erythema and where it began. Ask if he's had any associated pain or itching. Ask about recent fever, upper respiratory infection, or joint pain. Does he have a history of skin disease or other illnesses? Does he or anyone in his family have allergies, asthma, or eczema? Has he been exposed to someone who's had a similar rash or who's now ill?

Obtain a complete drug history, including recent immunizations. Ask about food intake and any exposure to chemicals.

## Physical exam
Assess the extent, distribution, and intensity of erythema. Look for edema and other skin lesions, such as hives, scales, papules, and purpura. Also check for warmth and tenderness.

## Causes
*Burns.* With thermal burns, erythema and swelling appear first, possibly followed by deep or superficial blisters and other signs of damage. Burns from ultraviolet rays, such as sunburn, cause delayed erythema and tenderness.

*Candidiasis.* When this fungal infection affects the skin, it produces erythema and a scaly, papular rash under the breasts and at the axillae, neck, umbilicus, and groin.

*Dermatitis.* Erythema commonly occurs with this family of inflammatory disorders. In *atopic dermatitis,* erythema and intense pruritus precede the development of small papules that may redden, weep, scale, and become lichenified. In *contact dermatitis,* erythema and vesicles, blisters, or ulcerations appear on exposed skin. In *seborrheic dermatitis,* erythema appears with dull red or yellow lesions. These sharply marginated lesions are sometimes ring-shaped and covered with greasy scales. Usually, they occur on the scalp, eyebrows, ears, and nasolabial folds.

*Erysipelas.* This infection causes rosy or crimson swollen lesions to appear suddenly, mainly on the head and neck. If severe, it may cause hemorrhagic pus-filled blisters.

*Rheumatoid arthritis.* In a flare-up of this disorder, erythema over the affected joints occurs with heat, swelling, pain, and stiffness.

*Rosacea.* This begins with scattered erythema across the center of the face, followed by superficial telangiectases, papules, pustules, and nodules. Rhinophyma may occur.

*Thrombophlebitis.* Erythema may appear over the inflamed vein. Fever, chills, and malaise may accompany localized pain, warmth, and induration; distal edema; and a positive Homans' sign.

*Other causes.* Acute febrile neutrophilic dermatosis; drugs, such as anticoagulants, antimetabolites, barbiturates, cephalosporins, corticosteroids, nonsteroidal anti-inflammatory drugs, oral contraceptives, salicylates, sulfonamides, sulfonylureas, tetracyclines, and thiazides; erythema ab igne; erythema annulare centrifugum; erythema chronicum migrans; erythema gyratum repens; frostbite; intertrigo; radiation therapy; Raynaud's disease; and thrombophlebitis.

## Nursing considerations
• Closely monitor and replace fluids and electrolytes, especially in patients with burns.
• Withhold all medications until after diagnosis. Then, expect to administer antibiotics and topical or systemic corticosteroids. For the patient with itchy skin, expect to give soothing baths or apply open wet dressings. Give antihistamines and analgesics as ordered.
• Prepare the patient for any diagnostic tests.

# Oliguria

A cardinal sign of renal and urinary tract disorders, oliguria is clinically defined as urine output of less than 400 ml/24 hours. Typically, it occurs abruptly and may herald serious, possibly life-threatening hemodynamic instability. Any disorder that decreases circulating fluid volume can produce oliguria.

## History

Ask the patient about his usual daily voiding pattern, including frequency and amount. When did he first notice changes in this pattern and in the color, odor, or consistency of his urine? Ask about pain or burning on urination. Note his normal daily fluid intake. Has it recently varied? Ask about recent episodes of diarrhea or vomiting. Explore associated complaints, especially fatigue, loss of appetite, thirst, dyspnea, chest pain, or recent weight gain.

Check for a history of renal, urinary tract, or cardiovascular disorders. Note recent traumatic injury, surgery, recent blood transfusions, or exposure to nephrotoxic agents or drugs.

## Physical exam

Weigh the patient and take his vital signs. Look for edema, especially in the flank area. Palpate both kidneys for tenderness and enlargement, and percuss for costovertebral angle (CVA) tenderness. Auscultate the heart and lungs for abnormal sounds, and the periumbilical area for renal artery bruits. As ordered, obtain a urine specimen and inspect it for abnormal color, odor, or sediment. Test for glucose, protein, and blood, and measure specific gravity.

## Causes

*Acute tubular necrosis.* Oliguria may occur abruptly (in shock) or gradually (in nephrotoxicity). It usually lasts for about 2 weeks and is followed by polyuria. Other findings may include hyperkalemia, uremia, and congestive heart failure (CHF).

*Benign prostatic hyperplasia.* Oliguria commonly results from urethral obstruction. Other findings include urinary frequency and incontinence, nocturia, and possibly hematuria.

*Calculi.* Oliguria or anuria may result from stones in the kidneys, ureters, or bladder outlet. Other findings may include renal colic, urinary urgency and frequency, dysuria, hematuria, and pyuria.

*Glomerulonephritis (acute).* This disorder produces oliguria or anuria. Other features are mild fever, fatigue, hematuria, generalized edema, elevated blood pressure, headache, nausea and vomiting, flank and abdominal pain, and pulmonary congestion.

*Pyelonephritis (acute).* Oliguria occurs suddenly, along with high fever, chills, fatigue, flank pain, CVA tenderness, weakness, nocturia, dysuria, hematuria, urinary frequency and urgency, and tenesmus. Urine may be cloudy.

*Renal failure (chronic).* Oliguria is a major sign of this disorder. Associated findings may include fatigue, irritability, uremic fetor, ecchymoses and petechiae, peripheral edema, hypertension, confusion, muscle twitching and cramps, peripheral neuropathies, anorexia, nausea and vomiting, constipation or diarrhea, stomatitis, pruritus, pallor, and yellow- or bronze-tinged skin.

*Urethral stricture.* Oliguria is accompanied by chronic urethral discharge, urinary frequency and urgency, dysuria, pyuria, and diminished urine stream.

*Other causes.* Bladder cancer; CHF; cirrhosis (severe); drugs, such as aminoglycosides, adrenergics, anticholinergics, diuretics, sulfonamides, and chemotherapeutic agents; hypovolemia; radiographic contrast media; renal artery or vein occlusion (bilateral); retroperitoneal fibrosis; sepsis; and toxemia of pregnancy.

## Nursing considerations

• Monitor vital signs, intake and output, and daily weight. Maintain fluid restrictions. Provide a diet low in sodium, potassium, and protein.
• Prepare the patient for any diagnostic tests.

Also called proptosis, exophthalmos is the abnormal protrusion of one or both eyeballs. This sign may result from hemorrhage, edema, or inflammation behind the eye; extraocular muscle relaxation; or space-occupying intraorbital lesions. It may occur suddenly or gradually, causing mild to dramatic protrusion. Sometimes, the eye pulsates.

Usually, exophthalmos is easily observed. However, lid retraction may mimic exophthalmos even though protrusion is absent. Similarly, ptosis in one eye may make the other appear exophthalmic. Fortunately, an exophthalmometer can differentiate these signs by measuring ocular protrusion.

## History

Ask when the patient first noticed exophthalmos. Is it associated with pain in or around the eye? If so, ask him about its severity and duration. Then ask about recent sinus infection or vision problems.

## Physical exam

Take the patient's vital signs, noting fever, which may accompany eye infection. Next, evaluate the severity of exophthalmos with an exophthalmometer. If the eyes bulge severely, look for cloudiness on the cornea, which may indicate ulcer formation. Describe any eye discharge and observe for ptosis. Then check visual acuity, with and without correction, and evaluate extraocular movements.

## Causes

*Dacryoadenitis.* Unilateral, slowly progressive exophthalmos is the most common sign. Assessment may also reveal limited extraocular movements, ptosis, eyelid edema and erythema, conjunctival injection, eye pain, and diplopia.

*Hemangioma.* Most common in young adults, this orbital tumor produces progressive exophthalmos, which may be mild or severe, unilateral or bilateral. Other signs and symptoms may include ptosis, limited extraocular movements, and blurred vision.

*Optic nerve meningioma.* Usually, this tumor produces unilateral exophthalmos and a swollen temple. Impaired visual acuity, visual field deficits, and headache may occur.

*Orbital cellulitis.* Often the result of sinusitis, this ocular emergency causes sudden onset of unilateral exophthalmos, which may be mild or severe. It may also produce fever, eye pain, headache, malaise, conjunctival injection, tearing, eyelid edema and erythema, purulent discharge, and impaired extraocular movements.

*Orbital choristoma.* A common sign of this benign tumor, progressive exophthalmos may be associated with diplopia and blurred vision.

*Scleritis (posterior).* Gradual onset of mild to severe unilateral exophthalmos is common. Other findings: severe eye pain, diplopia, papilledema, limited extraocular movements, and impaired visual acuity.

*Thyrotoxicosis.* Although a classic sign of this disorder, exophthalmos is absent in many patients. It's usually bilateral, progressive, and severe. Associated ocular features include ptosis, increased tearing, lid lag and edema, photophobia, conjunctival injection, diplopia, and decreased visual acuity. Elsewhere in the body, common findings include an enlarged thyroid, anxiety, heat intolerance, weight loss despite increased appetite, sweating, diarrhea, tremors, palpitations, and tachycardia.

*Other causes.* Cavernous sinus thrombosis, foreign body in the eye, Hodgkin's disease, lacrimal gland tumor, leiomyosarcoma, leukemia, lymphangioma, ocular tuberculosis, orbital emphysema or pseudotumor, and parasite infestation.

## Nursing considerations

• Because exophthalmos usually makes the patient self-conscious, provide privacy and support.
• Protect the exophthalmic eye from infection and other trauma, especially drying of the cornea. However, *never* place a gauze eye pad or other object over this eye; damage to the corneal epithelium may result when the pad is removed.
• If a slit lamp examination is ordered, explain the procedure to the patient. If necessary, refer him to an ophthalmologist for a complete examination.

Abnormally infrequent menstrual bleeding, oligomenorrhea is characterized by three to six menstrual cycles per year. When menstrual bleeding does occur, it's usually profuse (greater than 70 ml), prolonged (up to 10 days), and laden with clots and tissue. Although this sign may alternate with normal menstrual bleeding, it can progress to secondary amenorrhea.

Commonly associated with anovulation, oligomenorrhea is common in infertile, early postmenarchal, and perimenopausal women. It may result from ovarian, pituitary, and other metabolic disorders, certain drugs, and stress.

### History
After asking the patient how old she is, find out when menarche occurred. Has the patient ever had normal menstrual cycles? When did the abnormal cycles begin? Ask her to describe the pattern of bleeding, and ask if there are clots and tissue fragments in her menstrual flow. Note when she last had menstrual bleeding.

Ask about symptoms of ovulatory bleeding. Does she experience mild, cramping abdominal pain 14 days before she bleeds? Is the bleeding accompanied by premenstrual symptoms? Ask about the use of oral contraceptives, currently or in the past, and when she stopped taking them. Also ask about infertility and previous gynecologic disorders.

If the patient is breast-feeding, ask about problems with milk production. If she hasn't been breastfeeding, has she noticed milk leaking from her breasts? Ask about recent weight gain or loss. Is the patient less than 80% of her ideal weight? If so, does she claim that she's overweight? Ask if she's exercising more vigorously than usual.

Screen for metabolic disorders by asking about excessive thirst, frequent urination, or fatigue. Has the patient been jittery or had palpitations? Ask about headache, dizziness, and impaired peripheral vision. Finally, ask what drugs she's taking.

### Physical exam
Obtain weight and vital signs. Look for increased facial hair growth, sparse body hair, male distribution of fat and muscle, acne, and clitoral enlargement. Note if the skin is abnormally dry or moist, and check hair texture. Also watch for signs of psychological or physical stress.

### Causes
*Adrenal hyperplasia.* Oligomenorrhea may be accompanied by signs of androgen excess. If this disorder is congenital, the patient may have never had normal menses.

*Anorexia nervosa.* This is marked by a morbid fear of being fat, associated with loss of more than 20% of ideal body weight. Other findings include dramatic skeletal muscle atrophy and loss of fatty tissue, dry or sparse scalp hair, lanugo on the face and body, and blotchy or sallow, dry skin.

*Diabetes mellitus.* Oligomenorrhea may be an early sign in this disorder. In juvenile-onset diabetes, the patient may have never had normal menses. Other effects include excessive hunger, polydipsia, polyuria, weakness, dry mucous membranes, poor skin turgor, and weight loss.

*Drugs.* Oligomenorrhea may be caused by drugs that increase androgen levels, such as corticosteroids, adrenocorticotropic hormone, anabolic steroids, and danocrine, as well as phenothiazine derivatives and amphetamines. Oral contraceptives may be associated with delayed resumption of normal menses when their use is discontinued; however, 95% of women resume normal menses within 3 months.

*Other causes.* Polycystic ovary disease, prolactin-secreting pituitary tumor, Sheehan's syndrome, and thyrotoxicosis.

### Nursing considerations
• If the patient is recording her basal body temperature to track ovulatory cycles, give her blank charts and teach her how to keep them accurately.
• Prepare the patient for diagnostic tests, such as blood hormone levels, thyroid studies, and computed tomography scan.

Usually associated with conjunctivitis, eye discharge refers to the excretion of any substance other than tears. This common sign may occur in one or both eyes, producing scant to copious discharge. The discharge may be purulent, frothy, mucoid, cheesy, or ropy. Sometimes, discharge can be expressed by applying pressure to the tear sac, punctum, meibomian glands, or canaliculus.

Eye discharge commonly results from inflammatory and infectious eye disorders but may also result from certain systemic disorders. Because this sign may signal a vision-threatening disorder, it must be assessed and treated promptly.

## History

Find out when the discharge began. Does it occur at certain times of day or with certain activities? If the patient complains of pain, ask him to describe its character and location. Is it dull, continuous, sharp, or stabbing? Do his eyes itch or burn? Do they tear excessively? Are they sensitive to light? Does he feel like something is in them?

## Physical exam

After taking vital signs, carefully inspect the eye discharge. Note its amount and consistency. Then test visual acuity with and without correction. Examine external eye structures, beginning with the unaffected eye to prevent cross-contamination.

Observe for eyelid edema, entropion, crusts, lesions, or trichiasis. Next, ask the patient to blink as you watch for impaired lid movement. If the eyes seem to bulge, measure them with an exophthalmometer. Test the six cardinal fields of gaze. Examine for conjunctival injection and follicles, and for corneal cloudiness or white lesions.

## Causes

*Conjunctivitis.* In *allergic conjunctivitis,* itching and tearing accompany bilateral ropy discharge. *Bacterial conjunctivitis* causes purulent discharge that forms sticky crusts on eyelids during sleep. Itching, burning, tearing, and a foreign-body sensation may also occur. Eye pain indicates corneal involvement. *Fungal conjunctivitis* produces thick, purulent discharge and crusty, sticky eyelids. Also characteristic are eyelid edema, itching, burning, and tearing. Corneal involvement causes pain and photophobia. *Inclusion conjunctivitis* causes scant bilateral mucoid discharge, especially in the morning, with pseudoptosis and conjunctival follicles.

*Corneal ulcers.* Bacterial and fungal ulcers produce copious, purulent discharge. Related findings are crusty, sticky eyelids and, possibly, severe pain, photophobia, and impaired visual acuity.

*Dacryocystitis.* Lacrimal sac infection may produce scant but continuous purulent discharge that's easily expressed from the tear sac. Additional signs and symptoms include excessive tearing, pain, and tenderness near the tear sac. Eyelid inflammation and edema are most noticeable around the lacrimal punctum.

*Keratoconjunctivitis sicca.* Better known as dry eye syndrome, this disorder typically causes excessive, continuous mucoid discharge and insufficient tearing. Accompanying features may include eye pain, itching, burning, a foreign-body sensation, and dramatic conjunctival injection.

*Meibomianitis.* This disorder may produce continuous frothy eye discharge. Application of pressure on the meibomian glands yields a soft, foul-smelling, cheesy yellow discharge. The eyes look chronically red, with inflamed lid margins.

*Other causes.* Canaliculitis, dacryoadenitis, erythema multiforme major, herpes zoster ophthalmicus, orbital cellulitis, pemphigus, psoriasis vulgaris, and trachoma.

## Nursing considerations

• Apply warm soaks to soften crusts on eyelids and lashes. Gently wipe the eyes with a soft gauze pad. Carefully dispose of all materials to prevent possible spread of infection. Teach the patient how to avoid contaminating the unaffected eye.
• Sterilize ophthalmic equipment after use.
• Explain ordered diagnostic tests, including culture and sensitivity studies.

E

Abnormal eye movement that may be *conjugate* (both eyes move together) or *dysconjugate* (one eye moves differently from the other), ocular deviation is a common sign. It may result from ocular, neurologic, endocrine, and systemic disorders that interfere with the muscles, nerves, or brain centers governing eye movement. Occasionally, it signals a life-threatening disorder, such as ruptured cerebral aneurysm.

## ▶ Emergency interventions

If the patient displays ocular deviation, quickly take his vital signs and assess for altered level of consciousness (LOC), pupil changes, motor or sensory dysfunction, and severe headache. If possible, ask the patient's family about behavioral changes and recent head trauma. If you suspect an acute neurologic disorder, notify the doctor at once. Prepare to assist with respiratory support and ready the patient for emergency neurologic tests.

## History

If the patient is stable, find out how long he's had the ocular deviation, if he has noticed any motor or sensory changes, and if he has double vision, eye pain, fever, or headache. Check for a history of hypertension, diabetes, allergies, and thyroid, neurologic, or muscular disorders. Then obtain an ocular history. Has the patient ever had extraocular muscle imbalance, eye or head trauma, or eye surgery?

## Physical exam

Watch for partial or complete ptosis. Does the patient spontaneously tilt his head or turn his face to compensate for ocular deviation? Check for eye redness or periorbital edema. Assess visual acuity, then evaluate extraocular muscle function by testing the six cardinal fields of gaze.

## Causes

*Brain tumor.* Ocular deviation varies with the site and extent of the tumor. Other findings may include headache (most severe in the morning), behavioral changes, memory loss, dizziness, confusion, vision loss, motor and sensory dysfunction, aphasia, and possible hormonal imbalance.

*Cerebrovascular accident.* This life-threatening disorder may cause ocular deviation, depending on the site and extent of the stroke. Other findings may include altered LOC, contralateral hemiplegia and sensory loss, dysarthria, dysphagia, homonymous hemianopia, blurred vision, and diplopia.

*Diabetes mellitus.* A leading cause of isolated cranial nerve III palsy, this disorder may cause ocular deviation and ptosis. Typically, the patient also complains of sudden onset of diplopia and pain.

*Head trauma.* Ocular deviation varies with the site and extent of head trauma. The patient may have visible soft tissue injury, bony deformity, facial edema, and clear or bloody otorrhea or rhinorrhea. Other findings may include blurred vision, diplopia, nystagmus, behavioral changes, headache, motor and sensory dysfunction, increased intracranial pressure, and a decreased LOC that may progress to coma.

*Multiple sclerosis.* Ocular deviation may be an early sign of this disorder. Accompanying it are diplopia, blurred vision, and sensory dysfunction, such as paresthesia. Other features include nystagmus, constipation, muscle weakness, paralysis, spasticity, hyperreflexia, gait ataxia, intention tremor, dysphagia, dysarthria, impotence, and emotional instability.

*Orbital tumor.* Ocular deviation occurs as the tumor gradually enlarges. Other findings may include proptosis, diplopia, and blurred vision.

*Other causes.* Cavernous sinus thrombosis, cerebral aneurysm, encephalitis, myasthenia gravis, ophthalmoplegic migraine, orbital blow-out fractures, orbital cellulitis, and thyrotoxicosis.

## Nursing considerations

• Monitor the patient's vital signs and neurologic status if you suspect an acute neurologic disorder. Take seizure precautions, if necessary. Also prepare the patient for any diagnostic tests.

Eye pain may be described as burning, throbbing, aching, or stabbing in or around the eye. It may also be described as something in the eye—a foreign-body sensation. This symptom varies from mild to severe; its duration and location provide clues to the causative disorder. Most commonly, eye pain results from corneal abrasion. It may also result from glaucoma and other eye disorders, trauma, and neurologic and systemic disorders.

## ▶ Emergency interventions

If pain results from a chemical burn, notify the doctor immediately. Remove the patient's contact lenses, if present, and irrigate the eye with at least 1 liter of normal saline solution over 10 minutes. Evert the lids and wipe the fornices with a cotton swab to remove any particles or chemicals.

## History

If the patient's eye pain doesn't result from a chemical burn, have him describe it. Is it aching or sharp? How long does it last and when did it begin? Is it accompanied by burning or itching? Ask about recent trauma, surgery, or headaches.

## Physical exam

Don't manipulate the eye if you suspect trauma. Carefully assess the lids and conjunctiva for redness, inflammation, and swelling. Inspect for pto-sis or exophthalmos. Test visual acuity and assess extraocular movements. Characterize discharge.

## Causes

*Acute closed-angle glaucoma.* Blurred vision and sudden, excruciating pain in and around the eye characterize this disorder; pain may be severe enough to cause nausea and vomiting. Other findings: halo vision; a fixed, nonreactive, moderately dilated pupil; and rapidly decreasing visual acuity.

*Burns.* In *chemical burns,* sudden and severe eye pain may occur with erythema and blistering of the face and lids, photophobia, miosis, conjunctival injection, blurring, and inability to keep the eyelids open. In *ultraviolet radiation burns,* moderate to severe pain occurs about 12 hours after exposure along with photophobia and vision changes.

*Conjunctivitis.* *Allergic conjunctivitis* causes mild, burning, bilateral pain. *Bacterial and fungal conjunctivitis* cause pain only when they affect the cornea. *Viral conjunctivitis* produces itchy, red eyes accompanied by a foreign-body sensation.

*Corneal abrasions.* In this type of injury, eye pain is characterized by a foreign-body sensation. Excessive tearing, photophobia, and conjunctival injection are also common.

*Corneal ulcers.* Both bacterial and fungal corneal ulcers cause severe eye pain. They may also cause a purulent eye discharge, sticky eyelids, photophobia, and impaired visual acuity.

*Hordeolum (sty).* Localized pain increases as the sty grows. Eyelid erythema and edema occur.

*Iritis (acute).* Moderate to severe eye pain occurs with severe photophobia, dramatic conjunctival injection, and blurred vision.

*Ocular laceration and intraocular foreign bodies.* Penetrating eye injuries usually cause mild to severe unilateral eye pain and impaired visual acuity. Eyelid edema, conjunctival injection, and an abnormal pupillary response may also occur.

*Uveitis.* *Anterior uveitis* causes sudden severe pain, dramatic conjunctival injection, photophobia, and a small, nonreactive pupil. *Posterior uveitis* causes insidious onset of similar features, plus gradually blurred vision and distorted pupil shape.

*Other causes.* Blepharitis, chalazion, contact lenses, corneal erosion, dacryoadenitis, dacryo-cystitis, episcleritis, herpes zoster, hyphema, keratitis, keratoconjunctivitis sicca, lacrimal gland tumor, migraine headache, ocular surgery, optic neuritis, orbital blowout fracture, orbital cellulitis or pseudotumor, pemphigus, scleritis, sclerokeratitis, subdural hematoma, and trachoma.

## Nursing considerations

• To help ease eye pain, have the patient lie down in a dark, quiet environment and close his eyes.
• As ordered, prepare him for diagnostic studies.

E

# Nystagmus

The involuntary oscillations of one or — more commonly — both eyeballs, nystagmus is usually rhythmical and may be horizontal, vertical, or rotary. Nystagmus is easy to identify, but the patient may be unaware of it unless it affects his vision.

There are two types. *Pendular nystagmus* consists of horizontal (pendular) or vertical (seesaw) oscillations that are equal in both directions and resemble the movements of a clock's pendulum. *Jerk nystagmus* (convergence-retraction, downbeat, and vestibular) has a fast component and then a slow — perhaps unequal — corrective component in the opposite direction.

Nystagmus results from disease in the visual perceptual area, vestibular system, cerebellum, or brain stem rather than in the extraocular muscles or cranial nerves III, IV, and VI. Its causes vary and include brain stem or cerebellar lesions, multiple sclerosis, encephalitis, labyrinthine disease, and drug toxicity.

## History

Ask the patient how long he's had nystagmus. Does it occur intermittently? Does it affect his vision? Ask about recent infection, especially of the ear or respiratory tract, and about head trauma and cancer. Does the patient or anyone in his family have a history of cerebrovascular accident (CVA)? Also ask about vertigo, dizziness, tinnitus, nausea or vomiting, numbness, weakness, bladder dysfunction, and fever.

## Physical exam

Assess the patient's level of consciousness (LOC) and vital signs. Watch for signs of increased intracranial pressure. Next, test extraocular muscle function. Ask the patient to focus straight ahead, then follow your finger up, down, and in an "X" across his face. Note when nystagmus occurs, its velocity and direction. Finally, test reflexes, motor and sensory function, and cranial nerves.

## Causes

*Brain tumor.* Onset of jerk nystagmus may occur with tumors of the brain stem and cerebellum. Other symptoms may include deafness, dysphagia, nausea and vomiting, vertigo, and ataxia.

*Cerebrovascular accident.* A CVA involving the posterior inferior cerebellar artery may cause sudden horizontal or vertical jerk nystagmus that may be gaze-dependent. Other findings include dysphagia, dysarthria, numbness on the ipsilateral face and contralateral trunk and limbs, ipsilateral Horner's syndrome, ataxia, and vertigo.

*Encephalitis.* Jerk nystagmus is typically accompanied by altered LOC, ranging from lethargy to coma. Usually, it's preceded by sudden onset of fever, headache, and vomiting. Other findings include nuchal rigidity, seizures, aphasia, ataxia, photophobia, dysphagia, and ptosis.

*Head trauma.* Brain stem injury may cause jerk nystagmus, which is usually horizontal. Other findings include pupillary changes, altered respiratory pattern, coma, and decerebrate posture.

*Labyrinthitis (acute).* This inner ear inflammation causes sudden onset of jerk nystagmus, accompanied by dizziness, vertigo, tinnitus, nausea, and vomiting. Gradual sensorineural hearing loss may also occur.

*Ménière's disease.* This inner ear disorder is marked by acute attacks of jerk nystagmus, severe nausea and vomiting, dizziness, vertigo, gradual hearing loss, tinnitus, and diaphoresis.

*Multiple sclerosis.* Jerk or pendular nystagmus may occur intermittently. Usually, it's preceded by diplopia, blurred vision, and paresthesia. Other findings may include muscle weakness or paralysis, spasticity, hyperreflexia, intention tremors, gait ataxia, dysphagia, dysarthria, impotence, and emotional instability.

*Other causes.* Alcohol intoxication and barbiturate, carbamazepine, or phenytoin toxicity.

## Nursing considerations

• Prepare the patient for diagnostic tests, such as electronystagmography and a cerebral computed tomography scan.

This symptom may result from various neurologic, vascular, or infectious disorders. Its most common cause is trigeminal neuralgia, or tic douloureux. Pain can also be referred to the face from the ear, nose, paranasal sinuses, teeth, neck, and jaw.

Typically paroxysmal and intense, facial pain may occur along a facial nerve or its branch, usually cranial nerve V (trigeminal) or VII (facial). Differentiating facial pain from headache pain is sometimes difficult because many patients refer to all head and facial pain as headache.

## History

Characterize the facial pain. Is it stabbing, throbbing, or dull? When did it begin? How long has it lasted? What relieves it? Worsens it? Ask the patient to point to the painful area. If his facial pain is recurrent, have him describe a typical episode. Review his medical and dental history, noting head trauma, dental disease, and infection.

## Physical exam

Carefully examine the patient's face and head. Inspect the ear for vesicles and changes in the tympanic membrane to rule out referred ear pain. Inspect the nose for deformity or asymmetry. Assess the condition of the mucous membranes and septum, and turbinate size and shape. Characterize any secretions. Palpate frontal and maxillary sinuses for tenderness and swelling.

Evaluate oral hygiene by inspecting for caries, percussing any diseased teeth for pain, and asking the patient about sensitivity to hot, cold, or sweet liquids or foods. Have him open and close his mouth as you palpate the temporomandibular joint. Assess function in cranial nerves V and VII.

## Causes

*Dental caries.* Caries in the mandibular molars can produce ear, preauricular, and temporal pain. In contrast, caries in the maxillary teeth can produce orbital, retro-orbital, and parietal pain.

*Sinusitis. Acute maxillary sinusitis* produces unilateral or bilateral pressure, fullness, or burning pain behind the eyes and over the cheek, nose, and upper teeth. Other findings include nasal congestion and purulent discharge; red, swollen nasal mucosa and turbinates; facial and gingival swelling; trismus; fever; and malaise.

*Frontal sinusitis* commonly produces dull, aching pain above or around the eyes, which worsens with bending or stooping. It also causes nasal obstruction; red, swollen nasal mucosa; rhinorrhea; fever; and edema of the eyelids and face. In *sphenoid sinusitis,* dull pain persists behind the eyes and nose. Related findings include forehead and eye swelling, blurred vision, diplopia, fever, and chills.

*Temporomandibular joint syndrome.* Intermittent pain, usually unilateral, is described as a severe, dull ache or an intense spasm that radiates to the cheek, temple, lower jaw, ear, or mastoid area. Associated findings include trismus; malocclusion; and clicking, crepitus, and tenderness in the temporomandibular joint.

*Trigeminal neuralgia.* Paroxysms of intense pain, lasting up to 15 minutes, shoot along the superior maxillary or mandibular division of the trigeminal nerve. Pain can be triggered by touching the nose, cheek, or mouth; by hot or cold weather; by consuming hot or cold foods and beverages; or even by smiling or talking. Between attacks, pain may abate or vanish.

*Other causes.* Herpes zoster, multiple sclerosis, postherpetic neuralgia, sinus carcinoma, sphenopalatine neuralgia, and temporal arteritis.

## Nursing considerations

• If ordered, prepare the patient for tests, such as sinus, skull, or dental X-rays; sinus transillumination; and intracranial computed tomography.
• As ordered, give pain medications, and apply direct heat or administer a muscle relaxant to ease muscle spasms. Provide a humidifier, vaporizer, or decongestant to relieve nasal or sinus congestion.
• If appropriate, teach the patient to avoid stressful situations, hot or cold foods, and sudden jarring movements, which could trigger painful attacks.

Commonly an early sign of meningeal irritation, nuchal rigidity is profound stiffness of the neck that prevents flexion. This sign may herald life-threatening subarachnoid hemorrhage or meningitis. It may also be a late sign of cervical arthritis, in which joint mobility is gradually lost. Transient, mild neck stiffness may accompany muscle tension, muscle spasms, or myalgia and must be differentiated from true nuchal rigidity.

▶ **Emergency interventions**
To elicit nuchal rigidity, try to passively flex the patient's neck and touch his chin to his chest. A positive reaction triggers pain and muscle spasms. If you elicit this sign, notify the doctor immediately, and attempt to elicit Kernig's and Brudzinski's signs. Quickly assess the patient's level of consciousness (LOC) and take his vital signs. Note signs of increased intracranial pressure (ICP), such as increased systolic pressure, bradycardia, and widened pulse pressure. If these signs are present, start an I.V. line for drug administration and deliver oxygen, as necessary. Draw a sample for routine blood studies, as ordered.

**History**
Obtain a patient history, relying on family members if altered LOC prevents the patient from responding. Ask about the onset and duration of neck stiffness and associated symptoms, such as headache, fever, nausea, vomiting, and motor and sensory changes. Check for a history of hypertension, head trauma, cerebral aneurysm, arteriovenous malformation, endocarditis, recent infection (especially tooth abscess), or recent dental work. Then obtain a complete drug history.

If the patient has no other signs of meningeal irritation, ask about a history of arthritis or neck trauma.

**Physical exam**
Inspect the patient's hands for swollen, tender joints, and palpate the neck for pain or tenderness.

**Causes**
*Cervical arthritis.* Nuchal rigidity develops gradually. Initially, the patient may complain of neck stiffness in the early morning or after a period of inactivity. Stiffness then becomes increasingly severe and frequent. Pain on movement, especially with lateral motion or head turning, is common.

*Encephalitis.* This disorder may cause nuchal rigidity accompanied by other signs of meningeal irritation, such as positive Brudzinski's and Kernig's signs. Usually, nuchal rigidity appears abruptly, preceded by headache, vomiting, and fever. Other findings include seizures, ataxia, hemiparesis, nystagmus, and cranial nerve palsies.

*Meningitis.* Nuchal rigidity is an early sign in this disorder. It's accompanied by other signs of meningeal irritation — positive Brudzinski's and Kernig's signs, hyperreflexia, and possibly opisthotonos. Other early features include fever with chills, headache, photophobia, and vomiting. Later, the patient may become stuporous and seizure-prone or may slip into a coma.

*Subarachnoid hemorrhage.* In this acute disorder, nuchal rigidity develops immediately after bleeding into the subarachnoid space. Examination may detect positive Kernig's and Brudzinski's signs. Typically, the patient experiences abrupt onset of a severe headache, photophobia, fever, nausea and vomiting, dizziness, cranial nerve palsies, and focal neurologic signs. His LOC deteriorates rapidly, possibly progressing to coma.

**Nursing considerations**
• Prepare the patient for ordered diagnostic tests, such as a computed tomography scan and cervical spinal X-rays.
• Monitor the patient's vital signs, intake and output, and neurologic status. Avoid routine administration of narcotic analgesics, which may mask signs of increasing ICP.
• Enforce strict bed rest; keep the head of the patient's bed elevated at least 30 degrees to help reduce ICP.

**N**

# Fasciculations

## 110

Minor local muscle contractions, fasciculations represent the spontaneous discharge of a muscle fiber bundle innervated by a single motor nerve filament. These contractions cause visible dimpling or wavelike twitching of the skin but aren't strong enough to produce joint movement. They occur irregularly at frequencies ranging from once every several seconds to two or three times per second; infrequently, myokymia — continuous, rapid fasciculations that cause a rippling effect — may occur. Because fasciculations are brief and painless, they often go undetected or are ignored.

Benign, nonpathologic fasciculations are common and normal. They often occur in tense, anxious, or overtired persons and typically affect the eyelid, thumb, or calf. However, fasciculations may also indicate a severe neurologic disorder, most notably a diffuse motor neuron disorder that causes loss of control over muscle fiber discharge. They're also an early sign of pesticide poisoning.

▶ **Emergency interventions**

If onset is acute, ask about precipitating events, such as pesticide exposure. Remember that pesticide poisoning, although uncommon, requires prompt and vigorous intervention. You may need to maintain airway patency, monitor vital signs, administer oxygen, and perform gastric lavage or induce vomiting.

## History

If the patient isn't in severe distress, find out about any sensory changes, such as paresthesia, and any difficulty in speaking, swallowing, breathing, or controlling bowel or bladder function. Ask the patient if he's in pain. Explore his history for neurologic disorders, cancer, and recent infections. Also explore his life-style, asking especially about stress at home, on the job, or at school.

## Physical exam

Look for fasciculations while the affected muscle is at rest. Observe and test for motor and sensory abnormalities, particularly muscle atrophy and weakness, and decreased deep tendon reflexes. If you note these signs, suspect motor neuron disease and do a complete neurologic exam.

## Causes

*Amyotrophic lateral sclerosis.* Coarse fasciculations usually begin in the small muscles of the hands and feet, then spread to the forearms and legs. Widespread, symmetrical muscle atrophy and weakness occur.

*Herniated disk.* Fasciculations of the muscles innervated by compressed nerve roots may be widespread, but the chief symptom is severe low back pain that may radiate to one leg.

*Pesticide poisoning.* Ingestion of organophos-

phate or carbamate pesticides commonly produces acute onset of long, wavelike fasciculations and muscle weakness that rapidly progresses to flaccid paralysis. Other common effects include nausea, vomiting, diarrhea, loss of bowel and bladder control, hyperactive bowel sounds, and abdominal cramping. Cardiopulmonary findings may include bradycardia, dyspnea or bradypnea, and pallor or cyanosis. Other possible findings: seizures, visual disturbances, and increased secretions.

*Spinal cord tumors.* Fasciculations may develop, along with muscle atrophy and cramps, asymmetrically at first and then bilaterally as cord compression progresses. Motor and sensory changes distal to the tumor include weakness or paralysis, areflexia, paresthesia, and a tightening band of pain. Incontinence may occur.

*Other causes.* Bulbar palsy, Guillain-Barré syndrome, poliomyelitis, and syringomyelia.

## Nursing considerations

- Prepare the patient for tests, such as spinal X-rays, computed tomography, and electromyography with nerve conduction velocity tests.
- For the patient with progressive neuromuscular degeneration, focus your care on helping him cope with activities of daily living.
- Teach effective stress management techniques to the patient with stress-induced fasciculations.

F

# Nocturia

Excessive urination at night, nocturia may result from disruption of the normal diurnal pattern of urine concentration, or from overstimulation of the nerves and muscles that control urination. Usually caused by renal and lower urinary tract disorders, nocturia may also result from cardiovascular, endocrine, and metabolic disorders, drugs that induce diuresis, and overconsumption of fluids (especially those containing caffeine or alcohol) at bedtime.

## History
Ask the patient when his nocturia began, and about its frequency and pattern. What are precipitating factors? Also note the volume of urine voided, as well as changes in urine color, odor, or consistency. Has the patient changed his usual pattern or volume of fluid intake? Also ask about pain or burning on urination, difficulty initiating a urine stream, costovertebral angle (CVA) tenderness, and flank, upper abdominal, or suprapubic pain.

Does the patient or his family have a history of renal or urinary tract disorders or endocrine and metabolic disorders — especially diabetes? Check the drug history for diuretics, cardiac glycosides, and antihypertensives.

## Physical exam
Palpate and percuss the patient's kidneys, the CVA, and the bladder. Carefully inspect the urinary meatus. Inspect a urine specimen for color, odor, and sediment.

## Causes
*Benign prostatic hyperplasia.* Nocturia follows significant urethral obstruction, especially in men over age 50. This disorder causes frequency, hesitancy, incontinence, reduced urine stream, and possibly hematuria. Oliguria may also occur. Palpation reveals a distended bladder and enlarged prostate.

*Congestive heart failure.* Nocturia may develop early, caused by increased glomerular filtration associated with movement of edematous fluid from dependent areas during recumbency. Other early effects include fatigue, jugular vein distention, dyspnea, orthopnea, tachycardia, and a dry cough with wheezing.

*Cystitis.* All three forms of cystitis — bacterial, chronic interstitial, and viral — may cause nocturia marked by frequent, small voidings, dysuria, and tenesmus.

*Diabetes insipidus.* The result of antidiuretic hormone deficiency, this disorder usually produces nocturia early in its course.

*Diabetes mellitus.* Nocturia occurs early and involves frequent, large voidings. Associated findings include daytime polyuria, polydipsia, poly-

phagia, weakness, fatigue, and weight loss.

*Prostatic neoplasm.* Usually asymptomatic in early stages, this disorder later produces nocturia marked by infrequent voiding of moderate amounts of urine. Other findings include dysuria, bladder distention, urinary frequency, weight loss, pallor, weakness, perineal pain, and constipation. Palpation reveals a hard, irregularly shaped prostate.

*Pyelonephritis (acute).* Nocturia occurs frequently, usually marked by infrequent voiding of moderate amounts of urine, which may be cloudy. Other findings include high fever with chills, fatigue, flank pain, CVA tenderness, weakness, dysuria, hematuria, and tenesmus.

*Renal failure (chronic).* Nocturia is an early symptom, usually marked by infrequent voiding of moderate amounts of urine. Oliguria or possibly anuria develop later.

*Other causes.* Bladder neoplasm, cardiac glycosides, diuretics, and hypercalcemic or hypokalemic nephropathy.

## Nursing considerations
• Maintain the patient's fluid balance and ensure adequate rest. Monitor vital signs, intake and output, and daily weight. Continue to document frequency of nocturia, amount, and specific gravity. Give diuretics during daytime hours, if possible.
• Prepare the patient for any diagnostic tests.

**N**

# Fatigue

## 111

A feeling of excessive tiredness, lack of energy, or exhaustion, fatigue is accompanied by a strong desire to rest or sleep. This common symptom is distinct from weakness but may occur with it.

A normal response to physical overexertion, emotional stress, and sleep deprivation, fatigue can also result from psychological or physiologic disorders — especially viral infections and endocrine, cardiovascular, or neurologic disease.

## History

Try to identify the patient's fatigue pattern. Fatigue that worsens with activity and improves with rest generally indicates a physical disorder; the opposite pattern, a psychological disorder.

Ask the patient about recent stressful changes in his life-style, his nutritional habits, and weight changes. Review his medical, psychiatric, and family history for disorders that produce fatigue.

## Physical exam

Observe the patient's general appearance for overt signs of depression or organic illness. Assess his mental status.

## Causes

*Adrenocortical insufficiency.* Mild fatigue, the hallmark of this disorder, initially appears after exertion and stress but later becomes more severe and persistent. Typically, weakness and weight loss accompany GI disturbances.

*Anemia.* Fatigue after mild activity is often the first symptom of this disorder. Other findings include pallor, tachycardia, and dyspnea.

*Cancer.* Unexplained fatigue is often the earliest sign of cancer. Other findings include pain, nausea, vomiting, anorexia, weight loss, abnormal bleeding, and a palpable mass.

*Chronic infection.* Fatigue is often the most prominent symptom.

*Chronic obstructive pulmonary disease.* The earliest and most persistent symptoms of this disease are progressive fatigue and dyspnea.

*Congestive heart failure.* Persistent fatigue and lethargy are characteristic. Left ventricular failure produces exertional and paroxysmal nocturnal dyspnea, orthopnea, and tachycardia. Right ventricular failure produces distended neck veins.

*Depression.* Fatigue usually accompanies chronic depression. Other findings include anorexia, constipation, and sexual dysfunction.

*Diabetes mellitus.* Fatigue, the most common symptom in this disorder, may begin insidiously or abruptly. Related findings include weight loss, polyuria, polydipsia, and polyphagia.

*Hypothyroidism.* Fatigue begins early, along with forgetfulness, cold intolerance, weight gain, and constipation.

*Myasthenia gravis.* Cardinal symptoms are easy fatigability and muscle weakness, which worsen with exertion and abate with rest.

*Renal failure.* Acute renal failure commonly causes sudden fatigue. Oliguria is an early sign, followed by ammonia breath odor, nausea, vomiting, diarrhea or constipation, and dry skin and mucous membranes. In *chronic renal failure,* insidious fatigue and lethargy are accompanied by marked changes in all body systems.

*Valvular heart disease.* Progressive fatigue and cardiac murmur are common. Other findings are exertional dyspnea, cough, and hemoptysis.

*Other causes.* Anxiety; cirrhosis; drugs, notably antihypertensives and sedatives; hypercortisolism; hypopituitarism; malnutrition; myocardial infarction; rheumatoid arthritis; surgery; systemic lupus erythematosus; and thyrotoxicosis.

## Nursing considerations

• Help the patient set priorities — a reasonable schedule, good sleep habits, stress management.
• If fatigue results from organic illness, help the patient determine which activities he must accomplish, which of these he may need help with, and how to pace himself to ensure sufficient rest.
• If fatigue results from a psychogenic cause, refer the patient for psychological counseling.

The inward displacement of the nipple below the level of surrounding breast tissue, nipple retraction may indicate an inflammatory breast lesion or cancer. It results from scar tissue formation within a lesion or large mammary duct. As the scar tissue shortens, it pulls adjacent tissue in, causing nipple deviation, flattening, and finally retraction.

## History
Ask the patient when she first noticed retraction of the nipple. Has she experienced other nipple changes, such as itching, discoloration, discharge, or excoriation? Has she had breast pain, lumps, redness, swelling, or warmth? In taking the history, note risk factors of breast cancer, such as a family history or previous neoplasm.

## Physical exam
Examine both nipples and breasts with the patient sitting upright with her arms at her sides, with her hands pressing on her hips, and with her arms overhead; and with the patient leaning forward so that her breasts hang. Look for redness, excoriation, and discharge; nipple flattening and deviation; and breast asymmetry, dimpling, or contour differences.

Try to evert the nipple by gently squeezing the areola. With the patient supine, palpate both breasts for lumps, especially beneath the areola. Mold breast skin over the lump or gently pull it up toward the clavicle, looking for accentuated nipple retraction. Also palpate axillary lymph nodes.

## Causes
*Breast abscess.* Most common in lactating women, this disorder occasionally produces unilateral nipple retraction. More common findings include high fever with chills; breast pain, erythema, and tenderness; and cracked, sore nipples, possibly with purulent discharge.

*Breast cancer.* Unilateral nipple retraction is commonly accompanied by a hard, fixed nodule beneath the areola. Other nipple changes include itching, burning, erosion, and watery or bloody discharge. Breast changes commonly include dimpling, altered contour, peau d'orange, ulceration, tenderness (possibly pain), redness, and warmth. Axillary lymph nodes may be enlarged.

*Fat necrosis.* An unlikely cause of nipple retraction, fat necrosis closely mimics breast cancer, producing a firm, painless, irregular, fixed, benign nodule. Other findings include skin dimpling, tenderness, and ecchymoses.

*Mammary duct ectasia.* Nipple retraction commonly occurs along with an ill-defined, rubbery nodule beneath the areola and blue-green skin discoloration; areolar burning, itching, swelling, tenderness, and erythema; and nipple pain with a thick, sticky, grayish discharge.

*Mastitis.* Nipple retraction, deviation, cracking, or flattening may occur with a breast nodule, warmth, erythema, tenderness, and edema. Fatigue, high fever, and chills may be present.

## Nursing considerations
• Prepare the patient for ordered diagnostic tests, including mammography, cytology of nipple discharge, and biopsy.

The involuntary passage of stool, fecal incontinence follows any loss or impairment of external anal sphincter control. It can result from various GI, neurologic, and psychological disorders; laxative abuse; and surgery. In some patients, it may even be purposefully manipulative.

Fecal incontinence may be temporary or permanent; its onset may be gradual, as in dementia, or sudden, as in spinal cord trauma. Although usually not a sign of severe illness, it can greatly affect the patient's well-being.

## History

Ask the patient with fecal incontinence about its onset, duration, severity, and any discernible pattern — for instance, at night or with diarrhea. Note the frequency, consistency, and volume of stool passed within the last 24 hours and obtain a stool sample. Focus your history taking on GI, neurologic, and psychological disorders.

## Physical exam

If you suspect a brain or spinal cord lesion, perform a complete neurologic examination. If a GI disturbance seems likely, inspect the abdomen for distention, auscultate for bowel sounds, percuss, and palpate for a mass. Inspect the anal area for signs of excoriation or infection. If not contraindicated, check for fecal impaction.

## Causes

*Cerebrovascular accident.* Temporary fecal incontinence occasionally occurs but usually disappears with the restoration of muscle tone and deep tendon reflexes. Persistent fecal incontinence may reflect extensive neurologic damage. Other findings reflect the location and extent of damage.

*Dementias.* Any of these chronic degenerative brain diseases can produce fecal incontinence. Associated signs and symptoms include impaired judgment and abstract thinking, amnesia, emotional lability, hyperactive deep tendon reflexes, aphasia or dysarthria and, possibly, diffuse choreoathetotic movements.

*Gastroenteritis.* Severe infection may cause temporary fecal incontinence marked by explosive diarrhea. Nausea, vomiting, and colicky abdominal pain are typical. Other possible findings: headache, myalgia, and hyperactive bowel sounds.

*Head trauma.* Disruption of the neurologic pathways that control defecation can cause fecal incontinence. Additional findings depend on the location and severity of the injury.

*Inflammatory bowel disease.* Nocturnal fecal incontinence occurs occasionally with diarrhea. Related findings: abdominal pain, anorexia, weight loss, and hyperactive bowel sounds.

*Laxative abuse.* Chronic laxative abuse may cause insensitivity to a fecal mass or loss of the colonic defecation reflex.

*Multiple sclerosis.* Fecal incontinence occasionally appears as one of this disorder's extremely variable signs. Other effects depend on the area of demyelination and may include muscle weakness, ataxia, and paralysis; gait disturbances; sensory impairment, such as paresthesia; visual blurring, diplopia, or nystagmus; urinary disturbances; and emotional lability.

*Spinal cord lesions.* Any lesion that causes compression or transection of sensorimotor spinal tracts can lead to fecal incontinence. Incontinence may be permanent, especially with severe sacral segment lesions. Other signs and symptoms reflect motor and sensory disturbances below the lesion's level.

*Other causes.* GI surgery, rectovaginal fistula, and tabes dorsalis.

## Nursing considerations

• Maintain effective hygienic care, including control of foul odors. Also provide emotional support because the patient may feel deep embarrassment.
• For the patient with intermittent or temporary incontinence, encourage Kegel exercises to strengthen abdominal and perirectal muscles.
• For the neurologically capable patient with chronic incontinence, provide bowel retraining.

**F**

Nipple discharge can occur spontaneously or be elicited by nipple stimulation. It's characterized as intermittent or constant, unilateral or bilateral, and also by its color, consistency, and composition. Its incidence increases with age and parity. Rare in men and in nulligravid, regularly menstruating women, nipple discharge is relatively common — and often normal — in parous women and women in late pregnancy.

However, nipple discharge can signal serious underlying disease, particularly when accompanied by other breast changes. Significant causes include endocrine disorders, cancer, certain drugs, and blocked lactiferous ducts.

## History

Ask the patient when she first noticed the discharge, and determine its duration, extent, quantity, color, and consistency. Has she experienced pain, tenderness, itching, warmth, changes in contour, or lumps? If she reports a lump, ask about its onset, location, size, and consistency.

Obtain a gynecologic and obstetric history. Determine her normal menstrual cycle and the date of her last menses. Also check for any risk factors of breast cancer.

## Physical exam

Characterize the discharge. If the discharge isn't frank, try to elicit it by positioning the patient supine and gently squeezing her nipple between your thumb and index finger, noting any discharge. Then place your fingers on the areola and palpate the areolar surface, watching for any discharge.

Examine the nipples and breasts with the patient sitting with her arms at her sides, with her arms overhead, and with her hands pressing on her hips; and with the patient leaning forward so that her breasts hang. Check for nipple deviation, flattening, retraction, redness, asymmetry, thickening, excoriation, erosion, or cracking. Inspect the breasts for asymmetry, irregular contours, dimpling, erythema, and peau d'orange. With the patient supine, palpate the breasts and axilla for lumps, giving special attention to the areolae. Note the size, location, delineation, consistency, and mobility of any lump.

## Causes

*Breast abscess.* This disorder, most common in lactating women, may produce a thick, purulent discharge. Other findings include high fever with chills; breast pain, tenderness, and erythema; a palpable, soft nodule or generalized induration; and possibly nipple retraction.

*Breast cancer.* This may cause bloody, watery, or purulent discharge from a normal appearing nipple. Other findings include a hard, irregular, fixed lump; erythema; dimpling; peau d'orange; changes in contour; nipple deviation, flattening, or retraction; axillary lymphadenopathy; and possibly breast pain.

*Choriocarcinoma.* Galactorrhea may result from this highly malignant neoplasm, which can follow pregnancy. Other findings include persistent uterine bleeding and bogginess after delivery or curettage.

*Intraductal papilloma.* Unilateral serous, serosanguineous, or bloody nipple discharge is the predominant sign of this disorder. Discharge may be intermittent or profuse and constant. Subareolar nodules, breast pain, and tenderness may occur.

*Other causes.* Chest wall surgery; drugs, such phenothiazines, tricyclic antidepressants, antihypertensives, oral contraceptives, cimetidine, metoclopramide, and verapamil; herpes zoster; hypothyroidism; mammary duct ectasia; Paget's disease, prolactin-secreting pituitary tumors; proliferative (fibrocystic) breast disease; and trauma to the breasts.

## Nursing considerations

• Help relieve the patient's anxieties by clearly explaining the nature and origin of her discharge.
• If ordered, apply a breast binder, which may reduce discharge by eliminating nipple stimulation.
• Prepare the patient for ordered diagnostic tests.

A distinctive musty-sweet breath odor, fetor hepaticus characterizes hepatic encephalopathy, a life-threatening complication of severe liver disease. The odor results from the damaged liver's inability to metabolize and detoxify mercaptans produced by bacterial degradation of methionine, a sulfurous amino acid. These substances circulate in the blood, are expelled by the lungs, and flavor the breath.

▶ **Emergency interventions**
If you detect fetor hepaticus, quickly assess the patient's level of consciousness (LOC). If he's comatose, have another nurse notify the doctor while you assess respiratory status. Prepare to assist with intubation and provide ventilatory support, if necessary. As ordered, start a peripheral I.V. line for fluid administration, begin cardiac monitoring, and insert an indwelling urinary catheter to monitor output. Obtain arterial and venous samples for analysis of blood gases, ammonia, and electrolytes.

If the patient is conscious, closely observe him for signs of impending coma. Assess deep tendon reflexes, and attempt to elicit Babinski's sign. Be alert for signs of GI bleeding and shock, common complications of end-stage liver failure. Inform the doctor immediately if you note increased anxiety; restlessness; tachycardia; tachypnea; cool, moist, pale skin; hypotension; oliguria; hematemesis; or melena. Place the patient supine with his legs elevated 20 degrees, administer oxygen, and increase the infusion rate of I.V. fluids, as ordered. Draw blood samples for a complete blood count, type and cross match, and clotting profile. Be prepared to assist with intubation and ventilation or to begin cardiopulmonary resuscitation.

Continue your physical examination by assessing the degree of jaundice and abdominal distention and by palpating the liver for degree of enlargement.

## History
Obtain a complete medical history, relying on the patient's family if necessary. Focus on any factors that may have precipitated hepatic disease or coma, such as recent severe infection; overuse of sedatives, analgesics, or diuretics; excessive protein intake; and recent blood transfusion or surgery.

## Cause
*Hepatic encephalopathy.* Fetor hepaticus usually occurs in the final, comatose stage of this disorder but may occur earlier. Tremors progress to asterixis in the impending stage, accompanied by lethargy, aberrant behavior, and apraxia. Hyperventilation and stupor mark the stuporous stage, and the patient acts agitated when aroused. Seizures and coma herald the final stage, along with decreased pulse and respiratory rates, positive Babinski's sign, hyperactive reflexes, decerebrate posture, and opisthotonos.

## Nursing considerations
• Effective treatment of hepatic encephalopathy reduces blood ammonia levels by eliminating ammonia from the GI tract. You may be asked to administer neomycin or lactulose to suppress bacterial production of ammonia, give sorbitol solution to induce osmotic diuresis, give potassium supplements to correct alkalosis, provide continuous gastric aspiration of blood, or maintain the patient on a low-protein diet. If these methods aren't successful, hemodialysis or exchange transfusions may be employed.
• During treatment, closely monitor the patient's LOC, intake and output, and fluid and electrolyte balance.

Also called nyctalopia, night blindness refers to impaired vision in the dark, especially after entering a darkened room or while driving at night. Often difficult to detect, it is a symptom of choroidal and retinal degeneration that occurs in various ocular disorders and as an early indicator of vitamin A deficiency.

In some patients, night blindness occurs without an underlying disorder, simply reflecting poor adaptation to the dark, and is probably accompanied by myopia. Children, who generally lack adequate reserves of vitamin A, are especially prone to deficiency and resulting night blindness.

## History

If the patient complains of difficulty seeing at night, ask when he first noticed the problem. Is it intermittent or steadily worsening? Is it worse at certain times or in certain conditions? Also ask about other ocular symptoms, such as eye pain, blurred or halo vision, floaters or spots, and photophobia.

Explore any history of glaucoma, cataracts, and familial degeneration of vision. If no ocular problems are apparent, briefly evaluate the patient's nutritional status for possible vitamin A deficiency.

## Physical exam

Examine the eyes for ptosis, abnormal tearing, discharge, and conjunctival injection. Test visual acuity and visual fields in both eyes. If trained and equipped, measure intraocular pressure. Check pupillary response. Evaluate extraocular muscle function by testing the six cardinal fields of gaze.

## Causes

*Cataracts.* Night blindness and halo vision occur early in senile-type cataract formation. As the cataract matures, it causes gradual, painless visual blurring and vision loss, sometimes with visible lens opacity.

*Choroidal dystrophies.* Night blindness and decreased peripheral vision may occur early in choroidal dystrophies. Disease progression causes loss of central vision.

*Fundus albipunctatus.* Night blindness is the chief complaint in this retinal and choroidal disease. Multiple small, round, yellow-white dots are present on the retina.

*Fundus flavimaculatus.* In this disease, night blindness may be pronounced or may be an incidental finding. Irregular yellow or white lesions appear deep in the retina.

*Glaucoma.* Night blindness occurs late in chronic open-angle glaucoma, with halo vision, gradually impaired bilateral visual acuity, loss of peripheral vision, and possibly slight eye pain.

*Oguchi's disease.* This rare, hereditary retinal and choroidal degeneration produces night blind-ness and a retina with a yellowish metallic sheen.

*Optic nerve atrophy.* This disorder may cause night blindness, visual field and color vision defects, and decreased visual acuity. Pupillary reactions are sluggish, and optic disk pallor is evident.

*Retinitis pigmentosa.* Night blindness is typically the first symptom, usually arising in adolescence. Scattered black pigmentary bodies form in a characteristic "bone-spicule" arrangement on the retina. As the disease progresses, the visual field constricts, causing tunnel or "gun barrel" vision and eventually total blindness.

*Vitamin A deficiency.* Night blindness is typically the first symptom. Associated findings may include xerophthalmia (conjunctival dryness) and Bitot's spots (gray-white conjunctival plaques). The patient may complain of visual blurring or vision loss. His skin may be dry and scaly, and mucous membranes may be shrunken and hardened.

## Nursing considerations

• Because any visual impairment is frightening to the patient, you'll need to provide emotional support. Help decrease his anxiety and enhance cooperation by explaining scheduled diagnostic tests, such as electroretinography, in simple terms.

This common sign can arise from disorders affecting virtually every body system. As a result, fever alone has little diagnostic value. Persistent high fever, though, represents an emergency.

Fever can be classified as low (oral reading of 99° to 100.4° F [37.2° to 38° C]), moderate (100.5° to 104° F [38° to 40° C]), or high (above 104° F [40° C]). Fever over 108° F (42.2° C) causes unconsciousness and, if sustained, brain damage.

Fever can also be called remittent, intermittent, sustained, or relapsing. *Remittent fever,* the most common, refers to daily fluctuations above normal. In *intermittent fever,* daily temperature drops into the normal range, then rises back above normal. *Sustained fever* is persistent elevation with little fluctuation. *Relapsing fever* refers to alternating feverish and afebrile periods.

## ▶ Emergency interventions

If fever exceeds 106° F (41.1° C), notify the doctor. Take other vital signs and assess level of consciousness. Give antipyretic drugs and apply ice packs to axillae and groin, give tepid sponge baths, or apply a hypothermia blanket. These methods may evoke a hypothermic response; to avoid this, constantly monitor rectal temperature.

## History

If the patient's fever is low to moderate, ask when it began and how high it reached. Did the fever disappear, only to recur? Did he experience other symptoms? Obtain a full medical and surgical history. Ask about recent travel.

## Physical exam

Because fever can accompany diverse disorders, this examination may range from cursory to complete.

## Causes

*Drugs.* Fever and rash commonly result from hypersensitivity to anti-infectives, barbiturates, phenytoin, quinidine, iodides, methyldopa, procainamide, and some antitoxins. Fever can accompany chemotherapy or result from drugs that impair sweating, such as anticholinergics. It can also stem from toxic doses of salicylates, amphetamines, and tricyclic antidepressants. In susceptible patients, malignant hyperthermia can stem from inhaled anesthetics and muscle relaxants.

*Immune complex dysfunction.* When present, fever usually remains low. It may be remittent or intermittent, as in acquired immunodeficiency syndrome, or sustained, as in polyarteritis.

*Infectious and inflammatory disorders.* Fever ranges from low (in Crohn's disease and ulcerative colitis) to extremely high (in bacterial pneumonia). It may be remittent, as in infectious mononucleosis; sustained, as in meningitis; or relapsing, as in malaria. Fever may arise abruptly, as in Rocky Mountain spotted fever, or insidiously, as in mycoplasmal pneumonia.

*Neoplasms.* Primary neoplasms and metastases can produce prolonged fever of varying elevations. For instance, acute leukemia may present insidiously with low fever, pallor, and bleeding tendencies, or more abruptly with high fever, frank bleeding, and prostration.

*Thermoregulatory dysfunction.* Fever that rises rapidly and remains as high as 107° F (41.7° C) typically occurs in such life-threatening disorders as heatstroke, thyroid storm, malignant hyperthermia, and central nervous system lesions.

*Other causes.* Contrast media used in diagnostic tests, surgery, and transfusion reactions.

## Nursing considerations

• Regularly monitor temperature. Provide increased fluid and nutritional intake, as ordered.
• Minimize chills and diaphoresis by following a regular antipyretic dosage. Promote patient comfort by keeping room temperature stable and changing bedding and clothing frequently.
• Keep in mind that infants and young children experience higher and more prolonged fevers, more rapid temperature increases, and greater temperature fluctuations than older children and adults.

This pain may originate from any neck structure — from the meninges and cervical vertebrae to blood vessels, muscles, and lymphatic tissue. Neck pain can also be referred from other areas of the body but usually results from trauma or from degenerative, congenital, inflammatory, metabolic, or neoplastic disorders.

## ▶ Emergency interventions

If the patient's neck pain results from trauma, immediately ensure proper cervical spine immobilization, preferably with a long backboard and a Philadelphia collar. Take his vital signs and perform a quick neurologic assessment. Administer oxygen and assist with intubation and mechanical ventilation as necessary.

## History

Ask the patient or his companion how the injury occurred. If the patient hasn't sustained trauma, find out the severity, onset, and location of his neck pain. Ask about other symptoms, the patient's current and past illnesses, injuries, diet, medication use, and family health history.

## Physical exam

Inspect the patient's neck, shoulders, and cervical spine for abrasions, swelling, lacerations, masses, erythema, and ecchymoses. Assess range of motion in his neck by having him turn his head from side to side; note the degree of pain produced by these movements. Check sensation in his arms, and assess his hand grasp and arm reflexes. Try to elicit Brudzinski's and Kernig's signs, and palpate the cervical lymph nodes for enlargement.

## Causes

*Cervical extension injury.* Anterior or posterior neck pain may develop within hours or days after a whiplash injury. Anterior pain usually diminishes, but posterior pain persists and may intensify. Other findings may include tenderness, swelling and nuchal rigidity, headache, muscle spasms, visual blurring, and miosis.

*Cervical spine infection.* This disorder can cause moderate neck pain that restricts motion. Other findings: fever, muscle spasms, tenderness, dysphagia, paresthesia, and muscle weakness.

*Cervical spine tumor. Metastatic tumors* typically produce persistent neck pain that increases with movement and isn't relieved by rest. *Primary tumors* cause mild to severe pain along a specific nerve root. Other findings may include paresthesia, arm and leg weakness that progresses to atrophy and paralysis, and incontinence.

*Hemorrhage (subarachnoid).* This life-threatening condition may cause neck pain and rigidity, headache, and a decreased level of consciousness.

Kernig's and Brudzinski's signs are present.

*Herniated cervical disk.* This disorder characteristically causes variable neck pain that restricts movement and is aggravated by it. It also causes referred pain, paresthesia and other sensory disturbances, and arm weakness.

*Lymphadenitis.* Enlarged and inflamed cervical lymph nodes cause acute pain and tenderness. Fever, chills, and malaise may also occur.

*Meningitis.* Neck pain may accompany nuchal rigidity. Other findings include fever, headache, photophobia, positive Brudzinski's and Kernig's signs, and decreased level of consciousness.

*Spinous process fracture.* Fracture near the cervicothoracic junction produces acute pain radiating to the shoulders. Associated findings include swelling, exquisite tenderness, restricted range of motion, muscle spasms, and deformity.

*Other causes.* Ankylosing spondylitis; cervical fibrositis, spondylosis, and stenosis; cervical spine fracture; esophageal trauma; Hodgkin's lymphoma; laryngeal cancer; neck sprain; osteoporosis; Paget's disease; rheumatoid arthritis; torticollis; trauma to the trachea or thyroid.

## Nursing considerations

• Give anti-inflammatory drugs and analgesics, as ordered. Prepare the patient for ordered diagnostic tests.

**N**

A major indicator of renal and urinary tract disease or trauma, flank pain may vary from a dull ache to severe stabbing or throbbing pain. It may be unilateral or bilateral, constant or intermittent. Flank pain is aggravated by costovertebral angle (CVA) percussion and, in patients with renal or urinary tract obstruction, by increased fluid intake or ingestion of alcohol, caffeine, or diuretic drugs.

## ▶ Emergency interventions

If the patient has suffered trauma, assess for a visible or palpable flank mass, associated injuries, CVA pain, hematuria, Grey Turner's sign, and signs of shock. If you find any of these, notify the doctor immediately, and insert an I.V. line. As ordered, insert an indwelling urinary catheter.

## History

Ask the patient about the pain's onset, location, intensity, pattern, and duration, and find out if anything aggravates or alleviates it.

Ask the patient about any changes in fluid intake and urine output. Also ask about urinary tract infection or obstruction, recent streptococcal infection, and renal disease.

## Physical exam

During the physical examination, palpate the patient's flank area and percuss the CVA.

## Causes

*Bladder cancer.* Dull, constant flank pain may be unilateral or bilateral and may radiate to the leg, back, and perineum. The first sign of this neoplasm commonly is hematuria.

*Calculi.* Renal and ureteral calculi produce intense unilateral, colicky flank pain. Initial CVA pain radiates to the flank and suprapubic region.

*Cortical necrosis (acute).* Unilateral flank pain is usually severe and accompanied by gross hematuria, anuria, and fever.

*Cystitis (bacterial).* The patient may report unilateral or bilateral flank pain along with low back and suprapubic pain. Other effects include dysuria, nocturia, hematuria, frequency, and urgency.

*Perirenal abscess.* Intense unilateral flank pain and CVA tenderness accompany dysuria, persistent high fever, and chills.

*Polycystic kidney disease.* Dull, aching, bilateral flank pain is commonly the earliest symptom. The pain can become severe and colicky if cysts rupture and clots cause obstruction.

*Pyelonephritis (acute).* Intense, constant, unilateral or bilateral flank pain develops over a few hours or days along with typical urinary features. Other findings include persistent high fever, generalized myalgia, and CVA tenderness.

*Renal infarction.* Unilateral, constant, severe flank pain and tenderness typically accompany persistent, severe upper abdominal pain. The patient may also have CVA tenderness.

*Renal neoplasm.* Unilateral flank pain, gross hematuria, and a palpable flank mass form the classic clinical triad. Flank pain is usually dull and vague.

*Renal trauma.* Variable bilateral or unilateral flank pain is a common symptom. A palpable flank mass may also exist along with CVA or abdominal pain — possibly severe and radiating to the groin. Other findings include hematuria, oliguria, abdominal distention, Grey Turner's sign, and hypoactive bowel sounds.

*Renal vein thrombosis.* This causes severe unilateral flank and low back pain with CVA and epigastric tenderness. Other features may include fever, hematuria, and leg edema.

*Other causes.* Acute poststreptococcal glomerulonephritis, infantile polycystic kidney disease, nephroblastoma, obstructive uropathy, pancreatitis, and papillary necrosis.

## Nursing considerations

• Administer pain medication, as ordered. Continue to monitor vital signs, and maintain precise intake and output records. Prepare the patient for any diagnostic tests.

Nausea is a profound sense of revulsion to food, or a signal of impending vomiting. Commonly accompanied by autonomic signs, such as hypersalivation, diaphoresis, tachycardia, pallor, and tachypnea, nausea is closely associated with both anorexia and vomiting.

### History
If the patient isn't in distress, ask him to describe nausea's onset, duration, and intensity. Also ask about vomiting, abdominal pain, anorexia, weight loss, changes in bowel habits, and excessive belching or flatus. Inquire about GI, endocrine, and metabolic disorders; recent infections; and cancer, including any treatment. Find out if the patient takes medication or consumes alcohol. Ask the female patient if she is or could be pregnant.

### Physical exam
Inspect the patient's skin for jaundice, bruises, and spider angiomas, and assess skin turgor. Inspect the abdomen for distention, auscultate for bowel sounds and bruits, palpate for rigidity and tenderness, and test for rebound tenderness. Also percuss the abdomen.

### Causes
*Appendicitis.* Nausea and vomiting accompany vague epigastric or periumbilical discomfort that localizes in the right lower quadrant.

*Cholecystitis and cholelithiasis.* Nausea, vomiting, and severe right upper quadrant or epigastric pain occur after ingestion of fatty foods.

*Drugs.* Nausea-inducing drugs include anesthetics, antibiotics, antineoplastics, chloride replacements, digitalis (overdose), estrogens, ferrous sulfate, levodopa, opiates, oral potassium, quinidine, sulfasalazine, and theophylline (overdose).

*Gastroenteritis.* Nausea, vomiting, diarrhea, abdominal cramping, and hyperactive bowel sounds are common.

*Intestinal obstruction.* Nausea occurs with high small intestinal obstruction. Vomiting may be bilious or fecal, and abdominal pain is usually episodic and colicky.

*Migraine headache.* Nausea and vomiting may occur in the prodromal stage, along with photophobia, partial vision loss, and paresthesia.

*Motion sickness.* Nausea and vomiting are brought on by motion or rhythmic movement. Dizziness, headache, fatigue, diaphoresis, and dyspnea may also occur.

*Pancreatitis (acute).* Nausea — usually followed by vomiting — occurs early, along with steady, severe pain in the epigastrium or left upper quadrant that may radiate to the back.

*Peptic ulcer.* Nausea, vomiting, and epigastric pain occur when the stomach is empty or after ingestion of alcohol, caffeine, or aspirin.

*Peritonitis.* Nausea and vomiting usually accompany acute abdominal pain localized to the area of inflammation. Other findings may include high fever with chills, hypoactive or absent bowel sounds, and abdominal distention.

*Radiation and surgery.* Radiation therapy may cause nausea and vomiting. Postoperative nausea and vomiting are common, especially after abdominal surgery.

*Other causes.* Adrenal insufficiency, cirrhosis, congestive heart failure, diverticulitis, ectopic pregnancy, electrolyte imbalance, gastric cancer, gastritis, hepatitis, hyperemesis gravidarum, infection, irritable bowel syndrome, labyrinthitis, Ménière's disease, mesenteric artery ischemia, mesenteric venous thrombosis, metabolic acidosis, myocardial infarction, preeclampsia, renal and urologic disorders, thyrotoxicosis, and ulcerative colitis.

### Nursing considerations
- Have the patient breathe deeply to ease nausea and help prevent vomiting. Keep the air in his room clean-smelling, removing bedpans and emesis basins promptly after use. Elevate his head or place him on his side to prevent aspiration of vomitus.
- If possible, give medications by injection or suppository to avoid exacerbating nausea.

# Flatulence

A sensation of gaseous abdominal fullness, flatulence can result from GI disorders, abdominal surgery, and excessive intake of certain foods. It can also stem from stress and can be accompanied by belching, discomfort, and excessive passage of flatus. This symptom reflects slowed intestinal motility, which hampers the passage of gas; excessive swallowing of air (aerophagia), commonly brought on by stress; or increased intraluminal gas production caused by an excess of fermentable substrates, such as digested, unabsorbed carbohydrates and proteins.

Although usually not a serious symptom, flatulence and accompanying expulsion of flatus may cause the patient embarrassment and discomfort.

## History

Find out how long the patient has noticed the flatulence and if he also passes an excessive amount of flatus. Ask about frequent belching or snoring, and observe for overly rapid speech—all possible clues to aerophagia. Ask if he's undergoing unusual emotional stress. Obtain a medical history.

## Physical exam

Inspect the abdomen for distention and auscultate for abnormal bowel sounds. Percuss for increased tympany from gas accumulation, and palpate for tenderness and masses.

## Causes

*Cholecystitis.* Acute and chronic cholecystitis commonly produce flatulence with frequent passage of flatus. Colicky pain in the right upper quadrant becomes persistent and severe in an acute attack. Nausea, vomiting, and fever may occur.

*Cholelithiasis.* Complaints of flatulence and belching are common in this disorder. Abdominal pain develops in the right upper quadrant, usually after the patient eats fatty foods. With cystic duct obstruction, excruciating pain radiates to the back or the right shoulder, usually accompanied by nausea, vomiting, and fever.

*Cirrhosis.* Typically, flatulence develops early and insidiously, along with anorexia, dyspepsia, nausea, vomiting, diarrhea or constipation, abdominal pain, hepatomegaly, and splenomegaly.

*Colon cancer.* Obstruction of the colon by a tumor may cause flatulence; acute obstruction also produces abdominal distention and tympany on percussion. Abdominal pain may be present, with anorexia, weight loss, malaise, and altered bowel habits—constipation, diarrhea, or a change in the timing, frequency, or consistency of stools.

*Crohn's disease.* Flatulence accompanies other acute inflammatory signs and symptoms that mimic appendicitis: right lower quadrant pain, cramps, and tenderness; diarrhea; low-grade fever; nausea; and melena.

*Irritable bowel syndrome.* Findings include chronic flatulence, belching, and excessive flatus. Chronic constipation is typical, but diurnal diarrhea may also occur.

*Lactose intolerance.* Flatulence, cramping abdominal pain, and possibly diarrhea develop within several hours of ingesting dairy products.

*Malabsorption syndromes.* This group of syndromes may cause flatulence. Associated findings vary considerably, depending on which dietary constituent isn't absorbed, but may include passage of bulky, oily, malodorous, or slightly watery stools; abdominal pain; anorexia; and weight loss.

*Other causes.* Abdominal surgery.

## Nursing considerations

• Prepare the patient for blood tests, stool analysis, upper GI series, barium enema, or endoscopy.
• To aid expulsion of excessive flatus, position the patient on his left side; to prevent gas buildup, encourage frequent repositioning, ambulation, and normal fluid intake, as permitted. If these measures aren't effective, try inserting a rectal tube into the anus to relieve flatus or administering enemas, suppositories, antiflatulents, or anticholinergics, as ordered.
• As appropriate, provide the patient with a dietary plan that excludes gas-producing foods.

Abnormal dilation of the nostrils, nasal flaring usually occurs during inspiration but may occur during expiration or throughout the respiratory cycle. Nasal flaring indicates respiratory dysfunction, ranging from mild difficulty to potentially life-threatening respiratory distress.

## ▶ Emergency interventions

If you detect nasal flaring, assess the patient's respiratory status and notify the doctor. Inspiratory chest movement, absent breath sounds, cyanosis, diaphoresis, and tachycardia point to complete airway obstruction. As necessary, deliver back blows or abdominal thrusts, or assist with emergency intubation or tracheotomy and mechanical ventilation.

If the airway is open but breathing remains difficult, give oxygen by nasal cannula or face mask, and assist with intubation and mechanical ventilation as needed. Insert an I.V. line for fluid and medication access. Begin cardiac monitoring, and obtain a chest X-ray and samples for arterial blood gas and electrolyte studies.

## History

When the patient stabilizes, ask about cardiac and pulmonary disorders, allergies, trauma, or a recent illness, such as a respiratory infection.

## Causes

*Adult respiratory distress syndrome (ARDS).* Increased respiratory difficulty occurs with nasal flaring, dyspnea, tachypnea, diaphoresis, cyanosis, scattered crackles, and rhonchi. ARDS also causes tachycardia, anxiety, and decreased level of consciousness (LOC).

*Airway obstruction.* Complete obstruction produces sudden nasal flaring, absent breath sounds, tachycardia, diaphoresis, cyanosis, and decreasing LOC. Partial obstruction causes nasal flaring, gagging, wheezing, accessory muscle use, cyanosis, and hoarseness.

*Asthma (acute).* This disorder causes nasal flaring, dyspnea, tachypnea, expiratory wheezing, accessory muscle use, cyanosis, and a dry or productive cough.

*Chronic obstructive pulmonary disease.* Nasal flaring is accompanied by pursed-lip expiration, accessory muscle use, cyanosis, reduced chest expansion, crackles, rhonchi, wheezing, dyspnea, and a loose, rattling, productive cough.

*Pneumonia (bacterial).* Nasal flaring occurs with dyspnea, tachypnea, high fever, and sudden shaking chills. Initial dry, hacking cough later becomes productive. Stabbing chest pain worsens with movement and respirations. Auscultation reveals reduced or absent breath sounds, crackles, and pleural friction rub. Percussion reveals dullness.

*Pneumothorax.* Respiratory distress occurs with nasal flaring, dyspnea, tachypnea, shallow respirations, hyperresonance or tympany on percussion, agitation, distended neck veins, tracheal deviation, and cyanosis.

*Pulmonary edema.* Nasal flaring accompanies severe dyspnea, wheezing, and hemoptysis. Other findings include accessory muscle use with tachycardia, cyanosis, hypotension, crackles, distended neck veins, peripheral edema, and decreased LOC.

*Pulmonary embolus.* Nasal flaring accompanies dyspnea, tachypnea, wheezing, cyanosis, pleural friction rub, and productive cough. Other effects include sudden chest tightness or pleuritic pain, tachycardia, hypotension, low-grade fever, syncope, and restlessness.

*Other causes.* Anaphylaxis, pulmonary function tests, and respiratory treatments.

## Nursing considerations

• Place the patient in high Fowler's position. If he risks aspirating secretions, place him in a modified Trendelenburg or side-lying position.

• If necessary, suction the patient frequently. Administer humidified oxygen. Reposition him every hour and encourage coughing and deep breathing. Continually assess respiratory status, and check vital signs every 30 minutes or as needed.

• Prepare the patient for any diagnostic tests.

In a normal infant, the anterior fontanel, or "soft spot," is flat, soft yet firm, and well demarcated against surrounding skull bones. (The posterior fontanel, if not fused at birth, usually closes by age 2 months.) Subtle pulsations may be visible, reflecting the arterial pulse.

A bulging fontanel—widened, tense, and with marked pulsations—is a cardinal sign of potentially life-threatening increased intracranial pressure (ICP), a medical emergency. Because prolonged coughing, crying, or lying down can cause transient, physiologic bulging, the infant's head should be observed and palpated while he's upright and relaxed to detect pathologic bulging.

## ▶ Emergency interventions

If you detect a bulging fontanel, notify the doctor immediately. Measure fontanel size and head circumference, and note the overall shape of the head. Take vital signs, and assess level of consciousness (LOC) by observing spontaneous activity, postural reflex activity, and sensory responses. Note whether the infant assumes a normal, flexed posture or one of extreme extension, opisthotonos, or hypotonia. Observe movements of his arms and legs—excessive tremulousness or frequent twitching may herald the onset of a seizure. Look for other signs of increased ICP: abnormal respiratory patterns and a distinctive, high-pitched cry.

Ensure airway patency, and have size-appropriate emergency equipment on hand. Provide oxygen, establish I.V. access and, if the infant is having a seizure, stay with him to prevent injury. As ordered, administer anticonvulsants and antipyretics, osmotic diuretics to help reduce cerebral edema and ICP, and dexamethasone for edema secondary to head trauma. If the infant has an extremely high fever, give him a tepid sponge bath. If these measures fail to reduce ICP, neuromuscular blockade, intubation, mechanical ventilation, and, in rare cases, barbiturate coma and total body hypothermia may be necessary.

## History

Once the infant's condition is stabilized, you can begin investigating the underlying cause of increased ICP. Obtain his medical history from a parent or caretaker, paying particular attention to any recent infection or trauma, including birth trauma. Has the infant or any family member had a recent rash or fever? Ask about any changes in the infant's behavior, such as frequent vomiting, lethargy, or disinterest in feeding.

## Cause

*Increased ICP.* Besides a bulging fontanel and increased head circumference, other early signs and symptoms are often subtle and difficult to discern. They may include behavioral changes, irritability, and fatigue.

As ICP rises, the infant's pupils may dilate and his LOC may decrease to drowsiness and eventual coma. Seizures commonly occur.

## Nursing considerations

• Closely monitor the infant's condition, including urine output (via an indwelling urinary catheter, if necessary), and continue to observe for seizures. Restrict fluids, as ordered, and position the infant supine at a 30-degree head-up tilt to enhance cerebral venous drainage and reduce intracranial blood volume.

• Explain the purpose and procedure of diagnostic tests to the infant's parents or caretaker. Such tests may include intracranial computed tomography scan or skull X-ray, cerebral angiography, and a full sepsis workup, including blood and urine cultures.

# Myoclonus

Sudden, shocklike contractions of a single muscle or muscle group, myoclonus occurs in various neurologic disorders and commonly heralds onset of a seizure. Contractions may be isolated or repetitive, rhythmic or arrhythmic, symmetrical or asymmetrical, synchronous or asynchronous, and generalized or localized. In many cases, they're precipitated by a sensory stimulus, such as a bright light, a loud sound, or unexpected physical contact. One type, *intention myoclonus,* is evoked by intentional muscle movement, probably by a proprioceptive mechanism.

## ▶ Emergency interventions
If you observe myoclonus, notify the doctor immediately and assess the patient for seizure activity. If he has a seizure, help him lie down, providing soft support for his head. Loosen his clothing and turn his head to one side. Maintain airway patency; if necessary, provide ventilation using a manual resuscitation bag.

## History
If the patient is stable, assess his level of consciousness (LOC) and mental status. Then ask about the frequency, severity, location, and circumstances of the myoclonus. Has he ever had a seizure? If so, did myoclonus precede it? Is the myoclonus ever caused by a sensory stimulus?

## Physical exam
During the physical examination, check for muscle rigidity and wasting, and test deep tendon reflexes.

## Causes
*Creutzfeldt-Jakob disease.* Diffuse myoclonic jerks appear early in this rapidly progressive dementia. Associated effects may include ataxia, aphasia, hearing loss, muscle rigidity and wasting, fasciculations, hemiplegia, and visual disturbances or blindness.

*Encephalitis (viral).* Myoclonus is usually intermittent and either localized or generalized. Associated findings may include rapidly decreasing LOC, fever, headache, irritability, nuchal rigidity, vomiting, seizures, aphasia, ataxia, hemiparesis, facial muscle weakness, nystagmus, ocular palsies, and dysphagia.

*Epilepsy.* In *idiopathic epilepsy,* localized myoclonus affects an arm or leg and occurs singly or in short bursts, commonly upon awakening. It's more frequent and severe during the prodromal stage of a major generalized seizure, then becomes less so.

Myoclonic jerks are usually the first signs of *myoclonic epilepsy.* At first, myoclonus is uncommon and localized; but months later it occurs frequently, involving the entire body, disrupting voluntary movement (intention myoclonus), and eventually causing generalized seizures and dementia.

*Hypoxic encephalopathy.* Generalized myoclonus or convulsions may appear almost immediately after restoration of cardiopulmonary function. The patient may also have a residual intention myoclonus.

*Uremic encephalopathy.* This disorder commonly produces myoclonic jerks and seizures. Other findings include apathy, fatigue, irritability, headache, confusion, gradually decreasing LOC, nausea, vomiting, oliguria, edema, and papilledema.

*Other causes.* Alzheimer's disease, long-term hemodialysis (rare), and poisoning (bismuth, methyl bromide, strychnine).

## Nursing considerations
• In progressive myoclonus, take seizure precautions. Keep an oral airway, suction equipment, and padded tongue blade at the bedside, and pad the side rails. Protect the patient from harmful objects, and remain with him while he walks. Instruct the patient and his family about safety precautions.
• As ordered, administer drugs that suppress myoclonus: ethosuximide, 5-hydroxytryptophan, phenobarbital, clonazepam, or carbidopa. Prepare the patient for an EEG, as ordered.

M

# Fontanel depression

Normally, an infant's anterior fontanel is flat, soft yet firm, and well demarcated against the surrounding skull bones. Subtle pulsations reflect the infant's arterial pulse.

Depression of the anterior fontanel below the surrounding bony ridges of the skull is a sign of dehydration. A common disorder of infancy and early childhood, dehydration may result from insufficient fluid intake, but typically reflects excessive fluid loss from severe vomiting or diarrhea. It may also reflect insensible water loss, pyloric stenosis, or tracheoesophageal fistula.

### ▶ Emergency interventions

If you detect a markedly depressed fontanel, call the doctor immediately. Take the infant's vital signs, weigh him, and check for signs of shock, such as tachycardia, tachypnea, and cool, clammy skin. If these signs are present, insert an I.V. line and administer fluids, as ordered. Have size-appropriate emergency equipment on hand, and prepare to administer oxygen, as ordered. Apply a pediatric urine collection bag (or insert an indwelling urinary catheter, if necessary) to enable accurate output measurement.

### History

Obtain a thorough patient history from a parent or caretaker, focusing on recent fever, vomiting, diarrhea, and behavioral changes. Determine the infant's fluid intake and urine output over the last 24 hours. Ask about his preillness weight, and compare it with his current weight; weight loss in an infant virtually equals water loss.

### Cause

*Dehydration.* In *mild dehydration* (5% weight loss), the anterior fontanel appears slightly depressed. The infant has pale, dry skin and mucous membranes, reduced urine output, a normal or slightly elevated pulse rate, and possibly a decreased level of activity.

*Moderate dehydration* (10% weight loss) causes slightly more pronounced fontanel depression, gray skin with poor turgor, dry mucous membranes, and diminished urine output. The infant has normal or decreased blood pressure, an increased pulse rate, and possibly lethargy.

*Severe dehydration* (15% or greater weight loss) may result in a markedly depressed fontanel, extremely poor skin turgor, parched mucous membranes, marked oliguria, lethargy, and signs of shock.

### Nursing considerations

• Continue to monitor the infant's vital signs, intake, and output, and watch for signs of worsening dehydration.

• In mild dehydration, frequently provide small amounts of clear fluids. If the infant's unable to ingest sufficient fluid, begin total parenteral nutrition (TPN).

• In moderate or severe dehydration, your first priority is rapid restoration of extracellular fluid volume to treat or prevent shock. Continue to administer I.V. solution with sodium bicarbonate added, as ordered, to combat acidosis. As renal function improves, administer I.V. potassium replacements. Once the infant's fluid status stabilizes, begin to replace depleted fat and protein stores through diet. If the infant can't eat or if feeding aggravates diarrhea, provide TPN to prevent severe malnourishment.

• Tests to evaluate dehydration include urinalysis for specific gravity and possibly blood tests to determine electrolyte concentrations, blood urea nitrogen and serum creatinine levels, osmolality, and acid-base status.

**F**

Mydriasis—pupillary dilation caused by contraction of the dilator of the iris—is a normal response to decreased light, strong emotional stimuli, and topical administration of mydriatic and cycloplegic drugs. It can also result from ocular and neurologic disorders, eye trauma, and disorders that decrease level of consciousness. Mydriasis may be an adverse effect of antihistamines or other drugs.

### ▶ Emergency interventions

Mydriasis appears in two ocular emergencies: acute closed-angle glaucoma and traumatic iridoplegia. If a report of acute pain or trauma makes you suspect either disorder, call a doctor at once.

### History

Begin by asking the patient about other eye problems, such as pain, blurring, diplopia, or visual field defects. Obtain a health history, focusing on eye or head trauma, glaucoma and other ocular problems, and neurologic and vascular disorders. Also obtain a complete medication history.

### Physical exam

Perform a thorough eye and pupil examination. Inspect and compare the pupils' size, color, and shape. Also test each pupil for light reflex, consensual response, and accommodation. Check the eyes for ptosis, swelling, and ecchymosis. Test visual acuity in both eyes with and without correction. Evaluate extraocular muscle function by checking the six cardinal fields of gaze.

### Causes

*Aortic arch syndrome.* Bilateral mydriasis commonly occurs late in this syndrome. Other findings may include visual blurring, transient vision loss, and diplopia; dizziness and syncope; neck, shoulder, and chest pain; bruits; loss of radial and carotid pulses; paresthesia; and intermittent claudication.

*Botulism.* Botulinum toxin causes bilateral mydriasis, usually 12 to 36 hours after ingestion. Other early findings include loss of pupillary reflexes, visual blurring, diplopia, ptosis, strabismus and extraocular muscle palsies, anorexia, nausea, vomiting, diarrhea, and dry mouth. Vertigo, hearing loss, hoarseness, hypernasality, dysarthria, dysphagia, progressive muscle weakness, and loss of deep tendon reflexes soon follow.

*Carotid artery aneurysm.* Unilateral mydriasis may be accompanied by bitemporal hemianopia, decreased visual acuity, hemiplegia, decreased level of consciousness, headache, aphasia, behavioral changes, and hypoesthesia.

*Drugs.* Mydriasis can be caused by anticholinergics, antihistamines, sympathomimetics, barbiturates (in overdose), estrogens, and tricyclic antidepressants. It also commonly occurs early in anesthesia induction. Topical mydriatics and cycloplegics are administered specifically for their mydriatic effects.

*Glaucoma (acute closed-angle).* This ocular emergency is characterized by moderate mydriasis and loss of pupillary reflex in the affected eye, accompanied by abrupt onset of excruciating pain, decreased visual acuity, visual blurring, halo vision, conjunctival injection, and a cloudy cornea.

*Oculomotor nerve palsy.* Unilateral mydriasis is often the first sign of this disorder, followed by ptosis, diplopia, decreased pupillary reflexes, exotropia, and complete loss of accommodation.

*Traumatic iridoplegia.* Eye trauma often paralyzes the sphincter of the iris, causing mydriasis and loss of pupillary reflex; usually, this is transient. Associated findings may include a quivering iris (iridodonesis), ecchymosis, pain, and swelling.

*Other causes.* Adie's syndrome, brain stem infarction, and ocular surgery.

### Nursing considerations

- If the patient's mydriasis results from mydriatic drugs given during an eye examination, explain that he may have some temporary photophobia and loss of accommodation. Instruct him to wear dark glasses and to avoid bright light.
- Prepare the patient for ordered diagnostic tests.

The gag reflex—a protective mechanism that prevents aspiration of food, fluid, and vomitus—normally can be elicited by touching the posterior wall of the oropharynx with a tongue blade or by suctioning the throat. Prompt elevation of the palate, constriction of the pharyngeal musculature, and a sensation of gagging indicate a normal gag reflex. An abnormal gag reflex—either decreased or absent—interferes with the ability to swallow and, more important, increases susceptibility to life-threatening aspiration. An impaired gag reflex can result from any lesion affecting its mediators—cranial nerves IX (glossopharyngeal) and X (vagus) or the pons or medulla. It can also occur in coma or temporarily as a result of anesthesia.

### ▶ Emergency interventions
If you detect an abnormal gag reflex, immediately stop the patient's oral intake to prevent aspiration. Quickly evaluate his level of consciousness (LOC). If it's decreased, place him in a side-lying position to prevent aspiration; if not, place him in Fowler's position. Make sure you have suction equipment on hand.

### History
Ask the patient (or a family member, if the patient can't communicate) about the onset and duration of his swallowing difficulties. Determine if he has more difficulty swallowing liquids than solids, and if swallowing is more difficult at certain times of the day, as occurs in the bulbar palsy associated with myasthenia gravis. If the patient also has trouble chewing, suspect more widespread neurologic involvement because chewing involves different cranial nerves. Examine the patient's history for vascular and degenerative disorders.

### Physical exam
Assess respiratory status for evidence of aspiration, and perform a neurologic exam.

### Causes
*Anesthesia.* General and local (throat) anesthesia can produce temporary loss of the gag reflex.

*Basilar artery occlusion.* This disorder may suddenly diminish or obliterate the gag reflex. It also causes diffuse sensory loss, dysarthria, facial weakness, extraocular muscle palsies, quadriplegia, and decreased LOC.

*Brain stem glioma.* This lesion causes gradual loss of the gag reflex. Related symptoms reflect bilateral brain stem involvement and include diplopia and facial weakness. Common involvement of the corticospinal pathways causes extremity spasticity and paresis, and gait disturbances.

*Bulbar palsy.* Loss of the gag reflex reflects temporary or permanent paralysis of muscles supplied by cranial nerves IX and X. Similar indicators of this paralysis include jaw and facial muscle weakness, dysphagia, sensation loss at the tongue's base, increased salivation, difficulty articulating and breathing, and fasciculations.

*Wallenberg's syndrome.* Paresis of the palate and an impaired gag reflex usually develop within hours to days of thrombosis. The patient may have analgesia and thermanesthesia, occurring ipsilaterally on the face and contralaterally on the body, and he may have vertigo. He may also display nystagmus, ipsilateral ataxia of the arm and leg, and signs of Horner's syndrome.

### Nursing considerations
- Continually assess the patient's ability to swallow. If his gag reflex is absent, provide tube feedings; if it's merely diminished, try pureed foods.
- Advise the patient to take small amounts and eat slowly, while in a high Fowler's or sitting position. Stay with him while he eats and observe for choking. Remember to keep suction equipment handy in case of aspiration.
- Keep accurate intake and output records, and assess the patient's nutritional status daily.
- If ordered, prepare the patient for diagnostic studies, such as a computed tomography scan, EEG, and lumbar puncture.

**G**

# Muscle weakness

Muscle weakness can result from nerve degeneration or injury, or altered chemical regulation at the neuromuscular junction or within the muscle itself. It occurs in various neurologic and musculoskeletal disorders and certain metabolic, endocrine, and cardiovascular disorders. It may be caused by certain drugs or result from prolonged immobilization.

## History
Locate the patient's muscle weakness. Find out when he first noticed the weakness and whether it worsens with exercise or with time. Ask about muscle or joint pain, altered sensory function, and fatigue. Obtain a medical history, noting especially chronic disease, such as hyperthyroidism; musculoskeletal or neurologic problems; family history of chronic muscle weakness, especially in males; and alcohol and drug use.

## Physical exam
Evaluate the patient's muscle strength. Test all major muscles bilaterally. If the patient complains of pain, discontinue resistance and have him try the tests again. Also test sensory function and deep tendon reflexes bilaterally.

## Causes
*Amyotrophic lateral sclerosis.* Muscle weakness and atrophy progress from one hand to the arm, and then to the other hand and arm, then to the trunk, neck, tongue, larynx, pharynx, and legs, eventually resulting in respiratory insufficiency.

*Guillain-Barré syndrome.* Weakness rapidly ascends from the feet to the arms and facial nerves and may progress to total motor paralysis and respiratory failure. Associated findings include sensory loss or paresthesia, muscle flaccidity, loss of deep tendon reflexes, tachycardia, fluctuating hypertension and postural hypotension, diaphoresis, incontinence, facial diplegia, dysphagia, dysarthria, and hypernasality.

*Hodgkin's disease.* Muscle weakness may accompany lymphadenopathy. Other findings include paresthesia, fatigue, and weight loss.

*Hypercortisolism.* Limb weakness and eventually atrophy may occur. Related cushingoid features include buffalo hump, moon face, truncal obesity, purple striae, thin skin, acne, elevated blood pressure, fatigue, poor wound healing, and diaphoresis.

*Multiple sclerosis.* Muscle weakness in one or more limbs may progress to atrophy, spasticity, and contractures. Other findings may include blurred vision, nystagmus, hyperactive deep tendon reflexes, paresthesia, dysarthria, dysphagia, ataxic gait, intention tremors, emotional lability, impotence, and urinary dysfunction.

*Myasthenia gravis.* Progressive skeletal muscle weakness and fatigue mark this disorder. Other findings may include weak eye closure, ptosis, and diplopia; masklike facies; difficulty chewing and swallowing; nasal regurgitation of fluid with hypernasality; and a hanging jaw and bobbing head.

*Rheumatoid arthritis.* Muscle weakness may accompany pain, stiffness, and increased warmth, swelling, and tenderness in involved joints.

*Other causes.* Anemia, cerebrovascular accident, corticosteroids, dantrolene (overdose), digitalis toxicity, head trauma, herniated disk, hyperkalemia, hypokalemia, hypothyroidism, osteoarthritis, Paget's disease, Parkinson's disease, peripheral nerve trauma, peripheral neuropathy, poliomyelitis, polymyositis, prolonged immobilization in a cast, protein deficiency, seizure disorder, spinal trauma and disease, and thyrotoxicosis.

## Nursing considerations
• Provide assistive devices, and protect the patient from injury. If he has concomitant sensory loss, guard against decubitus ulcer formation and thermal injury. In chronic weakness, provide range-of-motion exercises or splint limbs as necessary. Give pain medications as ordered.
• Prepare the patient for blood tests, muscle biopsy, electromyography, nerve conduction studies, and X-rays or computed tomography scans.

**M**

# Gait, propulsive

Also called a festinating gait, a propulsive gait is characterized by a stooped, rigid posture. The patient's head and neck are bent forward; his flexed, stiffened arms are held away from the body; his fingers are extended; and his knees and hips are stiffly bent. During ambulation, this posture results in a forward shifting of the body's center of gravity and consequent impairment of balance, causing increasingly rapid, short, shuffling steps with involuntary acceleration (festination) and lack of control over forward motion (propulsion) or backward motion (retropulsion).

Propulsive gait is a cardinal sign of advanced Parkinson's disease, resulting from progressive degeneration of the ganglia, which are primarily responsible for smooth muscle movement. Because this sign develops gradually and its accompanying effects may be wrongly attributed to aging, propulsive gait may go unnoticed or unreported until severe disability results.

## History

Ask the patient when his gait impairment first developed and whether it has worsened recently. Because he may have difficulty remembering, having attributed the gait to "old age," you may gain information from family members or friends, especially those who see the patient only sporadically.

Also obtain a thorough drug history, including both medication type and dosage. Ask the patient if he's been taking any tranquilizers, especially phenothiazines. If the patient knows he has Parkinson's disease and has been taking levodopa, pay particular attention to the dosage because an overdose can cause acute exacerbation of signs and symptoms.

If Parkinson's disease isn't a known or suspected diagnosis, ask the patient if he's been acutely or routinely exposed to carbon monoxide or manganese.

## Causes

*Drugs.* Propulsive gait and possibly other extrapyramidal effects can also result from use of phenothiazines, other antipsychotics (notably haloperidol, thiothixene, and loxapine) and, infrequently, metoclopramide and metyrosine. Such effects are usually temporary, disappearing 1 to 2 weeks after cessation of therapy.

*Parkinson's disease.* The characteristic and permanent propulsive gait begins early as a shuffle. As the disease progresses, the gait slows. Cardinal signs of the disease are progressive muscle rigidity, which may be uniform (lead-pipe rigidity) or jerky (cogwheel rigidity); akinesia; and an insidious tremor that begins in the fingers, increases during stress or anxiety, and decreases with purposeful movement and sleep. Besides the gait, akinesia produces a high-pitched, monotone voice; drooling; masklike facies; stooped posture; and dysarthria, dysphagia, or both. Occasionally, it also causes oculogyric crises or blepharospasm.

*Other causes.* Acute carbon monoxide poisoning and chronic manganese poisoning.

## Nursing considerations

• Because of his gait and associated motor impairment, the patient may have problems performing activities of daily living. Assist him as appropriate, while at the same time encouraging his independence and self-reliance. Instruct the patient and his family to allow plenty of time for these activities, especially walking, because he's particularly susceptible to falls caused by festination and poor balance.

• Encourage the patient to maintain ambulation; for safety reasons, remember to stay with him while he's walking, especially if he's on unfamiliar or uneven ground.

• If appropriate, refer the patient to a physical therapist for exercise therapy and gait retraining.

# Muscle spasticity

Also known as muscle hypertonicity, spasticity is a state of excessive muscle tone with increased resistance to stretching and heightened reflexes, detected by evaluating a muscle's response to passive movement. A spastic muscle offers an initial resistance that suddenly gives way — a phenomenon known as the clasp-knife reflex. Caused by an upper motor neuron lesion, spasticity usually occurs in the arm and leg muscles. Long-term spasticity results in muscle fibrosis and contractures.

### ▶ Emergency interventions
Generalized spasticity and trismus in a patient with a recent skin puncture or laceration indicate tetanus. If you suspect this rare disorder, assess for signs of respiratory distress and notify the doctor. If necessary, provide ventilatory support and monitor the patient closely.

### History
Ask the patient about the onset, duration, and progression of spasticity. What, if any, events precipitated its onset? Has he experienced other muscle changes or related symptoms? Does his medical history reveal any incidence of trauma or degenerative or vascular disease?

### Physical exam
Take the patient's vital signs and perform a complete neurologic examination. Test reflexes and assess motor and sensory function in all limbs. Evaluate muscles for wasting and contractures.

### Causes
*Amyotrophic lateral sclerosis.* This disorder commonly produces spasticity, spasms, coarse fasciculations, hyperactive deep tendon reflexes, and a positive Babinski's sign. Earlier findings include progressive muscle weakness and flaccidity that begin in the hands and arms and spread to the trunk, neck, larynx, pharynx, and legs. Respiratory muscle weakness leads to respiratory insufficiency.

*Multiple sclerosis.* Muscle spasticity, hyperreflexia, and contractures may develop. Earlier muscle changes include progressive weakness and atrophy. Other findings may include diplopia, blurred vision, nystagmus, sensory loss or paresthesia, dysarthria, dysphagia, ataxic gait, intention tremors, emotional lability, impotence, and urinary dysfunction.

*Spinal cord injury.* Spasticity commonly results from cervical and high thoracic spinal cord injury, especially from incomplete lesions. Spastic paralysis in the affected limbs follows initial flaccid paralysis; typically, spasticity and muscle atrophy increase for up to 1½ to 2 years after the injury, then gradually regress to flaccidity. Other findings may include respiratory insufficiency or paralysis, sensory losses, bowel and bladder dysfunction, hyperactive deep tendon reflexes, positive Babinski's sign, sexual dysfunction, priapism, hypotension, anhidrosis, and bradycardia.

*Tetanus.* This rare, life-threatening disease produces varying degrees of spasticity. In generalized tetanus, the most common form, early findings include jaw and neck stiffness, trismus, headache, irritability, restlessness, low-grade fever with chills, tachycardia, diaphoresis, and hyperactive deep tendon reflexes. Painful involuntary spasms may cause abdominal rigidity, opisthotonos, and risus sardonicus. Glottal, pharyngeal, or respiratory muscle involvement can cause death by asphyxia or cardiac failure.

*Other causes.* Cerebral palsy (in children), cerebrovascular accident, epidural hemorrhage.

### Nursing considerations
• Prepare the patient for diagnostic tests, which may include electromyography, muscle biopsy, or intracranial or spinal computed tomography scan.
• Administer pain medications and antispasmodics, as ordered.
• Passive range-of-motion exercises, splinting, traction, and application of heat may help relieve spasms and prevent contractures.
• Encourage bed rest as appropriate.

Resulting from spastic hemiparesis, a scissors gait affects both legs and has little or no effect on the arms. The patient's legs flex slightly at the hips and knees, giving the appearance of crouching. With each step, his thighs adduct and his knees hit or cross in a scissorslike movement. His steps are short, regular, and laborious, as if he were wading through waist-deep water. His feet may be plantar-flexed and turned inward (equinovarus position), with a shortened Achilles tendon. As a result, he walks on his toes or the balls of his feet and may scrape his toes on the ground.

## History

Ask the patient (or a family member, if the patient can't answer) about the gait's onset and duration. Has it progressively worsened or remained constant? Ask about a history of trauma, including birth trauma and neurologic disorders.

## Physical exam

Thoroughly evaluate motor and sensory function and deep tendon reflexes in the legs.

## Causes

*Cervical spondylosis with myelopathy.* Scissors gait develops in the late stages of this degenerative disorder and steadily worsens. Associated signs and symptoms mimic those of herniated disk: se-

vere low back pain, which may radiate to the buttocks, legs, and feet; muscle spasms; sensorimotor loss; and muscle weakness and atrophy.

*Multiple sclerosis.* Progressive scissors gait usually develops gradually, with infrequent remissions. Characteristic weakness, most often in the legs, ranges from minor fatigue to paraparesis with urinary urgency and constipation. Related findings include facial pain, visual disturbances, paresthesia, incoordination, and loss of proprioception and vibration sensation in the ankle and toes.

*Spinal cord trauma.* Scissors gait may develop during recovery from partial spinal cord compression, especially with injury below C6. Associated findings depend on the injury's site and severity but may include sensory loss or paresthesia, weakness or paralysis distal to the injury, and bowel and bladder dysfunction.

*Spinal cord tumor.* Scissors gait can develop gradually from a thoracic or lumbar tumor. Other findings reflect the tumor's location and may include radicular, subscapular, shoulder, groin, leg, or flank pain; spasms or fasciculations; muscle atrophy; sensory deficits; hyperactive deep tendon reflexes; bilateral Babinski's reflex; spastic, neurogenic bladder; and sexual dysfunction.

*Other causes.* Cerebral palsy, cerebrovascular accident, hepatic failure, pernicious anemia, sy-

philitic meningomyelitis, and syringomyelia.

## Nursing considerations

• Because of the sensory loss associated with scissors gait, provide meticulous skin care to prevent pressure sores.
• Provide the patient and his family with complete skin care instructions. If appropriate, provide bladder and bowel retraining.
• Provide daily active and passive range-of-motion exercises.
• As appropriate, refer the patient to a physical therapist for gait retraining and for possible in-shoe splints or leg braces to maintain proper foot alignment for standing and walking.

# Muscle spasms

Strong, painful muscle spasms can occur in any muscle but are most common in the calf and foot. Spasms may result from simple muscle fatigue and exercise or may occur during pregnancy. They may also occur in electrolyte imbalances and neuromuscular disorders or as adverse reactions to certain drugs.

## ▶ Emergency interventions

If the patient reports frequent or unrelieved spasms in many muscles, with paresthesia in his hands and feet, attempt to elicit Chvostek's and Trousseau's signs. If these are present, suspect hypocalcemia and notify the doctor immediately. Assess respiratory function, watching for the development of laryngospasm; provide supplemental oxygen as necessary, and prepare to assist with intubation and mechanical ventilation. Draw blood for calcium levels and arterial blood gas analysis, and insert an I.V. line for administration of a calcium supplement, as ordered. Monitor cardiac status, and prepare to begin resuscitation if necessary.

## History

If the patient isn't in distress, ask when the spasms began. How long did they last? How painful were they? Did anything worsen or relieve the pain? Ask about other symptoms, such as weakness, sensory loss, or paresthesia.

## Physical exam

Evaluate the patient's muscle strength and tone. Then check all major muscle groups, and note movements that precipitate spasms. Test presence and quality of all peripheral pulses, and examine limbs for color and temperature changes. Test capillary refill time and inspect for edema. Also test reflexes and sensory function in all extremities.

## Causes

*Amyotrophic lateral sclerosis.* Muscle spasms may accompany progressive muscle weakness and atrophy that typically begin in one hand, spread to the arm, to the other hand and arm, and finally to the trunk, neck, tongue, larynx, pharynx, and legs.

*Arterial occlusive disease.* This usually produces spasms and intermittent claudication in the leg, with residual pain. Other findings include loss of peripheral pulses, pallor or cyanosis, decreased sensation, hair loss, dry or scaly skin, edema, and ulcerations.

*Dehydration.* Sodium loss may produce limb and abdominal cramps. Other findings include slight fever, decreased skin turgor, dry mucous membranes, tachycardia, postural hypotension, muscle twitching, seizures, nausea, vomiting, and oliguria.

*Hypocalcemia.* Tetany is the classic feature. Both Chvostek's and Trousseau's signs may also be elicited. Related findings include paresthesia of the lips, fingers, and toes; choreiform movements; hyperactive deep tendon reflexes; fatigue; palpitations; and cardiac arrhythmias.

*Hypothyroidism.* Spasms and stiffness may occur, along with leg muscle hypertrophy or proximal limb weakness and atrophy. Other findings include mental instability; fatigue; cold intolerance; dry, pale, cool skin; puffy face, hands, and feet; periorbital edema; sparse, brittle hair; bradycardia; and weight gain despite anorexia.

*Respiratory alkalosis.* Acute onset of muscle spasms may accompany twitching and weakness, carpopedal spasms, circumoral and peripheral paresthesia, vertigo, syncope, pallor, and extreme anxiety.

*Other causes.* Drugs, such as corticosteroids, diuretics, and estrogens; fractures; spinal injury or disease; and trauma.

## Nursing considerations

- Help alleviate the patient's spasms by slowly stretching the affected muscle in the direction opposite the contraction. Or have the patient stand, preferably on a cold surface, such as tile or marble. If necessary, administer a mild analgesic.
- Prepare the patient for diagnostic studies, as ordered.

**M**

Also called a hemiplegic gait, a spastic gait is a stiff, foot-dragging walk caused by unilateral leg muscle hypertonicity. The gait indicates focal damage to the corticospinal tract. The affected leg becomes rigid, with a marked decrease in flexion at the hip and knee and possibly plantar flexion and equinovarus deformity of the foot. Because the patient's leg doesn't swing normally at the hip or knee, his foot tends to drag or shuffle, scraping his toes on the ground. To compensate, the pelvis of the affected side tilts upward in an attempt to lift the toes, causing the patient's leg to abduct and circumduct. In addition, arm swing is hindered on the same side as the affected leg.

Spastic gait usually develops after a period of flaccidity (hypotonicity) in the affected leg. Once the gait develops, it's usually permanent.

## History
Find out when the patient first noticed the gait impairment and whether it developed suddenly or gradually. Ask if it waxes and wanes or has worsened progressively. Does fatigue, hot weather, or a warm bath or shower worsen the gait? Such exacerbation typically occurs in multiple sclerosis.

Examine the history for neurologic disorders, recent head trauma, and degenerative diseases.

## Physical exam
Test and compare strength, range of motion, and sensory function in all limbs. Also observe and palpate for muscle flaccidity or atrophy.

## Causes
*Brain abscess.* Spastic gait typically develops slowly after a period of muscle flaccidity and fever. Early signs and symptoms of abscess reflect increased intracranial pressure (ICP): headache, nausea, vomiting, and focal or generalized seizures. Later, site-specific features may include hemiparesis, tremors, visual disturbances, nystagmus, and pupillary inequality. The patient's level of consciousness may range from drowsiness to stupor.

*Brain tumor.* Depending on the tumor site and type, spastic gait usually develops gradually and worsens over time. Accompanying effects may include signs of increased ICP, papilledema, sensory loss on the affected side, dysarthria, ocular palsies, aphasia, and personality changes.

*Cerebrovascular accident.* Spastic gait usually appears after a period of weakness and hypotonicity on the affected side. Associated effects may include unilateral muscle atrophy, sensory loss, and footdrop; aphasia; dysarthria; dysphagia; visual field deficits; diplopia; and ocular palsies.

*Head trauma.* Spastic gait typically follows the acute stage of head trauma. The patient may also have focal or generalized seizures, personality changes, headache, and focal neurologic signs, such as aphasia and visual field deficits.

*Multiple sclerosis.* Spastic gait begins insidiously and follows this disorder's characteristic cycle of remission and exacerbation. The gait, as well as other signs and symptoms, usually worsens in warm weather or after a warm bath or shower. Characteristic weakness, most often affecting the legs, ranges from minor fatigability to paraparesis with urinary urgency and constipation. Other effects: facial pain, paresthesia, incoordination, loss of proprioception and vibration sensation in the ankle and toes, and visual disturbances.

## Nursing considerations
• Because leg muscle contractures are commonly associated with spastic gait, promote daily active and passive exercises.

• As appropriate, refer the patient to a physical therapist for gait retraining and possible in-shoe splints or leg braces to maintain proper foot alignment for standing and walking.

• The patient may have poor balance and a tendency to fall to the paralyzed side, so stay with him while he's walking. Provide a cane or a walker, as indicated.

# Muscle flaccidity

Also known as muscle hypotonicity, muscle flaccidity is characterized by profoundly weak and soft muscles, with decreased resistance to movement, increased mobility, and greater-than-normal range of motion. The result of disrupted muscle innervation, flaccidity can be localized to a limb or muscle group or generalized over the entire body. It may be acute, as in trauma, or chronic, as in neurologic disease. Muscle flaccidity may be life-threatening if it affects the respiratory system.

▶ **Emergency interventions**
If the patient's flaccidity results from trauma, stabilize the cervical spine and notify the doctor. Assess respiratory status. If you note signs of respiratory insufficiency, administer oxygen by nasal cannula or mask, and assist with intubation and mechanical ventilation.

### History
If the patient isn't in distress, ask about the onset and duration of muscle flaccidity and any precipitating factors. Also ask about associated symptoms, particularly weakness, other muscle changes, and sensory loss or paresthesia.

### Physical exam
Examine the affected muscles for atrophy, which indicates a chronic problem. Test muscle strength and check deep tendon reflexes in all limbs.

### Causes
*Amyotrophic lateral sclerosis.* Progressive muscle weakness and paralysis accompany generalized flaccidity. Typically, these effects begin in one hand, spread to the arm, the other hand and arm, and finally to the trunk, neck, tongue, larynx, pharynx, and legs. Progressive respiratory muscle weakness leads to respiratory insufficiency.

*Brain lesions.* Frontal and parietal lobe lesions may cause contralateral flaccidity, weakness or paralysis, and eventually spasticity. Other findings may include hyperactive deep tendon reflexes, positive Babinski's sign, loss of proprioception, analgesia, anesthesia, and thermanesthesia.

*Cerebellar disease.* Generalized muscle flaccidity is accompanied by ataxia, dysmetria, intention tremor, slight muscle weakness, fatigue, and dysarthria.

*Guillain-Barré syndrome.* Muscle flaccidity from rapidly progressive muscle deterioration is typically symmetrical and ascending, moving from the feet to the arms and facial nerves within 24 to 72 hours. Other findings include sensory loss or paresthesia, absent deep tendon reflexes, tachycardia, fluctuating hypertension and postural hypotension, diaphoresis, incontinence, dysphagia, dysarthria, hypernasality, and facial diplegia.

*Peripheral neuropathy.* This disorder may produce muscle flaccidity, usually in the legs, as a result of chronic progressive muscle weakness and paralysis. It may also cause mild to sharp burning pain, glossy red skin, anhidrosis, and loss of vibration sensation.

*Spinal cord injury.* Spinal shock can result in acute muscle flaccidity or spasticity below the level of injury. Associated signs and symptoms also occur below the level of injury and may include paralysis; absent deep tendon reflexes; analgesia; thermanesthesia; loss of proprioception and of vibration, touch, and pressure sensation; and anhidrosis. Injury in the C1 to C5 region causes respiratory paralysis and bradycardia.

*Other causes.* Generalized tonic-clonic seizures, Lowe's disease, muscular dystrophy, myelomeningocele, peripheral nerve trauma, poliomyelitis, and Werdnig-Hoffmann disease.

### Nursing considerations
• Provide passive range-of-motion exercises. Reposition a patient with generalized flaccidity every 2 hours, as ordered. Pad bony prominences and other pressure points, and prevent thermal injury by testing the patient's bathwater. Treat isolated flaccidity by supporting the affected limb in a sling or with a splint.
• Prepare the patient for any diagnostic tests.

Also called an equine or a prancing gait, steppage gait typically results from footdrop caused by weakness or paralysis of pretibial and peroneal muscles, usually from lower motor neuron lesions. In footdrop, the foot hangs with the toes pointing down, causing the toes to scrape the ground during ambulation. To compensate, the hip rotates outward and the hip and knee flex in an exaggerated way to lift the advancing leg off the ground. The foot is thrown forward, and the toes hit the ground first, producing an audible slap. The gait's rhythm is usually regular, with even steps and normal upper body posture and arm swing.

Steppage gait can be unilateral or bilateral and permanent or transient, depending on the site and type of neural damage.

## History

Ask about the onset of the gait and any recent changes in its character. Find out if any family member has a similar gait. Also find out if the patient has had any traumatic injury to the buttocks, hips, legs, or knees. Ask about a history of chronic disorders that may be associated with polyneuropathy, such as polyarteritis nodosa or alcoholism. While you're taking the history, note if the patient crosses his legs while sitting; this may put pressure on the peroneal nerve.

## Physical exam

Inspect and palpate the patient's calves and feet for muscle atrophy and wasting. Using a pin, test for sensory deficits along the length of both legs.

## Causes

*Guillain-Barré syndrome.* Typically occurring after recovery from the acute stage of this disorder, steppage gait can be mild or severe and unilateral or bilateral; it's invariably permanent.

*Multiple sclerosis.* Steppage gait and footdrop typically fluctuate in severity with this disorder's cycle of periodic exacerbation and remission. Muscle weakness, most often affecting the legs, can range from minor fatigability to paraparesis with urinary urgency and constipation.

*Peroneal muscle atrophy.* Bilateral steppage gait and footdrop begin insidiously in this disorder. Foot, peroneal, and ankle dorsiflexor muscles are affected first. Other early signs and symptoms include paresthesia, aching, and cramping in the feet and legs, along with coldness, swelling, and cyanosis. As the disorder progresses, all leg muscles become weak and atrophic, with hypoactive or absent deep tendon reflexes. Later, atrophy and sensory losses spread to the hands and arms.

*Peroneal nerve trauma.* Temporary ipsilateral steppage gait occurs suddenly but resolves with release of peroneal nerve pressure. It's associated with footdrop and weakness and sensory loss over the lateral surface of the calf and foot.

*Polyneuropathy.* In *polyarteritis nodosa with polyneuropathy,* unilateral or bilateral steppage gait is a late finding. Related findings include vague leg pain, abdominal pain, hematuria, fever, and increased blood pressure. In *alcoholic polyneuropathy,* steppage gait appears 2 to 3 months after onset of vitamin B deficiency. The gait may be bilateral, and it resolves with treatment of the deficiency. Early findings include paresthesia in the feet, leg weakness, and possibly sensory ataxia.

*Spinal cord trauma.* In the ambulatory patient, spinal cord trauma may cause steppage gait. Its other effects depend on the severity of injury.

*Other causes.* Diabetic polyneuropathy, herniated lumbar disk, and poliomyelitis.

## Nursing considerations

• The patient may tire rapidly when walking because of the extra effort he must expend to lift his feet off the ground. And when he tires, he may stub his toes, causing a fall. To prevent this, help the patient recognize his exercise limits, and encourage him to get adequate rest.

• Refer him to a physical therapist, if appropriate, for gait retraining and possible in-shoe splints or leg braces to maintain correct foot alignment.

**G**

Prolonged muscle immobility or disuse causes atrophy, or wasting. Atrophy most commonly results from neuromuscular disease or injury but may also stem from certain metabolic and endocrine disorders. Some muscle atrophy occurs with aging as well.

## History
Ask the patient when and where he first noticed the muscle wasting and how it has progressed. Also ask about any associated symptoms, particularly weakness and recent weight loss. Review the patient's medical history for chronic illnesses; musculoskeletal or neurologic disorders, including trauma; and endocrine and metabolic disorders. Also ask about alcohol consumption and drugs, particularly steroids.

## Physical exam
Visually evaluate small and large muscles. Check all major muscle groups for size, tonicity, and contractility. Test motor strength, measure the circumference of all limbs, and compare sides. Finally, palpate peripheral pulses for quality and rate, assess sensory function in and around the atrophied area, and test deep tendon reflexes.

## Causes
*Amyotrophic lateral sclerosis.* Muscle weakness and atrophy typically begin in one hand, spread to the arm, and then develop in the other hand and arm. Eventually these symptoms spread to the trunk, neck, tongue, larynx, pharynx, and legs.

*Cerebrovascular accident (CVA).* CVA may produce contralateral or bilateral weakness and, eventually, atrophy of the arms, legs, face, and tongue. Other findings may include dysarthria, aphasia, ataxia, apraxia, agnosia, and ipsilateral paresthesia or sensory losses.

*Multiple sclerosis.* Arm and leg atrophy can result from chronic progressive weakness. Spasticity and contractures may also develop. Other findings may include diplopia and blurred vision, nystagmus, hyperactive deep tendon reflexes, sensory loss or paresthesia, dysarthria, dysphagia, ataxic gait, intention tremors, emotional lability, impotence, and urinary dysfunction.

*Parkinson's disease.* Muscle rigidity, weakness, and disuse may produce muscle atrophy. Insidious tremors usually begin in the fingers (unilateral pill-rolling tremor), worsen with stress, and ease with purposeful movement and sleep.

*Peripheral neuropathy.* Muscle weakness progresses slowly to flaccid paralysis and eventually atrophy. Distal extremity muscles are generally affected first. Associated findings may include loss of vibration sense; paresthesia, hyperesthesia, or anesthesia in hands and feet; mild to sharp burning pain; anhidrosis; glossy red skin; and diminished or absent deep tendon reflexes.

*Spinal cord injury.* Spinal trauma can produce severe muscle weakness and flaccid, then spastic, paralysis, eventually leading to atrophy. Other findings may include respiratory insufficiency or paralysis, sensory losses, bowel and bladder dysfunction, hyperactive deep tendon reflexes, positive Babinski's reflex, sexual dysfunction, priapism, hypotension, and anhidrosis.

*Other causes.* Burns, compartment syndrome and Volkmann's contracture, herniated disk, hypercortisolism, hypothyroidism, meniscal tear, osteoarthritis, peripheral nerve trauma, prolonged immobilization, prolonged steroid therapy, protein deficiency, rheumatoid arthritis, and thyrotoxicosis.

## Nursing considerations
• Encourage the patient to perform frequent active range-of-motion exercises. If he can't actively move a joint, provide active-assistive or passive exercises, and apply splints or braces. If the muscle won't extend fully during exercises, use heat, pain medication, or relaxation techniques. Then slowly stretch it to full extension. If these techniques don't correct the contracture, use moist heat, a whirlpool bath, or ultrasound therapy.
• Prepare the patient for any diagnostic tests.

An atrial or presystolic gallop ($S_4$) is an extra heart sound that's heard or palpated immediately before the first heart sound. This low-pitched sound is best heard with the bell of the stethoscope pressed lightly against the cardiac apex. Some clinicians say an $S_4$ has the cadence of the "Ten" in Tennessee (Ten, $S_4$; nes, $S_1$; see, $S_2$).

Typically, this gallop results from myocardial infarction (MI), hypertension, valvular disorders, and other cardiac abnormalities. It results from abnormally forceful atrial contraction caused by augmented ventricular filling or by decreased left ventricular compliance. Usually, an $S_4$ originates from left atrial contraction, is heard at the apex, and doesn't vary with inspiration. It may also originate from right atrial contraction, in which case it's best heard at the lower left sternal border, intensifying with inspiration.

Although an $S_4$ seldom occurs in normal hearts, it may arise in elderly patients, in athletes with physiologic left ventricular hypertrophy, or during pregnancy from augmented ventricular filling.

▶ **Emergency interventions**

If you hear an $S_4$ in a patient with chest pain, suspect myocardial ischemia and notify the doctor. Take vital signs and assess for signs of heart failure, such as dyspnea and crackles. If you detect them, begin cardiac monitoring and give antianginal drugs, as ordered. If the patient has dyspnea, elevate the head of the bed and auscultate for abnormal breath sounds. If you hear coarse crackles, start an I.V. line and give oxygen and diuretics, as ordered. If he has bradycardia, give atropine and help insert a pacemaker, if ordered.

**History**

If his condition permits, ask about hypertension, valvular stenosis, cardiomyopathy, and the frequency and severity of anginal attacks.

**Causes**

*Angina.* An intermittent $S_4$ is characteristic during an anginal attack. It may occur with a paradoxical $S_2$ or a new murmur. Typically, the patient complains of anginal chest pain.

*Aortic insufficiency (acute).* This disorder causes an $S_4$; a soft, short diastolic murmur; tachycardia; $S_3$; dyspnea; neck vein distention; and crackles.

*Aortic stenosis.* This disorder usually causes an $S_4$ and a harsh, crescendo-decrescendo, systolic ejection murmur that's loudest at the right sternal border near the second intercostal space. Dyspnea, chest pain, and syncope are cardinal findings.

*Atrioventricular (AV) block. First-degree AV block* may cause an $S_4$ and a faint first heart sound ($S_1$). In *second-degree AV block,* an $S_4$ is easily heard. In *third-degree AV block,* $S_4$ varies in intensity with $S_1$ and is loudest when atrial systole coincides with early, rapid ventricular filling during diastole.

*Hypertension.* One of the earliest findings is an $S_4$. The patient may be asymptomatic or may experience headache, weakness, epistaxis, tinnitus, dizziness, syncope, fatigue, and facial flushing.

*Mitral insufficiency.* In acute mitral insufficiency, auscultation may reveal an $S_4$ (a harsh holosystolic murmur heard best at the apex or over the precordium) often accompanied by an $S_3$. Other features: fatigue, dyspnea, tachypnea, orthopnea, tachycardia, crackles, and neck vein distention.

*Mitral stenosis.* When associated with a normal sinus rhythm, mitral stenosis commonly causes an $S_4$. Cardinal findings: a loud apical $S_1$ and an opening snap with a diastolic murmur at the apex.

*Myocardial infarction.* A classic sign of MI, $S_4$ may persist even after the infarction heals. Typically, the patient reports crushing substernal chest pain that may radiate. Associated findings: dyspnea, restlessness, anxiety, a feeling of impending doom, diaphoresis, pallor, clammy skin, nausea, vomiting, and altered blood pressure.

*Other causes.* Anemia, cardiomegaly, pulmonary embolism, and thyrotoxicosis.

**Nursing considerations**

• Prepare the patient for tests, such as electrocardiography and echocardiography.

**G**

Murmurs are auscultatory sounds classified by their timing and duration in the cardiac cycle, location, loudness, configuration, pitch, and quality. They commonly result from organic heart disease.

## History
Ask the patient how long he's had a murmur. Also ask about palpitations, dizziness, syncope, chest pain, dyspnea, and fatigue. Obtain a medical history, noting incidence of rheumatic fever, heart disease, or cardiac surgery.

## Physical exam
Auscultate the chest systematically. Note especially the presence of cardiac arrhythmias, jugular vein distention, dyspnea, orthopnea, and crackles. Palpate the liver and check for peripheral edema.

## Causes
*Aortic regurgitation. Acute aortic regurgitation* typically produces a soft, short diastolic murmur over the left sternal border that's heard best when the patient sits and leans forward. $S_2$ may be soft or absent. *Chronic aortic regurgitation* causes a high-pitched, blowing, decrescendo diastolic murmur that's best heard over the second or third right intercostal space or over the left sternal border with the patient sitting, leaning forward, and hold-ing his breath after deep expiration.

*Aortic stenosis.* This murmur is systolic, beginning after $S_1$ and ending at or before aortic valve closure. It's harsh and grating, medium-pitched, and crescendo-decrescendo. Loudest over the second right intercostal space, this murmur may also be heard at the apex, at the suprasternal notch, and over the carotid arteries.

*Cardiomyopathy (hypertrophic obstructive).* A harsh late systolic murmur ends at $S_2$. Best heard over the left sternal border and at the apex, it's commonly accompanied by an audible $S_3$ or $S_4$.

*Complete heart block.* A short, crescendo-decrescendo diastolic murmur commonly occurs following atrial contraction. This murmur is heard best at the apex. $S_1$ may be paradoxical.

*Mitral prolapse.* This disorder causes a middle to late systolic click with a high-pitched late systolic crescendo murmur, best heard at the apex.

*Mitral regurgitation. Acute mitral regurgitation* is characterized by an early systolic or holosystolic decrescendo murmur at the apex, along with a widely split $S_2$ and often an $S_4$. *Chronic mitral regurgitation* produces a high-pitched, blowing, holosystolic plateau murmur that is loudest at the apex and usually radiates to the axilla or back.

*Mitral stenosis.* The murmur is soft, low-pitched, rumbling, decrescendo-crescendo, and diastolic. It's accompanied by a loud $S_1$ and an opening snap and is heard best at the apex with the patient in the left lateral position.

*Myxomas.* A *left atrial myxoma* usually produces a middiastolic murmur and a holosystolic murmur that's loudest at the apex, with an $S_4$, an early diastolic thudding sound, and a loud, widely split $S_1$. A *right atrial myxoma* causes a late diastolic rumbling murmur, a holosystolic crescendo murmur, and an early diastolic thudding sound heard best at the lower left sternal border. A *right ventricular myxoma* commonly generates a systolic ejection murmur with delayed $S_2$ and an early diastolic thudding sound heard best over the left sternal border.

*Papillary muscle rupture.* In this life-threatening complication of acute myocardial infarction, a loud holosystolic murmur occurs at the apex.

*Tricuspid regurgitation.* A soft, high-pitched, holosystolic blowing murmur increases with inspiration. It's heard best over the lower left sternal border and the xiphoid area.

*Tricuspid stenosis.* This produces a diastolic murmur resembling that of mitral stenosis, but louder with inspiration. $S_1$ may also be louder.

*Other cause.* Prosthetic valve replacement.

## Nursing considerations
• Prepare the patient for diagnostic tests, such as electrocardiography and echocardiography.

A ventricular gallop ($S_3$) is an extra heart sound associated with rapid ventricular filling in early diastole. This low-frequency sound occurs about 0.15 second after the second heart sound ($S_2$). It may originate in either ventricle. A right-sided gallop usually sounds louder on inspiration and is best heard along the lower left sternal border or over the xiphoid region. A left-sided gallop usually sounds louder on expiration and is best heard at the apex.

Ventricular gallops are easily overlooked because they're usually faint. Fortunately, certain techniques make their detection more likely. These include auscultating in a quiet environment; examining the patient in the supine, left lateral, and semi-Fowler's positions; and having the patient cough or raise his legs to augment the sound.

A *physiologic ventricular gallop* occurs during childhood, early adulthood, and the third trimester of pregnancy. It has the same timing as the pathologic $S_3$, but its intensity varies with respiration. A *pathologic ventricular gallop* may be one of the earliest signs of ventricular failure. Its intensity correlates with prognosis: the louder the gallop, the more ominous the prognosis. A gallop that persists despite therapy is also more significant.

## History
Ask the patient if he's had chest pain. If so, have him describe it. Ask about palpitations, dizziness, or syncope. Does he have difficulty breathing after exertion? While lying down? At rest? Does he have a productive cough? Ask about past cardiac disorders. Is he currently receiving treatment for heart failure? If so, what drugs is he taking?

## Physical exam
Auscultate for murmurs, $S_1$ and $S_2$ abnormalities, and crackles. Assess peripheral pulses, noting pulsus alternans. Check for liver enlargement or tenderness, neck vein distention, and edema. You may be able to palpate the gallop over the precordium.

## Causes
*Aortic insufficiency.* Acute and chronic insufficiency may produce an $S_3$. Typically, *acute insufficiency* also causes an $S_4$ and a soft, short diastolic murmur over the left sternal border. Related findings include tachycardia, dyspnea, neck vein distention, and crackles. *Chronic insufficiency* produces an $S_3$ and a high-pitched blowing, decrescendo diastolic murmur that's best heard over the second or third right intercostal space or the left sternal border. Typical related findings include palpitations, tachycardia, anginal pain, fatigue, dyspnea, orthopnea, and crackles.

*Cardiomyopathy.* A ventricular gallop is characteristic. When accompanied by pulsus alternans and altered $S_1$ and $S_2$, this gallop usually signals advanced heart disease. Other effects: fatigue, dyspnea, orthopnea, chest pain, palpitations, crackles, edema, neck vein distention, and $S_4$.

*Congestive heart failure (CHF).* A cardinal sign of CHF is an $S_3$. When it's loud and accompanied by sinus tachycardia, this gallop may indicate severe heart failure. Left-sided failure can also cause exertional dyspnea, paroxysmal nocturnal dyspnea, orthopnea, and possibly a dry cough; right-sided failure, neck vein distention.

*Mitral insufficiency.* Acute and chronic insufficiency may produce an $S_3$. In *acute insufficiency*, auscultation may also reveal an early or holosystolic decrescendo murmur at the apex, an $S_4$, and a widely split $S_2$. Typically, the patient will have sinus tachycardia, tachypnea, orthopnea, dyspnea, crackles, distended neck veins, and fatigue. In *chronic insufficiency*, a progressively severe $S_3$ is typical. Auscultation will also reveal a holosystolic, blowing, high-pitched apical murmur.

*Other causes.* Thyrotoxicosis.

## Nursing considerations
• Monitor the patient for tachycardia, dyspnea, crackles, or neck vein distention. As ordered, administer oxygen, diuretics, and other drugs.
• Prepare him for echocardiography, gated blood pool imaging, and cardiac catheterization.

**G**

Mouth lesions include ulcers, cysts, firm nodules, hemorrhagic lesions, papules, vesicles, bullae, and erythematous lesions. They may occur anywhere on the lips, cheeks, hard and soft palate, salivary glands, tongue, gingivae, or mucous membranes. Mouth lesions can result from trauma, infection, systemic diseases, drugs, and radiation therapy.

## History
Ask the patient when the lesions appeared and whether he's noticed any pain, odor, or drainage. Also ask if he's had any skin lesions. Ask about medications, including drug allergies. Obtain a medical history, noting especially cancer, sexually transmitted disease, recent infection, or trauma. Also obtain a dental history.

## Physical exam
Perform an oral examination, noting lesion sites and character. Examine lips for color and texture. Inspect and palpate the buccal mucosa and tongue for color, texture, and contour; note any painless ulcers on the sides or base of the tongue. Lift the tongue and examine its underside and the floor of the mouth. Examine the oropharynx. Also inspect teeth and gums, noting missing, broken, or discolored teeth; dental caries; excessive debris; and bleeding, inflamed, swollen, or discolored gums.

## Causes
*Candidiasis.* This disorder characteristically produces soft, elevated plaques on the buccal mucosa, tongue, and sometimes the palate, gingivae, and floor of the mouth; the plaques may be wiped away.

*Discoid lupus erythematosus.* Oral lesions are common, typically appearing on the tongue, buccal mucosa, and palate as erythematous areas with white spots and radiating white striae. Other findings include skin lesions on the face, possibly extending to the neck, ears, and scalp.

*Herpes simplex.* In primary infection, a brief period of prodromal tingling and itching, accompanied by fever and pharyngitis, is followed by eruption of vesicles on any part of the oral mucosa, especially the tongue, gums, and cheeks.

*Herpes zoster.* Painful vesicles appear on the buccal mucosa, tongue, uvula, pharynx, and larynx. Small red nodules often erupt unilaterally around the thorax or vertically on the arms and legs, and rapidly become vesicles filled with fluid or pus, forming scabs about 10 days after eruption.

*Stomatitis (aphthous).* Recurrent, painful ulcerations of the oral mucosa appear most often on the dorsum of the tongue, gingiva, and hard palate.

*Syphilis.* Primary syphilis produces a solitary painful ulcer (chancre) on the lip, tongue, palate, tonsil, or gingiva. Similar lesions may appear on the fingers, breasts, or genitals; regional lymph nodes may become enlarged and tender. In the *secondary* stage, painless ulcers may erupt on the tongue, gingivae, or buccal mucosa. At the *tertiary* stage, lesions develop on the skin and mucous membranes, especially the tongue and palate.

*Systemic lupus erythematosus.* Oral lesions commonly appear as erythematous areas associated with edema, petechiae, bleeding tendency, and a superficial ulcer with a red halo.

*Other causes.* Acute necrotizing ulcerative gingivitis; allergic reactions to penicillin, sulfonamides, gold, quinine, streptomycin, phenytoin, aspirin, or barbiturates; Behçet's syndrome; benign mucosal pemphigoid; cervicofacial actinomycosis; chemotherapeutic agents; epulis (giant cell); erythema multiforme; fibrous inflammatory hyperplasia; gonorrhea; lichen planus; mucous duct obstruction; oral mucosal tuberculosis; pemphigus; pyogenic granuloma; radiation therapy; squamous cell carcinoma; and trauma.

## Nursing considerations
• Provide a topical anesthetic, as ordered. Instruct the patient to avoid highly seasoned foods, citrus fruits, alcohol, and tobacco. Avoid using lemon-glycerin swabs for mouth care.
• Teach the patient proper oral hygiene. Tell him to notify his doctor if any mouth lesions don't heal within 2 weeks.

# Genital lesions in men

Genital lesions in men may result from infection, neoplasms, parasites, allergy, or the effects of drugs. In many cases, these lesions profoundly affect the patient's self-image, and he may hesitate to seek medical attention, fearing cancer or a sexually transmitted disease (STD). Unfortunately, self-treatment may alter the lesions, making diagnosis difficult.

## History

Ask the patient when he first noticed the lesion. Has he had similar lesions before? If so, were they treated? If he's treating the lesion himself, what measures is he using? Does he have any itching? Note if the lesion is painful. Take a complete sexual history.

## Physical exam

Examine the patient's entire skin, noting the location, size, color, and pattern of any lesions. Do the genital lesions resemble those on other parts of his body? Palpate for nodules, masses, and tenderness. Also look for bleeding, edema, and signs of infection, such as erythema.

## Causes

*Balanitis and balanoposthitis.* Typically, balanitis (glans infection) and posthitis (prepuce infection) occur together (balanoposthitis), causing painful ulceration. The patient may then develop features of acute infection. Without treatment, life-threatening sepsis can occur.

*Chancroid.* In this STD, one or more lesions erupt, usually on the groin, inner thigh, or penis. Within 24 hours, the lesion changes from a reddened area to a small papule. It then becomes an inflamed pustule that rapidly ulcerates. This ulcer bleeds easily and commonly has a purulent gray or yellow exudate.

*Fournier's gangrene.* In this life-threatening cellulitis, the scrotum suddenly becomes tense, swollen, painful, red, warm, and glossy. As gangrene develops, the scrotum also becomes moist.

*Genital herpes.* Caused by herpesvirus Type II, this infection produces fluid-filled vesicles on the glans penis, foreskin, or penile shaft. Usually painless at first, these vesicles may rupture and become extensive, shallow, painful ulcers with redness, edema, and tender inguinal lymph nodes.

*Lichen planus.* Small, polygonal, violet papules develop on the glans penis in this disorder. Usually, they're shiny and less than 3 cm in diameter and have milky striations.

*Lymphogranuloma venereum.* One to three weeks after sexual exposure, this disorder may produce a penile erosion or papule that heals rapidly and spontaneously; in fact, it commonly goes unnoticed. A few days or weeks later, the inguinal and subinguinal nodes enlarge, becoming painful, fluctuant masses.

*Penile cancer.* Usually, this cancer produces a painless, ulcerative lesion or enlarging "wart" on the glans or foreskin. Pain occurs if the foreskin becomes unretractable. Examination may reveal a foul-smelling discharge from the prepuce.

*Syphilis.* Two to four weeks after exposure to *Treponema pallidum*, one or more primary lesions, or chancres, may erupt on the genitalia. The chancre usually starts as a small, red, fluid-filled papule and then erodes to form a painless, firm, indurated, shallow ulcer with a clear base or, less commonly, a hard papule. This lesion gradually involutes and disappears.

*Other causes.* Bowen's disease; candidiasis; drugs, such as barbiturates, phenolphthalein, sulfonamides, and tetracycline; erythroplasia of Queyrat; folliculitis; furunculosis; genital warts; granuloma inguinale; impetigo; leukoplakia; pediculosis pubis; psoriasis; scabies; seborrheic dermatitis; tinea cruris (jock itch); and urticaria.

## Nursing considerations

• Expect to screen every patient with penile lesions for an STD. Also, prepare the patient for a biopsy to confirm or rule out penile cancer.
• Explain to the patient how to use prescribed ointments or creams.

A distinctive facial adiposity, moon face usually indicates hypercortisolism resulting from ectopic or excessive pituitary production of adrenocorticotropic hormone, adrenal adenoma or carcinoma, or long-term glucocorticoid therapy. Its typical characteristics include marked facial roundness, a double chin, prominent upper lip, and full supraclavicular fossae. Although the presence of moon face doesn't help pinpoint the cause of hypercortisolism, it does indicate a need for diagnostic testing.

### History

Ask the patient when he first noticed his facial adiposity, and try to obtain a preonset photograph to help evaluate the extent of the change.

Ask about weight gain and any personal or family history of endocrine disorders, obesity, or cancer. Has the patient noticed any fatigue, irritability, depression, or confusion? Ask a female patient for the date of her last menses and whether she has experienced any menstrual irregularities.

If the patient is receiving glucocorticoids, ask the name of the medication, dosage, route of administration, and reason for therapy. Also ask if the dosage has ever been modified and, if so, when and why.

### Physical exam

Take the patient's vital signs, weight, and height. Also assess the patient's overall appearance for other characteristic signs of hypercortisolism, including virilism in a female or gynecomastia in a male.

### Causes

*Hypercortisolism.* Moon face varies in severity, depending on the degree of cortisol excess and weight gain. The patient typically exhibits buffalo hump, truncal obesity with slender arms and legs, and thin, transparent skin with purple striae and ecchymoses. Other cushingoid features include acne, diaphoresis, fatigue, muscle wasting and weakness, poor wound healing, elevated blood pressure, and personality changes.

In addition to these findings, a woman may experience hirsutism and amenorrhea or oligomenorrhea; a man may experience gynecomastia and impotence.

*Other causes.* Moon face may result from prolonged use of glucocorticoids, such as cortisone, dexamethasone, hydrocortisone, and prednisone.

### Nursing considerations

• Relieve the patient's concern about his body image by explaining that moon face and other disconcerting cushingoid effects can usually be corrected by treating the underlying disorder or by discontinuing or modifying glucocorticoid therapy.

• Clearly explain to the patient any diagnostic tests the doctor orders. These may include serum and urine 17-hydroxycorticosteroid studies, and a 2-day, low-dose dexamethasone test followed by a 2-day, high-dose dexamethasone test.

Marked by a low-pitched grunting sound at the end of each breath, these respirations are a chief sign of respiratory distress in infants and children. They may be soft and heard only on auscultation, or loud and clearly audible without a stethoscope. The grunting coincides with closure of the glottis — an effort to increase end-expiratory pressure and prolong alveolar gas exchange, thereby enhancing ventilation and perfusion.

▶ **Emergency interventions**

If the patient has grunting respirations, quickly check for other signs of distress. These include tachypnea (respiratory rate of 60 breaths/minute in infants, 40 breaths/minute in children ages 1 to 5, or 30 breaths/minute in children over age 5); accessory muscle use; substernal, subcostal, or intercostal retractions; nasal flaring; tachycardia (160 beats/minute in infants, 120 to 140 beats/minute in children ages 1 to 5, or 120 beats/minute in children over age 5); cyanotic lips or nail beds; hypotension ($< 80/40$ mm Hg in infants, $< 80/50$ mm Hg in children ages 1 to 5, or $< 90/55$ mm Hg in children over age 5); and decreased level of consciousness. If you detect any of these signs, have another nurse notify the doctor while you gather suction apparatus, an airway, and oxygen setup. If the patient is a premature infant, assist with intubation and mechanical ventilation.

## History

Ask when the grunting respirations began. If the patient is a premature infant, find out his gestational age. Ask the parents if anyone in the home has had an upper respiratory infection (URI) recently. Has the patient had signs of a URI? Does he have a history of frequent colds or URIs? Has his activity level or alertness changed?

## Physical exam

Auscultate the lungs, especially the lower lobes. Note diminished or abnormal sounds, such as crackles or sibilant rhonchi, which may indicate mucus or fluid buildup. Note any cough, productive or nonproductive. Characterize the color, amount, and consistency of nasal discharge or sputum.

## Causes

*Respiratory distress syndrome.* The result of lung immaturity in a premature infant ($< 37$ weeks' gestation), this syndrome initially causes audible expiratory grunts along with intercostal, subcostal, or substernal retractions; tachycardia; and tachypnea. Later, as respiratory distress tires the infant, apnea or irregular respirations replace the grunting. Severe respiratory distress is characterized by cyanosis, dramatic nasal flaring, lethargy, bradycardia, and hypotension. Eventually, the infant becomes unresponsive. Auscultation reveals harsh, diminished breath sounds and crackles over the bases of the lungs on deep inspiration.

**Staphylococcus aureus *pneumonia.*** Life-threatening bacterial pneumonia primarily affects infants under age 1 and often follows URIs or colds. It causes grunting respirations accompanied by high fever, tachypnea, productive cough, anorexia, and lethargy. Auscultation reveals diminished breath sounds, scattered crackles, and sibilant rhonchi over the affected lung. As the disorder progresses, there may also be severe dyspnea, substernal and subcostal retractions, nasal flaring, cyanosis, and increasing lethargy.

*Other causes.* Congestive heart failure.

## Nursing considerations

• Closely monitor the patient's condition. Keep emergency equipment nearby in case respiratory distress worsens. Prepare to administer oxygen using an oxygen hood or tent, as ordered.
• Begin inhalation therapy with bronchodilators or antimicrobials, as ordered. Follow this with chest physiotherapy (CPT), as needed. Schedule CPT before meals to help prevent severe or spasmodic coughing and resultant vomiting.
• Prepare the patient for chest X-rays, as ordered.
• Sedatives are contraindicated in respiratory distress; restrain a restless child, if necessary.

**G**

Pupillary constriction caused by contraction of the sphincter muscle in the iris, miosis normally occurs as a response to fatigue, increased light, and administration of miotic drugs, as part of the eye's accommodation reflex, and with aging. It can also stem from ocular and neurologic disorders, trauma, systemic drugs, and contact lens overuse. A rare form of miosis—Argyll Robertson pupils—can stem from tabes dorsalis and diverse neurologic disorders. These miotic, unequal pupils don't react properly to light or mydriatic drugs, although they do constrict on accommodation.

## History
Ask the patient if he's experiencing other ocular symptoms, and have him describe their onset, duration, and intensity. Does he wear contact lenses? Also ask about trauma, serious systemic disease, and use of topical and systemic medications.

## Physical exam
Examine and compare both pupils for size, color, shape, reaction to light, accommodation, and consensual light response. Evaluate extraocular muscle function by assessing the six cardinal fields of gaze. Test visual acuity in each eye, with and without correction, paying particular attention to blurred or decreased vision in the miotic eye.

## Causes
*Cerebrovascular arteriosclerosis.* Miosis is usually unilateral. Other findings include blurring, slurred speech or aphasia, loss of muscle tone, memory loss, vertigo, and headache.

*Chemical burns.* An opaque cornea may make miosis hard to detect. However, chemical burns may also cause moderate to severe pain, diffuse conjunctival injection, inability to keep the eye open, and blistering.

*Cluster headache.* Ipsilateral miosis, tearing, conjunctival injection, and ptosis commonly accompany cluster headache, along with facial flushing and sweating, bradycardia, restlessness, and nasal stuffiness or rhinorrhea.

*Corneal foreign body.* Miosis in the affected eye occurs with pain, a foreign-body sensation, slight vision loss, conjunctival injection, photophobia, and profuse tearing.

*Corneal ulcer.* Miosis appears with moderate pain, blurring and some vision loss, and diffuse conjunctival injection.

*Hyphema.* Usually caused by blunt trauma, hyphema can cause miosis with pain, blurring, diffuse conjunctival injection, and slight eyelid swelling. The eyeball may feel harder than normal.

*Iritis (acute).* Miosis typically occurs in the affected eye along with decreased pupillary reflex, severe eye pain, photophobia, blurring, conjunctival injection, and possibly pus accumulation in the anterior chamber.

*Neuropathy.* In diabetic neuropathy, Argyll Robertson pupils may appear, along with paresthesia and other sensory disturbances, extremity pain, postural hypotension, impotence, incontinence, and leg muscle weakness and atrophy.

In alcoholic neuropathy, such pupils may also occur; related effects are progressive muscle weakness and wasting, sensory disturbances, and hypoactive deep tendon reflexes.

*Uveitis.* *Anterior uveitis* commonly produces miosis in the affected eye, with eye pain, conjunctival injection, and photophobia. In *posterior uveitis*, miosis is accompanied by gradual onset of eye pain, photophobia, floaters, blurring, conjunctival injection, and distorted pupil shape.

*Other causes.* Deep anesthesia; drugs, such as barbiturates, cholinergics, cholinesterase inhibitors, clonidine (overdose), guanethidine, opiates, reserpine, and topical drugs used for their miotic effect; Horner's syndrome; Parry-Romberg syndrome; pontine hemorrhage; and tabes dorsalis.

## Nursing considerations
• Reassure and support the patient. Explain any diagnostic tests, which may include an ophthalmologic examination or a neurologic workup.

# Gum bleeding

Bleeding gums usually result from dental disorders or, less often, from blood dyscrasias or the effects of certain drugs. Physiologic causes of this common sign include pregnancy, which can produce gum swelling in the first or second trimester; atmospheric pressure changes, which most commonly affect divers and aviators; and oral trauma. Bleeding ranges from slight oozing to hemorrhage. It may be spontaneous or may follow trauma. Occasionally, direct pressure can control it.

## History

Find out when the bleeding began. Has it been continuous or intermittent? Does it occur spontaneously or when the patient brushes his teeth? Have him show you the bleeding site, if possible.

Determine if the patient or his family has bleeding tendencies. How much does he bleed after a tooth extraction? Does he have a history of liver or spleen disease? Next, check the patient's dental history and ask how often he brushes his teeth and goes to the dentist. Note any prescription and over-the-counter drugs the patient takes.

## Physical exam

Examine the gums to determine bleeding site and amount. Gums normally appear pink and rippled with their margins snugly against the teeth. Check for inflammation, pockets around the teeth, swelling, retraction, discoloration, and gum hyperplasia. Note obvious decay, discoloration, foreign material, and absence of any teeth.

## Causes

*Drugs.* By disrupting blood clotting, coumadin and heparin may cause prolonged gum bleeding. Aspirin abuse may alter platelets, producing bleeding. Localized bleeding may result from "aspirin burn" caused by dissolving aspirin near an aching tooth.

*Gingivitis.* Reddened, edematous gums are characteristic. Gingivae between the teeth become bulbous and bleed easily. In *acute necrotizing ulcerative gingivitis*, bleeding is spontaneous. The gums also become so painful that the patient may be unable to eat. A characteristic grayish yellow pseudomembrane develops over punched-out gum erosions. Offensive halitosis is typical.

*Hemophilia.* Here, hemorrhage occurs from many sites in the oral cavity, especially the gums.

*Hereditary hemorrhagic telangiectasia.* This disorder is characterized by red to violet spiderlike hemorrhagic areas on the gums, which blanch on pressure and bleed spontaneously. These telangiectases may also occur on the lips, buccal mucosa, and palate as well as the face, ears, scalp, hands, arms, feet, and under the nails.

*Leukemia.* Easy gum bleeding is an early sign of acute monocytic, lymphocytic, or myelocytic leukemia. It's accompanied by gum swelling, necrosis, and petechiae. The soft, tender gums appear glossy and bluish. *Acute leukemia* causes severe prostration marked by high fever and bleeding tendencies, such as epistaxis and prolonged menses. Sometimes, it also causes dyspnea, tachycardia, palpitations, and abdominal or bone pain.

*Periodontal disease.* Typically, chewing, toothbrushing, or gum probing initiates gum bleeding, or bleeding occurs spontaneously. As gingivae separate from the bone, pus-filled pockets develop around the teeth and, occasionally, pus can be expressed. Other findings include unpleasant taste with halitosis, facial pain, loose teeth, and dental calculus and plaque.

*Other causes.* Agranulocytosis, benzene exposure, cirrhosis, Ehlers-Danlos syndrome, familial thrombasthenia, giant cell epulis, hypofibrinogenemia, idiopathic thrombocytopenic purpura, pemphigoid, pernicious anemia, polycythemia vera, pyogenic granuloma, thrombocytopenia, and vitamin C or K deficiencies.

## Nursing considerations

• When providing mouth care, avoid using lemon-glycerin swabs, which may burn or dry the gums. Teach the patient about mouth and gum care.
• Prepare the patient for diagnostic tests, such as blood studies or facial X-rays.

G

Uterine bleeding that occurs irregularly between menstrual periods, metrorrhagia is usually light, although it can range from staining to hemorrhage. Most often, this common sign reflects slight physiologic bleeding from the endometrium during ovulation. However, metrorrhagia may be the only indication of an underlying gynecologic disorder and can also result from stress, drugs, and treatments.

## History
Ask the patient when she began menstruating and about the duration of her menstrual periods, the interval between them, and the average number of tampons or pads she uses. When does metrorrhagia usually occur in relation to her period? Does she experience any other signs and symptoms? Find out the date of her last menses, and ask about any other recent changes in her normal menstrual pattern. Get details of any previous gynecologic problems. If applicable, obtain a contraceptive and obstetric history. Record the dates of her last Pap smear and pelvic examination. Next, ask the patient about her general health and any recent changes. Is she under emotional stress? If possible, obtain a pregnancy history of the patient's mother. Was the patient exposed to diethylstilbestrol (DES) in utero? (This drug has been linked to vaginal adenosis.)

## Causes
*Cervicitis.* This nonspecific infection may cause spontaneous bleeding, spotting, or posttraumatic bleeding. Assessment reveals red, granular, irregular lesions on the external cervix. Purulent vaginal discharge, lower abdominal pain, and fever may occur.

*Dysfunctional uterine bleeding.* Abnormal uterine bleeding not caused by pregnancy or major gynecologic disorders usually occurs as metrorrhagia, although menorrhagia is possible. Bleeding may be profuse or scant, intermittent or constant.

*Endometrial polyps.* This disorder may produce metrorrhagia, but most patients are asymptomatic.

*Endometriosis.* Metrorrhagia may be the only indication of this disorder, or it may accompany pelvic discomfort and dyspareunia.

*Endometritis.* Infection of the endometrium results in metrorrhagia and purulent vaginal discharge. It also produces fever, lower abdominal pain, and abdominal muscle spasm.

*Gynecologic carcinoma.* Metrorrhagia commonly occurs as an early sign of these carcinomas. Later, the patient may experience weight loss, pelvic pain, fatigue, and possibly an abdominal mass.

*Syphilis.* Primary- or secondary-stage syphilis may cause metrorrhagia and postcoital bleeding. In primary syphilis, one or more usually painless chancres erupt on the genitalia and possibly other areas. In secondary syphilis, generalized lymphadenopathy may appear, along with a rash on the arms, trunk, palms, soles, face, and scalp. Other features of this stage include headache, malaise, anorexia, weight loss, nausea, vomiting, sore throat, and possibly low fever.

*Vaginal adenosis.* This disorder commonly produces metrorrhagia. Palpation reveals roughening or nodules in affected vaginal areas.

*Other causes.* Drugs, such as anticoagulants and oral contraceptives; and surgery and procedures, such as cervical conization and cauterization.

## Nursing considerations
• As ordered, obtain blood and urine samples for pregnancy testing and assist with pelvic examination. Encourage bed rest to reduce bleeding, and administer analgesics if metrorrhagia is accompanied by discomfort. Monitor the amount of bleeding by recording the number of pads or tampons used.
• Girls who have recently begun menstruating may mistake irregular periods for metrorrhagia.

**M**

# Gum swelling

## 129

Gum swelling may result from one of two mechanisms: an increase in the size of existing gum cells (hypertrophy) or an increase in their number (hyperplasia). This common sign may involve one or many papillae — the triangle-shaped bits of gum between adjacent teeth. Occasionally, the gums swell markedly, obscuring the teeth altogether. Usually, the swelling is most prominent on the labia and bucca.

Most commonly, gum swelling results from the effects of phenytoin. It may also result from nutritional deficiency and certain systemic disorders. Physiologic gum swelling and bleeding may occur during the first or second trimester of pregnancy when hormonal changes make the gums highly vascular; even slight irritation causes swelling and gives the papillae a characteristic raspberry hue (pregnancy epulis). Irritating dentures may also cause swelling associated with red, soft, movable masses on the gums.

## History

After ruling out pregnancy or the use of phenytoin or similar prescription drugs as the cause of gum swelling, take a history. Have the patient describe the swelling fully. Has he had it before? Is it localized or generalized? Find out when the swelling began and ask about any aggravating or alleviating factors. Note if the swelling is painful. Then explore the patient's medical and dental history. Does he wear dentures? If so, are they new? Ask about use of alcohol and tobacco, which are gum irritants. Then have the patient describe his diet to assess nutritional status.

## Physical exam

Inspect the patient's mouth in a good light. As you examine the gums, characterize their color and texture, and note any ulcers, lesions, masses, lumps, or debris-filled pockets around the teeth. Then inspect the teeth for discoloration, obvious decay, and looseness.

## Causes

*Crohn's disease.* Granular or cobblestone gum swelling occurs in this disorder, which is characterized by cramping abdominal pain and diarrhea.

*Drugs.* A common adverse effect of phenytoin is gum swelling. Cyclosporine also produces this sign in about 15% of patients.

*Fibrous hyperplasia (idiopathic).* In this disorder, the gums become diffusely enlarged and may even cover the teeth. Large, firm, painless masses of fibrous tissue form on the gums.

*Leukemia.* Gum swelling is commonly an early sign, especially in acute monocytic, lymphocytic, or myelocytic leukemia. Usually, the swelling is localized and accompanied by necrosis. The tender gums appear blue and glossy and bleed easily. *Acute leukemia* also causes severe prostration, high fever, and signs of abnormal bleeding.

*Vitamin C deficiency.* The gums are spongy, tender, and edematous, and the papillae appear red or purple. The gums bleed easily, and inspection may reveal pockets filled with clotted blood around loose teeth. Associated findings include anorexia, pallor, dry mouth, scaly dermatitis, weakness, lethargy, insomnia, and abnormal bleeding.

## Nursing considerations

• Because gum swelling may affect the patient's appearance, offer emotional support and reassure him that swelling usually resolves with treatment. For phenytoin-induced swelling, substitute another anticonvulsant, such as ethotoin, and prepare the patient for surgery, as ordered.
• When providing mouth care, avoid using lemon-glycerin swabs, which can irritate the gums. Instead, use a soft toothbrush or one that's padded with sponge or gauze.
• To prevent further swelling, teach the patient the basics of good nutrition. Remind him to eat foods high in vitamin C daily. Also encourage him to avoid gum irritants, such as commercial mouthwashes, alcohol, and tobacco.
• Advise semiannual periodontal checkups.

Profuse or extended menstrual bleeding, menorrhagia may occur as a single episode or a chronic sign. Normal menstrual flow lasts about 5 days and produces a total blood loss of 60 to 250 ml. In menorrhagia, however, the menstrual period may be prolonged, and total blood loss can range from 80 ml to overt hemorrhage. Usually a result of gynecologic disorders, this common sign can also result from endocrine and hematologic disorders, stress, and certain drugs and procedures.

## ▶ Emergency interventions

Evaluate hemodynamic status by taking orthostatic vital signs. Immediately call the doctor if the patient shows an increase of 10 beats/minute in pulse rate, a decrease of 10 mm Hg in systolic blood pressure, or other signs of hypovolemic shock — pallor, tachycardia, tachypnea, and cool, clammy skin. Insert a large-gauge I.V. catheter to begin fluid replacement. Place the patient in a supine position with her feet raised. Give oxygen as needed. Prepare her for a pelvic examination.

## History

Try to determine the patient's age at menarche, the duration of menstrual periods, and the interval between them. Establish the date of her last menses, and ask about recent changes in her normal menstrual pattern. Have her describe the bleeding, and ask about other signs and symptoms before and during the menstrual period.

Ask if the patient is sexually active and if she practices birth control. Could she be pregnant? Ask about past pregnancies, noting any complications. Find out the dates of her most recent pelvic examination and Pap smear and the details of previous gynecologic infections or neoplasms. Ask about abnormal bleeding and any treatment. If possible, obtain a pregnancy history of the patient's mother to determine possible exposure to diethylstilbestrol in utero.

Note if the patient or her family has a history of thyroid, adrenal, or hepatic disease; blood dyscrasias; or tuberculosis, which may predispose to menorrhagia. Ask about past surgery, X-ray or other radiation therapy, and emotional stress.

## Physical exam

Prepare the patient for a pelvic examination if one hasn't already been performed.

## Causes

*Blood dyscrasias.* Menorrhagia is one of several possible signs of bleeding, such as epistaxis, bleeding gums, purpura, hematemesis, hematuria, and melena.

*Dysfunctional uterine bleeding.* Menorrhagia is a less common sign than metrorrhagia. The bleeding can be constant or intermittent.

*Endometriosis.* Menorrhagia is the most common sign of this disorder. Typically, the patient also reports pain in the lower abdomen, vagina, posterior pelvis, and back.

*Hypothyroidism.* Menorrhagia is a common early sign, along with fatigue, cold intolerance, constipation, and weight gain despite anorexia. As hypothyroidism progresses, intellectual and motor activity decrease. The skin becomes dry and cool, the hair dry and sparse, the nails thick and brittle.

*Uterine fibroids.* Menorrhagia is the most common sign, but other forms of abnormal uterine bleeding, as well as dysmenorrhea or leukorrhea, can also occur. Other findings may include abdominal pain, backache, constipation, urinary urgency or frequency, and an enlarged uterus.

*Other causes.* Cervical conization or cauterization; congestive heart failure; drugs, such as oral contraceptives and anticoagulants; and intrauterine contraceptive devices.

## Nursing considerations

• Monitor the patient for signs of hypovolemia. Monitor intake and output, and estimate uterine blood loss by recording the number of sanitary napkins or tampons used.
• Obtain blood and urine samples for pregnancy testing.

**M**

# Gynecomastia

## 130

This term refers to excessive development of one or both mammary glands in males, resulting in breast enlargement. This size change may be barely palpable or immediately obvious. Usually bilateral, gynecomastia may be associated with breast tenderness and milk secretion.

Normally, estrogens, growth hormone, and corticosteroids stimulate ductal growth, while progesterone and prolactin stimulate growth of the alveolar lobules. Although the pathophysiology of gynecomastia isn't fully understood, hormonal imbalance — particularly the estrogen-androgen ratio and increased prolactin — is a likely contributing factor. Normal hormone changes may cause physiologic gynecomastia in neonatal, pubertal, and geriatric males.

## History

Ask the patient when he first noticed his breast enlargement. Since then, have his breasts changed size? Is gynecomastia accompanied by breast tenderness or discharge? Next, take a thorough drug history and explore associated symptoms, such as a testicular mass or pain, loss of libido, decreased potency, or loss of chest, axillary, and facial hair.

## Physical exam

Examine the breasts for any asymmetry, dimpling, abnormal pigmentation, or ulceration. Observe the testicles for size and symmetry. Then palpate them to detect nodules, tenderness, or unusual consistency. Look for normal penile development after puberty, and note hypospadias.

## Causes

*Adrenal carcinoma.* Estrogen production by an adrenal tumor may produce a feminizing syndrome in males characterized by bilateral gynecomastia, loss of libido, impotence, testicular atrophy, reduced facial hair growth, and cushingoid signs.

*Breast cancer.* Painful unilateral gynecomastia develops rapidly. Palpation may reveal a hard or stony breast lump. Breast examination may also detect changes in breast symmetry; thickening, dimpling, peau d'orange, or ulceration of the skin; and a warm, reddened area. The patient's nipple may produce a watery, bloody, or purulent discharge and may itch or burn. He may also have nipple erosion, deviation, flattening, or retraction.

*Drugs.* Estrogens used to treat prostatic cancer, such as diethylstilbestrol, directly affect the estrogen-androgen ratio. Drugs with an estrogen-like effect, such as digitalis, may do the same. Regular marijuana or heroin use reduces plasma testosterone levels, causing gynecomastia. Other drugs, such as spironolactone and cimetidine, produce this sign by interfering with androgen production or action. Phenothiazines, tricyclic antidepressants, and antihypertensives produce gynecomastia in an unknown way.

*Pituitary tumor.* Effects of this hormone-secreting tumor include bilateral gynecomastia, galactorrhea, impotence, and decreased libido.

*Testicular failure (secondary).* Commonly associated with mumps or other infections, this disorder causes bilateral gynecomastia after normal puberty. It may also cause sparse facial hair, decreased libido, impotence, and testicular atrophy.

*Testicular tumors.* These tumors typically cause bilateral gynecomastia, nipple tenderness, and decreased libido.

*Other causes.* Cirrhosis, hepatic carcinoma, hermaphroditism, hypothyroidism, Klinefelter's syndrome, malnutrition, Reifenstein's syndrome, renal failure (chronic), thyrotoxicosis, and treatments (such as hemodialysis, major surgery, and testicular irradiation).

## Nursing considerations

• To promote comfort, apply cold compresses to the breasts and give analgesics, as ordered.
• Because gynecomastia alters the patient's body image, provide emotional support. Reassure him that treatment can correct the gynecomastia.
• Prepare the patient for diagnostic tests, including chest and skull X-rays and blood hormone levels.

**G**

A common sign of upper GI bleeding, melena is the passage of black, tarry stools. The distinctive color results from hydrochloric acid acting on the blood as it travels through the GI tract. At least 60 ml of blood is needed to produce this sign. Severe melena can signal acute bleeding and life-threatening hypovolemic shock. Usually, melena indicates bleeding from the esophagus, stomach, or duodenum, but it can also indicate bleeding from the jejunum, ileum, or ascending colon.

▶ **Emergency interventions**

If the patient is experiencing severe melena, quickly take orthostatic vital signs to detect hypovolemic shock, while another nurse immediately notifies the doctor. A decrease of 10 mm Hg or more in systolic pressure, or an increase of 10 beats/minute or more in pulse rate, indicates volume depletion. Quickly look for other signs of shock, such as tachycardia, tachypnea, and cool, clammy skin. Insert a large-bore I.V. catheter to administer replacement fluids and allow blood transfusion. Place the patient flat with his head turned to the side and his feet elevated. Administer oxygen as needed.

## History

If the patient's condition permits, ask when he first noticed that his stools had become black and tarry. Has this happened before? Ask about other signs and symptoms, particularly hematemesis or hematochezia, and about use of anti-inflammatory drugs, alcohol, or other GI irritants. Find out if the patient has a history of GI lesions, such as hemorrhoids.

## Physical exam

Inspect the patient's mouth and nasopharynx for evidence of bleeding. Auscultate, palpate, and percuss the abdomen.

## Causes

*Colon cancer.* On the right side of the colon, early tumor growth may cause melena accompanied by abdominal aching, pressure, or dull cramps. The patient later develops weakness, fatigue, exertional dyspnea, and vertigo.

On the left side, melena is a later sign. Early tumor growth commonly causes rectal bleeding accompanied by intermittent abdominal fullness or cramping and rectal pressure.

*Diverticulitis.* Melena may occur as occult blood in the stool or as acute hemorrhage. Other findings may include left lower quadrant pain and tenderness, constipation, and a palpable abdominal mass.

*Esophageal varices (ruptured).* This life-threatening disorder can produce melena. It's usually preceded by signs of shock, such as tachycardia, tachypnea, hypotension, and cool, clammy skin.

*Gastritis.* Melena and hematemesis are common. The patient may also experience mild epigastric or abdominal discomfort, belching, nausea, vomiting, fever, and malaise.

*Mesenteric vascular occlusion.* This life-threatening disorder produces slight melena with 2 to 3 days of persistent, mild abdominal pain. The pain becomes more severe and may be accompanied by tenderness, distention, guarding, and rigidity.

*Peptic ulcer.* Melena may signal life-threatening hemorrhage from vascular penetration. The patient may also have nausea, vomiting, hematemesis, hematochezia, and diffuse epigastric pain that's gnawing, burning, or sharp.

*Other causes.* Alcohol; drugs, such as aspirin and other nonsteroidal anti-inflammatory agents; esophageal or gastric carcinoma; malaria; Mallory-Weiss syndrome; thrombocytopenia; typhoid fever; and yellow fever.

## Nursing considerations

• Monitor the patient's vital signs, and watch for signs of hypovolemic shock.
• Encourage bed rest. Keep the patient's perianal area clean and dry to prevent skin irritation.
• Prepare the patient for diagnostic tests, including blood studies, gastroscopy or other endoscopic studies, barium swallow, and upper GI series.

Halitosis describes any breath odor that's unpleasant, disagreeable, or offensive. Certain types of halitosis characterize specific disorders; for example, a fruity breath odor typifies ketoacidosis. Other types of halitosis include putrid, foul, fetid, and musty breath odors.

This common sign may result from oral, nasal, sinus, or respiratory disorders. Halitosis may also stem from GI disorders associated with belching, regurgitation, or vomiting. It may be an adverse effect of oral or inhalant drugs.

Usually, halitosis stems from cigarette smoking and ingestion of alcohol and certain foods, such as onions. Poor oral hygiene—especially in the patient with an orthodontic device, dentures, or dental caries—commonly causes halitosis.

## History

If you detect halitosis, try to characterize the odor. Is it fruity? Fecal? Musty? If the patient is aware of the halitosis, find out how long he's had it. Does he have a bad taste in his mouth? Difficulty swallowing or chewing? Pain or tenderness?

Find out if the patient smokes or chews tobacco. Have him describe his diet and daily oral hygiene. Does he wear dentures? Ask about chronic disorders and recent respiratory infection. If the patient reports a cough, find out if it's productive.

## Physical exam

Assess the patient's mouth, throat, and nose. Look for lesions, bleeding, drainage, obstruction, or signs of infection. Assess for tenderness by percussing and palpating over the sinuses. Auscultate for abnormal breath sounds and take vital signs.

## Causes

*Bowel obstruction.* Halitosis is a late sign of small- and large-bowel obstruction. In *small-bowel obstruction,* vomiting of gastric, bilious, then fecal material produces a related odor. In *large-bowel obstruction,* fecal vomiting produces breath odor.

*Bronchiectasis.* Usually, this disorder produces foul or putrid halitosis; however, some patients may have sickeningly sweet breath. Typically, the patient also has a chronic productive cough.

*Gastrojejunocolic fistula.* In this disorder, fecal vomiting causes fecal breath odor. Typically, halitosis follows intermittent diarrhea.

*Gingivitis.* Characterized by red, edematous gums, this disorder may also cause halitosis. The gingivae between the teeth become bulbous and bleed easily with slight trauma.

*Hepatic encephalopathy.* A characteristic late sign is a musty, sweet, or mousy (new-mown hay) breath odor called fetor hepaticus. Other late effects include coma, asterixis, hyperactive reflexes, and positive Babinski's reflex.

*Ketoacidosis.* Both diabetic and starvation ketoacidosis produce a fruity breath odor, orthostatic hypotension, weakness, anorexia, abdominal pain, and altered level of consciousness.

*Periodontal disease.* Halitosis is accompanied by an unpleasant taste. Typically, the gums bleed spontaneously or with slight trauma and are marked by pus-filled pockets around the teeth.

*Pharyngitis (gangrenous).* Halitosis is a chief sign of this disorder. The patient also complains of a foul taste in the mouth, an extremely sore throat, and a choking sensation.

*Renal failure (chronic).* A urinous or ammonia breath odor accompanies widespread effects.

*Zenker's diverticulum.* This esophageal disorder causes halitosis and a bad taste in the mouth associated with regurgitation.

*Other causes.* Common cold, esophageal cancer, gastric carcinoma, inhaled anesthetics, lung abscess, necrotizing ulcerative mucositis (acute), and sinusitis.

## Nursing considerations

• If mouth and sinus examination doesn't reveal the cause of halitosis, prepare the patient for upper GI and chest X-rays or endoscopy, as ordered.

• Encourage good oral hygiene. If halitosis is drug-induced, reassure the patient that it will subside when his body eliminates the drug.

Commonly an indicator of meniscal injury, Mc-Murray's sign is a palpable, audible click or pop elicited by manipulating the leg. It results when gentle manipulation of the leg traps torn cartilage and then lets it snap free. Because eliciting this sign forces the surface of the tibial plateau against the femoral condyles, it's contraindicated in patients with suspected fractures of the tibial plateau or femoral condyles.

Eliciting McMurray's sign requires special training and gentle manipulation of the patient's leg to avoid extending a meniscal tear or locking the knee.

A positive McMurray's sign augments other findings commonly associated with meniscal injury, such as severe knee pain and decreased range of motion.

## History

After McMurray's sign has been elicited, find out if the patient is experiencing acute knee pain. Then ask him to describe any recent knee injury. For example, did his injury place twisting external or internal force on the knee, or did he experience blunt knee trauma from a fall? Also ask about previous knee injury, surgery, or prosthetic replacement and about other joint problems, such as arthritis, which could have weakened the knee. Ask if anything aggravates or relieves the pain and if he needs assistance to walk.

## Physical exam

Have the patient point to the exact area of pain. Assess the leg's range of motion, both passive and with resistance. Next, check for cruciate ligament stability by noting anterior or posterior movement of the tibia on the femur. Finally, measure the quadriceps muscles in both legs for symmetry.

To elicit McMurray's sign, place the patient in a supine position and flex his affected knee until his heel nearly touches his buttock. Place your thumb and index finger on either side of the knee joint space, and grasp his heel with your other hand. Then rotate the foot and lower leg laterally to test the posterior meniscus. Keeping his foot in a lateral position, extend the knee to a 90-degree angle to test the anterior meniscus. A palpable or audible click — a positive McMurray's sign — indicates a meniscal tear.

## Cause

**Meniscal tear.** McMurray's sign can commonly be elicited in this injury. Associated signs and symptoms may include acute knee pain at the medial or lateral joint line (depending on the injury site) and decreased range of motion or locking of the knee joint. Quadriceps weakening and atrophy commonly occur.

## Nursing considerations

- Prepare the patient for knee X-rays, arthroscopy, and arthrography, as ordered, and obtain any previous X-rays for comparison. If trauma precipitated the knee pain and McMurray's sign, an effusion or hemarthrosis may occur. Prepare the patient for aspiration of the joint. Immobilize and apply ice to the knee, and assist with application of a cast or a knee immobilizer.
- Instruct the patient to elevate the affected leg and to perform straight leg-raising exercises up to 200 times a day. As appropriate, teach him how to use crutches. Also tell him the prescribed dosage of analgesics and anti-inflammatory drugs.
- Help the patient adjust to life-style changes by providing support and including his family or friends in teaching.
- McMurray's sign in adolescents is elicited most commonly in meniscal tears from sports injuries. It also may be elicited in children with congenital discoid lateral meniscus.

**M**

# Halo vision

Halo vision refers to seeing rainbowlike, colored rings around lights or bright objects. The rainbowlike effect can be explained by this physical principle: As light passes through water (in the eye, through tears or the cells of various anteretinal media), it breaks up into spectral colors.

Usually, halo vision develops suddenly; its duration depends on the causative disorder. This symptom may occur in disorders associated with excessive tearing and corneal epithelial edema. Among these causes, the most common and significant is acute closed-angle glaucoma, which can lead to blindness. Here, increased intraocular pressure (IOP) forces fluid into corneal tissues anterior to Bowman's membrane, causing edema. Halos are also an early symptom of cataracts and result from dispersion of light by abnormal opacities on the lens.

Nonpathologic causes of excessive tearing associated with halos include poorly fitted or overworn contact lenses, emotional extremes, and exposure to intense light, as in snow blindness.

## History
Ask the patient, "How long have you been seeing halos around lights?" Find out when halos are most frequently seen. Patients with glaucoma typically see halos most frequently in the morning, when IOP is most severely elevated. Ask the patient if light bothers his eyes. Does he have any eye pain? If so, have him describe it. Remember that halos associated with excruciating eye pain or severe headache may point to acute closed-angle glaucoma—an ocular emergency. Note a history of glaucoma or cataracts.

## Physical exam
Examine the patient's eyes, noting conjunctival injection, excessive tearing, and lens changes. Assess pupil size, shape, and response to light. Then test visual acuity and assist the doctor with an ophthalmoscopic examination.

## Causes
*Cataract.* Halos may be an early symptom of painless, progressive cataract formation. The glare of headlights may blind the patient, making nighttime driving impossible. Other features include blurred vision, impaired visual acuity, and lens opacity, all of which develop gradually.

*Corneal endothelial dystrophy.* Typically, halos are a late symptom. Impaired visual acuity may also occur.

*Glaucoma.* Halos characterize all types of glaucoma. *Acute closed-angle glaucoma* also causes blurred vision followed by severe headache or excruciating pain in and around the affected eye. Examination will reveal a moderately dilated fixed pupil that doesn't respond to light, conjunctival injection, a cloudy cornea, and impaired visual acuity. Nausea and vomiting may also occur. Usually, *chronic closed-angle glaucoma* is asymptomatic until pain and blindness occur in advanced disease. Sometimes, halos and blurred vision develop slowly. In *chronic open-angle glaucoma,* halos are a late symptom accompanied by mild eye ache, peripheral vision loss, and impaired visual acuity.

## Nursing considerations
• To help minimize halos, remind the patient not to look directly at bright lights.

**H**

A telltale indicator of localized peritoneal inflammation in appendicitis, McBurney's sign is tenderness elicited by palpating the right lower quadrant over McBurney's point. Before McBurney's sign is elicited, the abdomen is inspected for distention and auscultated for hypoactive or absent bowel sounds.

## History
Ask the patient about abdominal pain. When did it begin? Does coughing, movement, eating, or elimination worsen or help relieve it? Also ask about the development of any other signs and symptoms.

## Physical exam
To elicit McBurney's sign, position the patient supine with his knees slightly flexed and his abdominal muscles relaxed. Then palpate deeply and slowly in the right lower quadrant over McBurney's point, which is located one-third of the distance from the anterior superior iliac spine to the umbilicus. Point tenderness, a positive McBurney's sign, indicates appendicitis. Continue light palpation of the patient's abdomen to detect additional tenderness, rigidity, guarding, or pain. Observe the patient's facial expression for signs of pain, such as grimacing or wincing.

## Cause
*Appendicitis.* McBurney's sign appears within the first 2 to 12 hours, after initial pain in the epigastric and periumbilical area shifts to the right lower quadrant (specifically, over McBurney's point). This persistent point pain increases with walking or coughing. Nausea and vomiting are present from the start. Boardlike abdominal rigidity and rebound tenderness accompany cutaneous hyperalgesia, fever, constipation or diarrhea, tachycardia, retractive respirations, anorexia, and moderate malaise.

Rupture of the appendix causes a sudden cessation of pain. Then, as peritonitis develops, abdominal pain recurs, together with pallor, hypoactive or absent bowel sounds, diaphoresis, and a high fever.

## Nursing considerations
• As ordered, draw blood for laboratory tests and prepare the patient for abdominal X-rays to confirm appendicitis.
• If appendicitis is suspected, prepare the patient for appendectomy. Administer I.V. fluids to prevent dehydration. *Never* administer cathartics or enemas, as they may rupture the appendix. Give the patient nothing by mouth, and administer analgesics judiciously, since they may lessen symptoms.

To reduce pain, place the patient in Fowler's position. (This is also helpful postoperatively.) *Never* apply heat to the lower right abdomen; this may cause the appendix to rupture.
• McBurney's sign is also elicited in children with appendicitis.

A headache is the most common neurologic symptom, producing mild to severe pain. About 90% of all headaches are benign. A generalized, pathologic headache may result from disorders associated with intracranial inflammation, increased intracranial pressure (ICP), meningeal irritation, or vascular disturbance. It may also result from the effects of drugs, tests, and treatments.

## History
Ask the patient to describe the character, location, and duration of his headaches. How often does he get them? What are the precipitating factors?

Take a drug history, and ask about head trauma within the last 4 weeks. Has the patient had nausea, vomiting, photophobia, or any visual changes? Does he feel drowsy, confused, or dizzy? Does he have insomnia? Also ask about seizures.

## Physical exam
Assess the patient's level of consciousness (LOC). Then check vital signs. Watch for signs of increased ICP. Check pupil size and response to light. Also note any neck stiffness.

## Causes
*Encephalitis.* A severe, generalized headache is characteristic. The patient's LOC usually deteriorates within 48 hours. Other findings include fever, nuchal rigidity, irritability, and seizures.

*Epidural hemorrhage (acute).* Usually, head trauma and immediate, brief loss of consciousness precede this hemorrhage, which causes a progressively severe headache. It's accompanied by nausea and vomiting, bladder distention, confusion, and then a rapid decrease in LOC.

*Influenza.* A severe headache usually begins suddenly with the flu. Accompanying signs and symptoms may last for 3 to 5 days and include stabbing retro-orbital pain, weakness, diffuse myalgia, fever, chills, coughing, and rhinorrhea.

*Meningitis.* A severe, generalized headache occurs suddenly and worsens with movement. Other signs include nuchal rigidity, positive Kernig's and Brudzinski's signs, hyperreflexia, and possibly opisthotonos. Fever occurs early and may be accompanied by chills.

*Psittacosis.* A severe headache begins abruptly, with fever, chills, malaise, and myalgia. An early dry cough later produces small amounts of mucoid sputum with blood streaks.

*Subarachnoid hemorrhage.* Commonly, this hemorrhage produces a sudden, violent headache. Related signs and symptoms include nuchal rigidity, rapidly deteriorating LOC, nausea, vomiting, seizures, dizziness, and ipsilateral pupil dilation.

*Subdural hematoma.* In *acute subdural hematoma*, head trauma produces immediate loss of consciousness followed by a headache, drowsiness, confusion, and agitation that may progress to coma.

*Chronic subdural hematoma* produces a dull, pounding headache that fluctuates in severity and is located over the hematoma. Weeks or months after head trauma, this disorder may cause giddiness, personality changes, confusion, seizures, and altered LOC that progressively worsens. Late signs may include unilateral pupil dilation, sluggish pupil reaction to light, and ptosis.

*Other causes.* Cervical traction, intracerebral hemorrhage, lumbar puncture, myelography, vasodilators, and withdrawal from vasopressors or sympathomimetic drugs.

## Nursing considerations
• Monitor vital signs and LOC. Watch for any change in the headache's severity or location.
• Give analgesics, as ordered. Darken the patient's room and minimize other stimuli.

# Masklike facies

A total loss of facial expression, masklike facies results from bradykinesia, usually caused by extrapyramidal damage. Even the rate of eye blinking is reduced—to one to four blinks per minute—producing a characteristic "reptilian" stare. Although a neurologic disorder is the most common cause, masklike facies can also result from certain systemic diseases and the effects of drugs and toxins. The sign often develops insidiously and may at first be mistaken for depression or apathy.

## History
Ask the patient and his family or friends when they first noticed the masklike facial expression and any other signs or symptoms. Find out which medications the patient is taking, if any, and ask about any changes in dosage.

## Physical exam
Determine the degree of facial muscle weakness by asking the patient to smile and to wrinkle his forehead. Typically, the patient's responses are slowed.

## Causes
*Carbon monoxide poisoning.* Masklike facies usually develops several weeks after acute poisoning. The patient may also have rigidity, dementia, impaired sensory function, choreoathetosis, generalized seizures, and myoclonus.

*Dermatomyositis.* Masklike facies reflects muscle soreness and weakness extending from the face and neck to the shoulder and pelvic girdle. Dysphagia and dysphonia develop. Characteristic cutaneous signs include edema and dusky lilac suffusion of the eyelid margin or periorbital tissue; an erythematous rash on the face, neck, upper back, chest, arms, and nail beds; and violet (Gottron's) papules dorsal to the interphalangeal joint.

*Drugs.* Phenothiazines (particularly piperazine derivatives) and other antipsychotics commonly cause masklike facies as well as other extrapyramidal effects. Metoclopramide and metyrosine infrequently cause masklike facies. This sign usually improves when the drug is reduced or discontinued.

*Manganese poisoning (chronic).* Masklike facies develops gradually, along with a resting tremor and personality changes. The patient also experiences chorea, propulsive gait, dystonia, and rigidity. Later, extreme muscle weakness and fatigue occur.

*Parkinson's disease.* Masklike facies occurs early but is often overlooked. More noticeable signs include muscle rigidity and an insidious tremor. The patient exhibits stooped posture and propulsive gait, and speaks in a high-pitched monotone. He may have drooling, dysphagia, and dysarthria.

*Scleroderma.* A late sign, masklike facies develops along with a smooth, wrinkle-free appearance, "pinching" of the mouth, and possibly contractures, as facial skin becomes tight and inelastic. Other later features include pain, stiffness, and swelling of joints and foreshortened fingers. Skin on the fingers and then on the hands and forearms thickens, and becomes taut and shiny.

## Nursing considerations
• If the patient's masklike facies results from Parkinson's disease, explain to his family that the sign may hide facial clues to depression—a common symptom of Parkinson's disease.

M

# Headache, localized

A headache is the most common neurologic symptom, producing mild to severe pain. About 90% of all headaches are benign. A localized headache may result from disorders associated with intracranial inflammation, increased intracranial pressure (ICP), meningeal irritation, vascular disturbance, or muscle contraction (tension). It may also result from ocular or sinus disorders and from the effects of treatments.

## History
Ask the patient to describe his headaches, especially their location and duration. How often does he get them? What precipitates them? Ask about head trauma within the last 4 weeks, nausea, vomiting, photophobia, visual changes, and seizures. Does he feel drowsy, confused, or dizzy? Does he have insomnia?

## Physical exam
Assess level of consciousness (LOC) and check vital signs. Be alert for signs of increased ICP. Check pupil size and response to light. Also note any neck stiffness.

## Causes
*Brain abscess.* Headache localizes to the abscess site. It usually intensifies gradually and is aggravated by straining. Nausea, vomiting, and focal or generalized seizures may also occur. The patient's LOC will vary from drowsiness to deep stupor.

*Brain tumor.* Initially, a headache develops near the tumor site, becoming generalized as the tumor grows. Usually, the headache is intermittent, deep-seated and dull, and most intense in the morning. It's aggravated by coughing, stooping, Valsalva's maneuver, and changes in head position.

*Cerebral aneurysm (ruptured).* Headache is sudden and excruciating. It may be unilateral and usually peaks within minutes of aneurysmal rupture. The patient may lose consciousness. He may also experience nausea and vomiting, and signs of meningeal irritation.

*Glaucoma (acute closed-angle).* This ophthalmic emergency may cause an excruciating headache. It also causes acute eye pain, blurred vision, halo vision, nausea, and vomiting.

*Hypertension.* This disorder may cause a slightly throbbing occipital headache on awakening, its severity decreasing during the day. If diastolic blood pressure exceeds 120 mm Hg, the headache remains constant.

*Migraine.* Severe, throbbing headache may follow a 5- to 15-minute prodrome of visual disturbances; tingling of the face, lips, or hands; dizziness; or unsteady gait. Other signs include anorexia, nausea, vomiting, and photophobia.

*Muscle-contraction (tension) headache.* Aching or painful tightness around the head occurs, especially in the neck and occipital and temporal areas.

*Postconcussional syndrome.* One to 30 days after head trauma, a headache may develop and last for 2 to 3 weeks. Neurologic status is normal, but the patient may have dizziness, blurred vision, fatigue, insomnia, and an inability to concentrate.

*Sinusitis (acute).* A dull periorbital headache is aggravated by bending over or touching the face. It's relieved by sinus drainage.

*Temporal arteritis.* A throbbing, unilateral headache in the temporal or frontotemporal region may be accompanied by vision loss, hearing loss, confusion, and fever.

*Typhoid fever.* This begins with a severe frontal headache, steadily increasing fever, abdominal discomfort, and constipation.

*Other causes.* Cervical traction and localized intracerebral hemorrhage.

## Nursing considerations
- Monitor vital signs and LOC. Watch for any change in the headache's severity or location.
- Give analgesics, as ordered. Darken the patient's room and minimize other stimuli.

**H**

Enlargement of one or more lymph nodes, lymphadenopathy may result from increased production of lymphocytes or reticuloendothelial cells, or from infiltration of foreign cells. This sign may be generalized (involving three or more node groups) or localized. Generalized lymphadenopathy may be caused by bacterial or viral infection, connective tissue disease, endocrine disorders, or neoplasms. Localized lymphadenopathy most commonly results from infection or trauma.

### History
Ask the patient when he first noticed the swelling and if it's on one side of his body or both. Are the swollen areas sore, hard, or red? Ask about recent colds or viruses and any other health problems. Also ask if he's had a nodal biopsy. Find out if the patient has a family history of cancer.

### Physical exam
Palpate the entire lymph node system. If you detect enlarged nodes, note their size in centimeters and whether they're fixed or mobile, tender or nontender. Also note nodal texture. If you detect tender, erythematous lymphadenopathy, check the area drained by that part of the lymph system for signs of infection.

### Causes
*Brucellosis.* Generalized lymphadenopathy usually affects cervical and axillary lymph nodes, making them tender. The disease usually begins insidiously with easy fatigability, headache, backache, anorexia, and arthralgias. It may also begin abruptly with chills, fever, and diaphoresis.

*Cytomegalovirus infection.* Generalized lymphadenopathy occurs in the immunocompromised patient. It's accompanied by fever, malaise, rash, and hepatosplenomegaly.

*Hodgkin's disease.* Usually, lymph nodes in the neck enlarge first and become hard, swollen, movable, and discrete. Other findings include pruritus and, in older patients, fatigue, weakness, night sweats, malaise, weight loss, and unexplained fever (usually to 101° F [38.3° C]).

*Infectious mononucleosis.* Painful lymphadenopathy involves cervical, axillary, and inguinal nodes. Prodromal symptoms (headache, malaise, and fatigue) occur 3 to 5 days before the classic triad of lymphadenopathy, sore throat, and temperature fluctuations with an evening peak of about 102° F (38.9° C).

*Leukemia (acute lymphocytic).* Generalized lymphadenopathy accompanies fatigue, malaise, pallor, and low fever. Other findings include prolonged bleeding time, swollen gums, weight loss, bone or joint pain, and hepatosplenomegaly.

*Leukemia (chronic lymphocytic).* Generalized lymphadenopathy appears early, along with fatigue, malaise, and fever. Later, hepatosplenomegaly, fatigue, and weight loss occur. Other findings include bone tenderness, edema, dyspnea, palpitations, bleeding, and skin lesions.

*Rheumatoid arthritis.* Lymphadenopathy is an early, nonspecific finding associated with fatigue, malaise, continuous low fever, weight loss, and vague arthralgias and myalgias.

*Systemic lupus erythematosus.* Generalized lymphadenopathy commonly accompanies butterfly rash, photosensitivity, Raynaud's phenomenon, and joint pain and stiffness.

*Other causes.* Drugs such as phenytoin; leptospirosis; mycosis fungoides; non-Hodgkin's lymphoma; sarcoidosis; Sjögren's syndrome; syphilis (secondary); tuberculous lymphadenitis; typhoid vaccination; Waldenström's macroglobulinemia.

### Nursing considerations
• If the patient has a fever above 101° F (38.3° C), provide antipyretics, tepid sponge baths, or a hypothermia blanket, as ordered.
• Expect to obtain blood for routine tests, a platelet count, and liver and renal function studies. Prepare the patient for other tests, as ordered. If they reveal an infection, or if the patient has draining wounds or lesions, observe isolation precautions.

Hearing loss can be classified as conductive, sensorineural, mixed, and functional. *Conductive loss* results from external and middle ear disorders that block sound transmission. *Sensorineural loss* results from disorders of the inner ear or cranial nerve VIII. *Mixed loss* combines aspects of both conductive and sensorineural loss. *Functional loss* results from psychological factors.

Hearing loss may result from trauma, infection, tumors, systemic and hereditary disorders, and the effects of ototoxic drugs and treatments. Most commonly, it results from presbycusis—a sensorineural loss that usually affects those over age 50. Other physiologic causes of hearing loss include cerumen impaction, barotitis media, and chronic exposure to noise over 90 decibels.

## History
If the patient reports hearing loss, ask him to describe it fully. Is it unilateral or bilateral? Continuous or intermittent? Ask about a family history of hearing loss. Then ask about his medical and drug history and work environment. Explore associated signs and symptoms: pain, discharge, ringing, buzzing, hissing, or other unusual noises in one or both ears.

## Physical exam
Inspect the external ear for inflammation, boils, foreign bodies, or discharge. Then apply pressure to the tragus and mastoid to elicit tenderness. If you detect tenderness or external ear abnormalities, perform an otoscopic examination. Note any color change, perforation, bulging, or retraction of the tympanic membrane. Use the ticking watch and whispered voice tests to assess gross hearing. Initially evaluate the type and degree of hearing loss with the Weber and Rinne tests.

## Causes
*Acoustic neuroma.* This tumor causes unilateral, progressive, sensorineural loss. The patient may have tinnitus, vertigo, and facial paralysis.

*Cholesteatoma.* Gradual hearing loss occurs along with vertigo and facial paralysis.

*Drugs.* Chloroquine, cisplatin, vancomycin, and aminoglycosides may cause irreversible hearing loss. Loop diuretics, such as furosemide, usually produce a brief, reversible hearing loss. Quinine, quinidine, or high doses of erythromycin or salicylates may also cause reversible loss.

*Ménière's disease.* Initially, this disease produces intermittent, unilateral sensorineural hearing loss that involves only low tones. Later, hearing loss becomes constant and affects other tones. Associated findings: intermittent severe vertigo, nausea, vomiting, ear fullness, a roaring or hollowseashell tinnitus, diaphoresis, and nystagmus.

*Otitis externa.* Conductive loss characterizes both acute and malignant otitis externa and results from ear canal debris.

*Otitis media.* Typically, this middle ear inflammation produces transient unilateral conductive loss. In *acute suppurative* and *chronic otitis media*, hearing loss develops gradually over a few hours.

*Otosclerosis.* In this hereditary disorder, unilateral conductive loss usually begins in the early twenties and may gradually progress to bilateral mixed loss. The patient may report tinnitus and improved hearing in a noisy environment.

*Other causes.* Adenoid hypertrophy, allergies, aural polyps, external ear canal cyst or tumor, furuncle, glomus jugulare tumor, glomus tympanium, granuloma, head trauma, hypothyroidism, multiple sclerosis, myringitis, nasopharyngeal cancer, osteoma, radiation therapy or surgery (local), Ramsay Hunt syndrome, skull fracture, temporal arteritis, temporal bone fracture, tertiary syphilis, tuberculosis, tympanic membrane perforation, and Wegener's granulomatosis.

## Nursing considerations
• Remember to face the patient and speak slowly.
• As ordered, prepare him for audiometric tests.
• He may require a hearing aid or cochlear implant to improve hearing. Tell him to avoid exposure to loud noises to prevent further hearing loss.

H

A cardinal symptom of vision-threatening retinal detachment, light flashes can occur locally or throughout the visual field. Usually, the patient reports seeing spots, stars, or lightning streaks. Light flashes can arise suddenly or gradually, indicating temporary or permanent vision impairment.

Most often, light flashes signal the splitting of the posterior vitreous membrane into two layers; the inner layer detaches from the retina while the outer layer remains fixed to it. The sensation of light flashes may result from vitreous traction on the retina, hemorrhage caused by a tear in the retinal capillary, or strands of solid vitreous floating in a local pool of liquid vitreous.

▶ **Emergency interventions**
Until retinal detachment is ruled out, restrict the patient's eye and body movement. Have another nurse immediately call an ophthalmologist, who will perform a funduscopic examination to rule out retinal detachment or gauge its extent.

**History**
Ask the patient when the light flashes began. Can he pinpoint their location or do they occur throughout the visual field? Find out if he's experiencing eye pain or headache, and have him describe it. Ask if he wears or has ever worn corrective lenses and if he or a family member has a history of eye or vision problems. Also ask if he has any other medical problems — especially hypertension or diabetes mellitus, which can cause retinopathy and possibly retinal detachment. Obtain an occupational history, too, because the patient's light flashes may be related to job stress or eyestrain.

**Physical exam**
Perform a complete eye and vision examination, especially if trauma is apparent or suspected. First, inspect the external eye, lids, lashes, and tear puncta for any abnormalities and the iris and sclera for signs of bleeding. Observe pupil size and shape, and check for reaction to light, for accommodation, and for the consensual light response. Next, test visual acuity in each eye. Then test visual fields; be sure to document any light flashes the patient reports during this test.

**Causes**
*Head trauma.* A patient who has sustained minor head trauma may report "seeing stars" when the injury occurs. He may also complain of localized pain at the injury site, generalized headache, and dizziness. Later, he may develop nausea, vomiting, and decreased level of consciousness.

*Migraine headache.* Light flashes — possibly accompanied by an aura — may herald a classic migraine headache. As these symptoms subside, the patient typically experiences a severe, throbbing, unilateral headache that usually lasts 1 to 12 hours and may be accompanied by numbness and tingling of the lips, face, or hands; slight confusion; dizziness; photophobia; nausea; and vomiting.

*Retinal detachment.* Light flashes described as floaters or spots are localized in the portion of the visual field where the retina is detaching. With macular involvement, the patient may experience painless visual impairment resembling a curtain covering the visual field.

*Vitreous detachment.* Sudden onset of light flashes may be accompanied by visual floaters. Usually both eyes are affected, one at a time.

**Nursing considerations**
• If the patient has retinal detachment, prepare him for reattachment surgery. Explain that after surgery, he may need to continue wearing bilateral eye patches and may have activity and position restrictions until the retina heals completely.
• If the patient doesn't have retinal detachment, reassure him that his light flashes are temporary and don't indicate eye damage. For the patient with migraine headache, maintain a quiet, darkened environment; encourage sleep; and administer analgesics as ordered.

**L**

Heat intolerance refers to the inability to withstand high temperatures or to maintain a comfortable body temperature. It produces a continuous feeling of being overheated and, at times, profuse diaphoresis. Usually, this symptom develops gradually and is chronic.

Most often, heat intolerance results from thyrotoxicosis. In this disorder, excess thyroid hormone stimulates peripheral tissues, increasing basal metabolism and producing excess heat. Although rare, hypothalamic disease may also cause heat — and cold — intolerance by disrupting normal temperature control.

## History

As you begin the assessment, notice how much clothing the patient is wearing. Then ask him when he first noticed his heat intolerance. Did he gradually use fewer blankets at night? Does he have to turn up the air conditioning to keep cool? Is it hard for him to adjust to warm weather? Find out if the patient's appetite or weight has changed. Also ask about unusual nervousness or other personality changes.

Take a drug history, especially noting use of amphetamines or amphetamine-like drugs. Ask the patient if he takes prescribed thyroid drugs. If so, what is the daily dosage? When did he last take a dose?

## Physical exam

After taking vital signs, inspect the patient's skin for flushing and diaphoresis. Also note tremors and lid lag.

## Causes

*Drugs.* Amphetamines and amphetamine-like appetite suppressants may increase basal metabolism, resulting in heat intolerance. Excessive doses of thyroid hormone may also cause heat intolerance.

*Hypothalamic disease.* Among the causes of this rare disease are pituitary adenoma and hypothalamic and pineal tumors. Here, body temperature fluctuates dramatically, causing alternating heat and cold intolerance. Related features include amenorrhea, disturbed sleep patterns, increased thirst and urination, increased appetite with weight gain, impaired visual acuity, headache, and personality changes, such as bursts of rage or laughter.

*Thyrotoxicosis.* A classic symptom of thyrotoxicosis, heat intolerance may be accompanied by an enlarged thyroid, nervousness, weight loss despite increased appetite, diaphoresis, diarrhea, tremors, and palpitations. Although exophthalmos is characteristic, many patients don't display this sign. Associated findings may affect virtually every body system. Some common findings include irritability, difficulty concentrating, mood swings, weakness, fatigue, lid lag, tachycardia, full and bounding pulse, widened pulse pressure, dyspnea, and amenorrhea or gynecomastia. Typically, the patient's skin is warm and flushed; premature graying and alopecia occur in both sexes.

## Nursing considerations

- Adjust room temperature to make the patient comfortable.
- If the patient has diaphoresis, change his clothing and bed linens, as necessary, and encourage fluids.

# Lid lag

Also known as Graefe's sign, lid lag — the inability of the upper eyelid to follow the eye's downward movements — is a cardinal sign of thyrotoxicosis. Testing for lid lag involves holding a finger, penlight, or other target above the patient's eye level, then moving it downward and observing eyelid movement as his eyes follow the target. This sign is demonstrated when a rim of sclera appears between the upper lid margin and the iris when the patient lowers his eyes, when one lid closes more slowly than the other, or when both lids close slowly and incompletely with jerky movements. Lid lag results from chronic contraction of Müller's muscle in the upper eyelid.

## History
Ask the patient when he first noticed lid lag or its possible manifestation — incomplete closure of the eyelid. Explore other signs and symptoms, and ask about a history of thyroid disease.

## Physical exam
Perform a physical examination, focusing on the effects of thyrotoxicosis, such as an enlarged thyroid, diaphoresis, tremors, and exophthalmos.

## Cause
*Thyrotoxicosis.* This disorder may produce bilateral lid lag and other ocular effects, including exophthalmos, decreased blinking, eye dryness and discomfort, and conjunctival injection. Restricted eye movement may produce diplopia. Assessment also reveals the classic effects of thyrotoxicosis: enlarged thyroid, nervousness, heat intolerance, weight loss despite increased appetite, diaphoresis, diarrhea, tremors, and palpitations.

Because thyrotoxicosis affects virtually every body system, it can produce many additional findings. For example, central nervous system effects include clumsiness, shaky handwriting, and emotional lability. Integumentary effects may include smooth, warm, flushed, and thickened skin with itchy patches; fine, soft hair with premature graying and increased loss; friable nails; and onycholysis.

Cardiopulmonary involvement causes constant dyspnea; tachycardia; full, bounding pulse; widened pulse pressure; visible point of maximal impulse; and, occasionally, a systolic murmur.

Besides nausea and vomiting, GI findings may include anorexia, diarrhea, and hepatomegaly. Musculoskeletal findings may include weakness, fatigue, atrophy, paralysis and, occasionally, clubbed fingers and toes.

Women may report oligomenorrhea or amenorrhea; men may show gynecomastia; and both sexes may experience decreased libido.

## Nursing considerations
• If lid lag is accompanied by exophthalmos, provide privacy to ease the patient's self-consciousness. Don't cover the affected eye with a gauze pad or other object because removal could destroy the corneal epithelium.
• Children may have lid lag associated with aberrant regeneration of cranial nerve III or, rarely, thyrotoxicosis.

Painless, irregular, bony enlargements of the distal finger joints, Heberden's nodes range in diameter from 2 to 3 mm. They develop on one or both sides of the dorsal midline. Usually, the dominant hand has larger nodes, which affect one or more fingers but not the thumb.

Repeated fingertip trauma may cause Heberden's nodes in only one joint ("baseball finger"). However, osteoarthritis is the most common cause; in fact, Heberden's nodes occur in more than half of all osteoarthritic patients. Because the nodes aren't associated with pain or loss of function, they're not a primary indicator of osteoarthritis but are a helpful adjunct to diagnosis.

Heberden's nodes reflect degeneration of articular cartilage, which irritates the bone and stimulates osteoblasts, causing bony enlargement.

## History
Begin by asking the patient if anyone else in his family has had Heberden's nodes or osteoarthritis. Also ask about repeated fingertip trauma on the job or associated with sports. Are the patient's joints stiff? Does stiffness disappear with movement? Ask him which hand is dominant.

## Physical exam
Carefully palpate the nodes, noting any signs of inflammation, such as redness and tenderness. Then assess range of motion in the fingers of each hand. As you do so, listen and feel for crepitation.

## Cause
*Osteoarthritis.* This disorder commonly causes Heberden's nodes and, possibly, nodes in the proximal interphalangeal joints (Bouchard's nodes). The most common arthritis type, osteoarthritis also goes by the names osteoarthrosis, degenerative joint disease, and hypertrophic arthritis. A progressive, nonsystemic, noninflammatory disorder, it causes bone and joint degeneration. Its chief symptom is joint pain that's aggravated by movement or weight bearing. Joints may also be tender and display restricted range of motion. The disorder commonly affects joints of the hand (distal and proximal interphalangeals and the first carpometacarpal), knee, hip, cervical and lumbar vertebrae, and great toe (metatarsophalangeal). Typically, joint stiffness is triggered by disuse and is relieved by brief exercise. Stiffness may be accompanied by bony enlargement and crepitus.

## Nursing considerations
• Remind the patient to take anti-inflammatory drugs, as ordered, and to exercise regularly to minimize joint pain and stiffness.
• Encourage him to avoid joint strain, for example, by maintaining a healthy weight.

• Teach the patient proper body mechanics, and advise him to use appropriate supports to maintain good body alignment. Also instruct him to use properly sized and adjusted furniture and work equipment. If he's obese, urge him to lose weight.

**H**

Decreased level of consciousness (LOC) — from lethargy to stupor to coma — usually results from neurologic disorders and commonly signals life-threatening complications of hemorrhage, trauma, or cerebral edema. This sign can also result from metabolic, GI, musculoskeletal, urologic, and cardiopulmonary disorders; nutritional deficiency; the effects of toxins; and drug use.

▶ **Emergency interventions**

Use the Glasgow Coma Scale to determine the severity of decreased LOC and obtain baseline data. If the patient's score is 13 or less, notify the doctor. Insert an artificial airway, elevate the head of the bed 30 degrees and, if a spinal cord injury has been ruled out, turn the patient's head to the side. Be prepared to suction the patient. Assess breathing and circulation. As necessary, support breathing with a manual resuscitation bag. If the patient's score is 7 or less, expect to assist with intubation and emergency resuscitation.

**History**

Ask the patient or his family about headache, dizziness, personality changes, memory loss, neurologic disease, cancer, trauma, and drug and alcohol use.

**Physical exam**

Perform a neurologic examination.

**Causes**

*Brain abscess.* Decreased LOC can vary from drowsiness to stupor. Early findings are intractable headache, nausea, vomiting, and seizures.

*Brain tumor.* LOC decreases slowly. The patient may also experience behavior changes, memory loss, morning headache, dizziness, and vision loss.

*Cerebral aneurysm (ruptured).* Somnolence, confusion and, at times, stupor characterize moderate bleeding. Deep coma occurs in often-fatal severe bleeding. Onset is abrupt, with severe headache, nausea, and vomiting.

*Cerebral contusion.* Usually unconscious for a time, the patient may develop dilated, nonreactive pupils and assume a decorticate or decerebrate posture. Conscious, he may be confused or violent.

*Diabetic ketoacidosis.* This potentially fatal disorder produces a rapid decrease in LOC, along with anorexia, abdominal pain, nausea, vomiting, fruity breath odor, and Kussmaul's respirations.

*Epidural hemorrhage (acute).* This life-threatening disorder produces momentary loss of consciousness followed by a lucid interval, rapidly deteriorating consciousness, and possibly coma.

*Hyperosmolar nonketotic syndrome.* LOC decreases rapidly to coma. Early findings include polyuria, polydipsia, weight loss, and weakness.

*Intracerebral hemorrhage.* This life-threatening disorder causes rapid loss of consciousness, often with severe headache, dizziness, nausea, and vomiting.

*Pontine hemorrhage.* LOC decreases to coma within minutes, to death within hours.

*Shock.* Decreased LOC occurs late, progressing to stupor and coma. Associated findings include restlessness, hypotension, tachycardia, weak pulse, oliguria, and cool, clammy skin.

*Subdural hematoma (chronic).* LOC deteriorates slowly. Other findings include confusion, decreased ability to concentrate, and personality changes.

*Subdural hemorrhage (acute).* This potentially fatal disorder causes agitation, confusion, and decreased LOC leading to coma.

*Other causes.* Adrenal crisis, alcohol intoxication, cerebrovascular accident, drug overdose, encephalitis, encephalopathies (hepatic, hypoxic, hypertensive, hypoglycemic, and uremic), heatstroke, hypercapnia with pulmonary disease, hypernatremia, hyperventilation syndrome, hypokalemia, hyponatremia, hypothermia, meningitis, myxedema crisis, poisoning, postvaccinal encephalomyelitis, seizures, thyroid storm, transient ischemic attack.

**Nursing considerations**

• Check the patient's neurologic status hourly. Monitor intake and output, and check for increasing intracranial pressure. Ensure airway patency, proper nutrition, and safety.

L

The vomiting of blood, hematemesis usually indicates GI bleeding above the ligament of Treitz. Bright red or blood-streaked vomitus indicates fresh or recent bleeding. Dark red, brown, or black vomitus — about the color and consistency of coffee grounds — indicates that blood has been retained in the stomach and partially digested.

Most often, hematemesis results from GI disorders. It may also stem from coagulation disorders and from treatments that irritate the GI tract. Always an important sign, hematemesis varies in severity depending on the amount and source of bleeding. Massive hematemesis (vomiting of 500 to 1,000 ml of blood) may be rapidly fatal.

## ▶ Emergency interventions

If the patient has massive hematemesis, quickly check vital signs. If signs of shock appear, notify the doctor. Place the patient in a supine position and elevate his feet 20 to 30 degrees. Start a large-bore I.V. line for fluid replacement. Send a blood sample for typing and cross matching, and give oxygen. As ordered, assist with endoscopy to locate the bleeding site. Prepare to insert a nasogastric (NG) or Sengstaken-Blakemore tube to perform suction or iced lavage or to compress bleeding sites.

## History

If the patient's hematemesis isn't life-threatening, have him describe the amount, color, and consistency of the vomitus. When did it begin? Has it ever happened before? Has he had bloody or black tarry stools? Is the hematemesis preceded by nausea, flatulence, diarrhea, or weakness? Has he had recent bouts of retching? Ask about a history of ulcers or liver or coagulation disorders. Ask about alcohol consumption. Is he taking any drug?

## Physical exam

Check for postural hypotension, an early warning sign of hypovolemia. Take blood pressure and pulse with the patient supine, sitting, then standing. After obtaining other vital signs, inspect the mucous membranes, nasopharynx, and skin for any abnormalities. Palpate the abdomen for tenderness, pain, or masses. Note lymphadenopathy.

## Causes

*Coagulation disorders.* These may cause GI bleeding and moderate to severe hematemesis.

*Esophageal varices (ruptured).* Life-threatening rupture of esophageal varices may produce "coffee ground" or massive, bright red vomitus. Signs of shock may follow or even precede hematemesis if the stomach fills with blood before vomiting. Melena or painless hematochezia may occur.

*Gastritis (acute).* Hematemesis and melena are the most common signs; mild epigastric discomfort, nausea, fever, and malaise may occur. Common causes include alcohol abuse, severe illness, and use of nonsteroidal anti-inflammatory drugs.

*Peptic ulcers.* Hematemesis may occur when a peptic ulcer penetrates an artery, a vein, or highly vascular tissue. Massive hematemesis is typical with arterial penetration. Other features: melena or hematochezia, shock, and dehydration.

*Other causes.* Achalasia, esophageal carcinoma, esophageal injury by caustics, esophageal rupture, gastric carcinoma, gastroesophageal reflux disease, GI leiomyoma, Mallory-Weiss syndrome, nose or throat surgery, traumatic NG or endotracheal intubation.

## Nursing considerations

• Monitor vital signs every 15 minutes; watch for shock. Keep accurate intake and output records.
• Place the patient on bed rest in low- or semi-Fowler's position to prevent aspiration of emesis. Use suctioning equipment as needed.
• Provide frequent oral hygiene and emotional support. As ordered, give epinephrine or vasopressin to control bleeding. As the bleeding tapers off, give hourly doses of antacids by NG tube.
• Explain diagnostic tests, such as endoscopy and barium swallow. Check stools often for occult blood.

Although it commonly signifies a musculoskeletal disorder, leg pain can also result from more serious vascular or neurologic disorders. It may arise suddenly or gradually and may be localized or affect the entire leg. Constant or intermittent, it may be dull, burning, or sharp. Severe leg pain that follows cast application for a fracture may signal limb-threatening compartment syndrome.

### ▶ Emergency interventions
If the patient has acute leg pain and a history of trauma, take his vital signs and assess the leg's neurovascular status. Observe leg position and check for swelling, gross deformities, or abnormal rotation. Check distal pulses, and note skin color and temperature. Inform the doctor immediately if the leg is pale, cool, and pulseless.

### History
When the patient's condition permits, ask him when the pain began and have him describe its intensity, character, and pattern. Must he use a crutch or another assistive device?

Obtain a history of leg injury or surgery and of joint, vascular, or back problems. Also ask the patient about medications and whether they've helped to relieve his leg pain.

### Physical exam
If his condition permits, watch the patient walk. Observe how he holds his leg while standing and sitting. Palpate the legs, buttocks, and lower back. If the doctor has ruled out a fracture, test range of motion in the hip and knee. Also check reflexes with the patient's leg straightened and raised. Compare both legs for symmetry, movement, and range of motion. If the patient wears a cast or splint, check distal circulation, sensation, and mobility, and stretch his toes to elicit associated pain.

### Causes
*Bone neoplasm.* Continuous deep or boring pain, often worse at night, may be the first symptom. Later, skin breakdown and impaired circulation may occur.

*Compartment syndrome.* Intense lower leg pain that increases with passive muscle stretching marks this limb-threatening disorder. Restrictive dressings or traction may aggravate the pain.

*Fracture.* Severe pain accompanies swelling and ecchymosis in the affected leg. Movement or weight bearing produces extreme pain. Neurovascular status distal to the fracture may be impaired, causing paresthesia, absent pulse, mottled cyanosis, and cool skin.

*Infection.* Local leg pain, erythema, swelling, and warmth characterize soft tissue and bone infections. Fever and tachycardia may be present with other systemic signs.

*Occlusive vascular disease.* Continuous cramping pain in the legs and feet may worsen with walking, inducing claudication. The patient may report cold feet, cold intolerance, and increased pain at night.

*Thrombophlebitis.* Discomfort may range from tenderness to severe pain, along with swelling, warmth, and a feeling of heaviness in the affected leg. Other findings include fever, chills, malaise, muscle cramps, and a positive Homans' sign.

*Other causes.* Sciatica, strains and sprains, varicose veins, and venous stasis ulcers.

### Nursing considerations
• If the patient has acute leg pain, monitor neurovascular status by frequently checking distal pulses and assessing the temperature and color of both legs. Also monitor thigh and calf circumference. Prepare him for X-rays. Use sandbags to immobilize the leg; apply ice and possibly skeletal traction, as ordered.

• If a fracture isn't suspected, prepare the patient for laboratory tests.

• If the patient has *chronic* leg pain, teach him how to use anti-inflammatory drugs and perform range-of-motion exercises. If necessary, teach him how to use an assistive device. If physical therapy is ordered, establish a daily exercise regimen.

A cardinal sign of renal and urinary tract disorders, hematuria is the abnormal presence of blood in the urine (three or more red blood cells per high-powered microscopic field in a urine specimen). Microscopic hematuria is confirmed by an occult blood sample; macroscopic hematuria is visible. Dark or brownish blood generally indicates renal or upper urinary tract bleeding; bright red blood, lower tract bleeding. Nonpathologic hematuria may result from fever and hypercatabolic states and may follow strenuous exercise.

## History

Ask the patient when he noticed the hematuria, if he had it before, and if it varies between or during voidings. Is he passing clots? Ask about bleeding hemorrhoids, recent trauma, strenuous exercise, and the onset of menses (in women). Note a history of renal, urinary, prostatic, or coagulation disorders. Obtain a drug history.

## Physical exam

Palpate and percuss the abdomen and flanks. Percuss the costovertebral angle (CVA) to elicit tenderness. Check the urinary meatus for bleeding or other abnormalities.

## Causes

*Bladder cancer.* Commonly causing gross hematuria in men, this disorder may produce pain in the bladder, rectum, pelvis, flank, back, or leg. Symptoms of urinary tract infection (UTI) may occur.

*Calculi. Bladder calculi* usually cause gross hematuria and referred pain to the penile or vulvar area. It may cause bladder distention. *Renal calculi* may produce microscopic or gross hematuria.

*Coagulation disorders.* Macroscopic hematuria is commonly the first sign of hemorrhage in coagulation disorders. Other signs include epistaxis, purpura, and signs of GI bleeding.

*Cortical necrosis (acute).* Gross hematuria is accompanied by intense flank pain, anuria, and fever.

*Cystitis.* Hematuria occurs in all types of cystitis. Symptoms of UTI may also occur.

*Glomerulonephritis.* Usually, *acute glomerulonephritis* begins with gross hematuria tapering off to microscopic hematuria. It may produce oliguria or anuria, and flank and abdominal pain. *Chronic glomerulonephritis* usually causes microscopic hematuria accompanied by proteinuria.

*Nephritis (interstitial).* The acute form causes microscopic hematuria, fever, and a maculopapular rash. In *chronic interstitial nephritis,* expect dilute, almost colorless urine with polyuria.

*Pyelonephritis (acute).* This infection typically produces microscopic or macroscopic hematuria that progresses to gross hematuria. Other effects are high fever, flank pain, and symptoms of UTI.

*Renal infarction.* Gross hematuria is typical. Other findings include severe flank and upper abdominal pain, CVA tenderness, and anorexia.

*Renal neoplasm.* Gross hematuria occurs with aching flank pain and a smooth, firm, flank mass.

*Renal papillary necrosis (acute).* Gross hematuria may be accompanied by intense flank pain, CVA tenderness, and abdominal rigidity.

*Renal vein thrombosis.* Macroscopic hematuria usually occurs with this thrombosis. Abrupt obstruction produces flank and lumbar pain, and epigastric and CVA tenderness.

*Other causes.* Appendicitis; benign prostatic hyperplasia; bladder trauma; diagnostic tests, such as cystoscopy and renal biopsy; diverticulitis; drugs, such as anticoagulants, cyclophosphamide, metyrosine, oxyphenbutazone, phenylbutazone, and thiabendazole; obstructive nephropathy; polycystic kidney disease; prostatitis; renal trauma; renal tuberculosis; schistosomiasis; sickle cell anemia; subacute infective endocarditis; treatments involving instrumentation of the urinary tract; urethral trauma; vaginitis; and vasculitis.

## Nursing considerations

- Check vital signs at least every 4 hours, and monitor intake and output.
- Administer prescribed pain drugs, as ordered.

**H**

An early indicator of meningeal irritation, Kernig's sign is combined resistance and hamstring muscle pain that results when the examiner attempts to extend the supine patient's flexed leg.

This sign usually appears in meningitis or subarachnoid hemorrhage. In these potentially life-threatening disorders, hamstring muscle pain results from stretching the blood- or exudate-irritated meninges surrounding spinal nerve roots.

Kernig's sign can also indicate a herniated disk or spinal cord tumor; the pain results from disk or tumor pressure on spinal nerve roots.

## ▶ Emergency interventions
If you elicit Kernig's sign and suspect life-threatening meningitis or subarachnoid hemorrhage, inform the doctor immediately. Take the patient's vital signs, then test for Brudzinski's sign to obtain further evidence of meningeal irritation. Next, ask the patient or his family to describe the onset of illness. Typically, progressive onset of headache, fever, nuchal rigidity, and confusion suggests meningitis. Conversely, sudden onset of severe headache, nuchal rigidity, photophobia, and possibly loss of consciousness usually indicates subarachnoid hemorrhage.

## History
If meningeal irritation isn't suspected, ask the patient if he feels back pain radiating down one or both legs. Does he feel leg numbness, tingling, or weakness? Ask about other signs and symptoms, and note a history of cancer or back injury.

## Physical exam
During the physical examination, focus on motor and sensory function.

## Causes
*Lumbosacral herniated disk.* Kernig's sign may appear in this disorder, but the cardinal and earliest feature is unilateral or bilateral sciatic pain. Other findings include postural deformity, paresthesia, hypoactive deep tendon reflexes in the involved leg, and dorsiflexor muscle weakness.

*Meningitis.* Usually, Kernig's sign is present early in meningitis. Fever also occurs early, possibly with chills. Other findings may include nuchal rigidity, hyperreflexia, Brudzinski's sign, and opisthotonos. As intracranial pressure (ICP) increases, headache and vomiting may occur. In severe meningitis, the patient may experience stupor, coma, and seizures. Cranial nerve involvement may produce ocular palsies, facial weakness, deafness, and photophobia.

*Spinal cord tumor.* Kernig's sign can be elicited occasionally, but the earliest symptom is commonly pain felt locally or along the spinal nerve, frequently in the leg. Associated findings may include weakness or paralysis distal to the tumor, paresthesia, urine retention or incontinence, fecal incontinence, and sexual dysfunction.

*Subarachnoid hemorrhage.* Kernig's sign and Brudzinski's sign can be elicited within minutes after the initial bleed. The patient experiences sudden onset of severe headache, nuchal rigidity, and decreased level of consciousness. Photophobia, fever, nausea, vomiting, dizziness, and seizures are possible. Focal signs may include hemiparesis or hemiplegia, aphasia, and sensory or visual disturbances. Increasing ICP may produce bradycardia, increased blood pressure, respiratory pattern change, and rapid progression to coma.

## Nursing considerations
• Prepare the patient for diagnostic tests, such as computed tomography scan, spinal X-ray, and myelography. Closely monitor his vital signs, ICP, and cardiopulmonary and neurologic status. Ensure bed rest, quiet, and minimal stress.
• If the patient has subarachnoid hemorrhage, darken the room and elevate the head of the bed at least 30 degrees to reduce ICP. If he has a herniated disk or spinal cord tumor, he may require pelvic traction.

Hemianopia is loss of vision in half the visual field (usually the vertical half) of one or both eyes. Its cause? A lesion affecting the optic chiasm, tract, or radiation. If field defects are identical in both eyes but affect less than half the field of vision in each eye (incomplete homonymous hemianopia), the lesion may be in the occipital lobe; otherwise, it probably involves the parietal or temporal lobe. Reduced visual perception caused by cerebral lesions is usually associated with impaired color vision.

## History

Suspect a visual field defect if the patient seems startled when you approach him from one side or if he fails to see objects placed directly in front of him. To help determine the type of defect, compare the patient's visual fields with your own—assuming yours are normal. First, ask the patient to cover his right eye while you cover your left eye. Then, move a pen or similar-shaped object from the periphery of his (and your) uncovered eye into his field of vision. Ask the patient to indicate when he first sees the object. Does he see it at the same time you do? After you do? Repeat this test in each quadrant of both eyes. Then, for each eye, plot the defect by shading the area of a circle that corresponds to the area of vision loss.

## Physical exam

Evaluate the patient's level of consciousness (LOC), take his vital signs, and check his pupillary reaction and motor response. Ask if he's experienced headache, dysarthria, or seizures. Does he have ptosis or facial or extremity weakness? Hallucinations or loss of color vision? When did neurologic symptoms start? Obtain a medical history, noting especially eye disorders, hypertension, and diabetes mellitus.

## Causes

*Carotid artery aneurysm.* An aneurysm in the internal carotid artery can cause contralateral or bilateral defects in the visual fields. It can also cause hemiplegia, decreased LOC, headache, aphasia, behavior disturbances, and unilateral hypoesthesia.

*Cerebrovascular accident (CVA).* Hemianopia can result when a hemorrhagic, thrombotic, or embolic CVA affects any part of the optic pathway. Associated signs and symptoms depend on the CVA's location and size.

*Occipital lobe lesion.* The most common symptoms arising from a lesion on one occipital lobe include incomplete homonymous hemianopia, scotomas, and impaired color vision. The patient may also experience visual hallucinations: flashes of light or color or visions of objects, people, animals, or geometric forms. These may appear in the defective field or may move toward it from the intact field.

*Parietal lobe lesion.* This disorder produces homonymous hemianopia and sensory deficits, such as an inability to perceive body position or passive movement or to localize tactile, thermal, or vibratory stimuli. It may also cause apraxia and visual or tactile agnosia.

*Pituitary tumor.* A tumor that compresses nerve fibers supplying the nasal half of both retinas causes complete or partial bitemporal hemianopia that occurs first in the upper visual fields but later can progress to blindness. Related findings include blurred vision, diplopia, and headache.

## Nursing considerations

• If the patient's visual field defect is significant, prepare him for further visual field testing, such as perimetry or a tangent screen examination.

• Advise him to scan his surroundings frequently, turning his head in the direction of the defective visual field so he can directly view objects he'd normally notice peripherally. Also, approach him from the unaffected side.

• Position his bed so his unaffected side faces the door; if he's ambulatory, remove objects that could cause falls and alert him to other possible hazards.

A cardinal sign of hemorrhage within the peritoneal cavity, Kehr's sign is referred left shoulder pain caused by diaphragmatic irritation from intraperitoneal blood. Usually, the pain arises when the patient lies supine or lowers his head. Such positioning increases the contact of free blood or clots with the left diaphragm, involving the phrenic nerve.

Kehr's sign usually develops right after a hemorrhage, although onset is sometimes delayed up to 48 hours. A classic sign of a ruptured spleen, it also occurs with a ruptured ectopic pregnancy.

▶ **Emergency interventions**
After you detect Kehr's sign, quickly take the patient's vital signs and have another nurse immediately notify the doctor. If the patient shows signs of hypovolemia, elevate his feet 30 degrees. Insert a large-bore I.V. catheter for fluid and blood replacement and an indwelling urinary catheter. Begin monitoring intake and output. Draw blood to determine hematocrit, and give supplemental oxygen.

If the doctor suspects internal abdominal injuries, he may order peritoneal lavage. Assemble appropriate equipment, including a peritoneal dialysis tray, I.V. pole and macrodrip I.V. tubing, 3- to 5-ml syringe with 25G needle, lactated Ringer's or normal saline solution, and a local anesthetic.

Next, measure the patient's abdominal girth and insert a nasogastric tube, if ordered. If your patient's a woman, assess for pregnancy. Shave, prepare, and drape the abdomen.

After the doctor inserts the catheter into the peritoneal cavity and introduces the lavage solution through the I.V. tubing, clamp the tubing and tape the catheter to your patient's abdomen. Unless contraindicated, gently turn the patient from side to side or manually manipulate his abdomen, as ordered, to mix the lavage solution and the peritoneal fluids.

Now open the clamp to the bag, as ordered, so that peritoneal fluid drains by gravity. Drain 25 to 30 ml of peritoneal fluid.

Place about 10 ml of the fluid in a sterile and labeled culture and sensitivity container, then divide the rest of the fluid into labeled tubes, and send the specimens to the laboratory.

After the doctor removes the catheter and sutures the incision, apply an antibiotic ointment and sterile dressing. Monitor urine output for hematuria, which suggests bladder perforation. Observe for worsened abdominal pain, which may indicate bowel perforation. Monitor vital signs frequently, and periodically check abdominal girth against the baseline measurement.

**Physical exam**
Inspect the patient's abdomen for bruises and distention, and palpate for tenderness. Percuss for Ballance's sign—an indicator of massive perisplenic clotting and free blood in the peritoneal cavity from a ruptured spleen.

**Cause**
*Intra-abdominal hemorrhage.* Kehr's sign usually accompanies intense abdominal pain, abdominal rigidity, and muscle spasm. Other findings vary with the cause of bleeding.

**Nursing considerations**
• If surgery is indicated, withhold oral intake, and prepare the patient for abdominal X-rays, computed tomography and ultrasound scans, and possibly, paracentesis and culdocentesis.
• Give analgesics as prescribed.
• If you suspect Kehr's sign in a child, keep in mind that he may have difficulty describing the pain. Watch for nonverbal clues, such as rubbing the shoulder.

Expectoration of blood or bloody sputum from the lungs or tracheobronchial tree, hemoptysis is sometimes confused with bleeding from the mouth, throat, nasopharynx, or GI tract. Usually frothy and bright red, it commonly results from chronic bronchitis, bronchogenic carcinoma, or bronchiectasis. It can also result from inflammatory, infectious, cardiovascular, or coagulation disorders.

## ► Emergency interventions
If hemoptysis is copious, prepare to suction the patient and assist with endotracheal intubation. Insert an I.V. line, monitor vital signs, and draw an arterial blood sample.

## History
Ask the patient when hemoptysis began, if it's happened before, how much blood or sputum he's coughing up now, and how often. Ask about cardiac, respiratory, or bleeding disorders. If he's receiving anticoagulant therapy, find out the drug, its dosage, and the duration of therapy. Is he taking other prescription drugs?

## Physical exam
Take vital signs and examine the nose, mouth, and pharynx for sources of bleeding. Inspect the chest for abnormal movement. Check respiratory rate, depth, and rhythm. Examine the skin for lesions. Palpate the chest for tenderness, respiratory excursion, fremitus, and abnormal pulsations. Then percuss and auscultate the lungs. Also auscultate the heart.

## Causes
*Bronchiectasis.* Sputum can vary from blood-tinged to frank blood and may also be copious, foul-smelling, and purulent.

*Bronchitis (chronic).* A productive cough that lasts at least 3 months can lead to blood-streaked sputum. Other respiratory effects include dyspnea, prolonged expiration, and wheezing.

*Laryngeal cancer.* Hemoptysis occurs, but hoarseness is the usual early sign. Other findings may include dysphagia, dyspnea, and stridor.

*Lung abscess.* Common findings include blood-streaked sputum or large amounts of purulent, foul-smelling sputum; fever; dyspnea; and pleuritic or dull chest pain.

*Lung cancer.* Ulceration of the bronchus commonly causes recurring hemoptysis (an early sign), varying from blood-streaked sputum to blood.

*Pneumonia.* *Klebsiella* pneumonia begins abruptly and may produce tenacious, dark brown or red sputum. Pneumococcal pneumonia causes pinkish or rusty mucoid sputum. It begins with a sudden, shaking chill and rising temperature.

*Pulmonary contusion.* Blunt chest trauma commonly causes a cough with hemoptysis. Other effects include dyspnea, chest pain, crackles, and decreased or absent breath sounds.

*Pulmonary edema.* Frothy, blood-tinged pink sputum occurs with severe dyspnea, orthopnea, diffuse crackles, and a ventricular gallop.

*Pulmonary embolism with infarction.* Hemoptysis commonly occurs. Typical early symptoms are dyspnea and anginal or pleuritic chest pain.

*Pulmonary tuberculosis.* Blood-streaked or -tinged sputum is common; massive hemoptysis may occur in advanced cavitary tuberculosis. Other findings: chronic productive cough, fine crackles after coughing, dyspnea, and night sweats.

*Other causes.* Bronchial adenoma, coagulation disorders, cystic fibrosis, Goodpasture's syndrome, lung or airway injury from diagnostic procedures, primary pulmonary hypertension, ruptured aortic aneurysm, silicosis, systemic lupus erythematosus, tracheal trauma, and Wegener's granulomatosis.

## Nursing considerations
• Place the patient in a slight Trendelenburg position to promote drainage of blood from the lung. If necessary to protect the nonbleeding lung, place him in the lateral decubitus position, with the bleeding lung facing down.
• Tell the patient to report recurring hemoptysis.

**H**

Engorged, distended internal or external jugular veins reflect increased venous pressure in the right side of the heart. When the supine patient's head is elevated 45 degrees, a pulse wave higher than 10 cm above the angle of Louis (sternal angle) indicates distention. This common sign usually occurs in congestive heart failure and other cardiovascular disorders.

## ▶ Emergency interventions

If you detect jugular vein distention in a patient with pale, clammy skin who suddenly appears anxious and dyspneic, take his blood pressure. If you note hypotension and pulsus paradoxus, suspect cardiac tamponade and notify the doctor immediately. Elevate the foot of the bed 20 to 30 degrees, give supplemental oxygen, and monitor cardiac status. Start an I.V. line for fluid administration, and keep cardiopulmonary resuscitation equipment close by. Assemble equipment for emergency pericardiocentesis. Monitor the patient's blood pressure, heart rhythm, and respirations.

## History

If the patient isn't in distress, ask him about chest pain, shortness of breath, paroxysmal nocturnal dyspnea, anorexia, nausea, vomiting, recent weight gain, and any history of cancer or heart, pulmonary, or renal disease.

## Physical exam

Obtain vital signs and weigh the patient. Tachycardia, tachypnea, and increased blood pressure indicate fluid overload that is stressing the heart. Inspect and palpate the extremities and face for edema. Then auscultate the lungs for crackles and the heart for gallops and a pericardial friction rub. Inspect the abdomen for distention, and palpate and percuss for an enlarged liver. Finally, monitor urine output and note any decrease.

To visualize and evaluate venous pulsations, use the internal jugular vein. Shine a flashlight across the patient's neck to create shadows that highlight his venous pulse. Be sure to distinguish jugular venous pulsations from carotid venous pulsations. Next, locate the highest point along the vein where you can see pulsations. Measure in centimeters the distance between that high point and the sternal angle; measure as well the angle of the bed. A finding greater than 10 cm above the sternal angle, with the head of the bed at a 45-degree angle, indicates jugular vein distention.

## Causes

*Cardiac tamponade.* This life-threatening condition produces jugular vein distention along with anxiety, restlessness, cyanosis, chest pain, and clammy skin.

*Congestive heart failure.* Right ventricular failure causes jugular vein distention along with possible weakness and anxiety, cyanosis, dependent edema of the legs and sacrum, weight gain, confusion, and hepatomegaly.

*Hypervolemia.* Markedly increased intravascular fluid volume causes jugular vein distention along with rapid weight gain, elevated blood pressure, bounding pulse, peripheral edema, dyspnea, and crackles.

*Pericarditis (chronic constrictive).* Progressive signs and symptoms of restricted heart filling cause jugular vein distention that's more prominent on inspiration (Kussmaul's sign). Other features include chest pain, fluid retention with dependent edema, hepatomegaly, ascites, and pericardial friction rub.

*Other causes.* Superior vena cava obstruction.

## Nursing considerations

• If ordered, monitor central venous pressure to assess right ventricular function, and administer pain medication and diuretics. Restrict fluids and monitor intake and output. Routinely change the patient's position to avoid skin breakdown from peripheral edema.

• Teach the patient about diet restrictions and possible drug adverse effects.

# Hepatomegaly

This sign indicates potentially reversible primary or secondary liver disease. It may stem from diverse pathophysiologic mechanisms: dilated hepatic sinusoids (in congestive heart failure), persistently high venous pressure leading to liver congestion (in chronic constrictive pericarditis), dysfunction and engorgement of hepatocytes (in hepatitis), and fatty infiltration of parenchymal cells causing fibrous tissue (in cirrhosis).

Hepatomegaly may be confirmed by palpation, percussion, or radiologic tests. It may be mistaken for displacement of the liver by the diaphragm in a respiratory disorder; by an abdominal tumor; by a spinal deformity such as kyphosis; by the gallbladder; or by fecal material or colonic neoplasm.

## History
Hepatomegaly is seldom a patient's major complaint. It usually comes to light during palpation and percussion of GI structures. If you suspect hepatomegaly, ask the patient about alcohol use and exposure to hepatitis. Also ask if he's currently ill or taking any prescribed drugs. If he complains of abdominal pain, ask him to locate and describe it.

## Physical exam
Inspect the skin and sclera for jaundice, dilated veins (suggesting generalized congestion), scars from previous surgery, and spider angiomas (common in cirrhosis). Next, inspect the abdominal contour. Is it protuberant over the liver or distended (possibly from ascites)? Measure abdominal girth. Percuss the liver. During the patient's deep inspiration, palpate the liver's edge. Take vital signs and assess nutritional status and level of consciousness.

## Causes
*Cirrhosis.* Late in this disorder, the liver becomes enlarged, nodular, and hard. Other late signs and symptoms affect the entire body.

*Congestive heart failure.* This disorder produces hepatomegaly along with jugular vein distention, cyanosis, dependent edema of the legs and sacrum, steady weight gain, confusion, and possible nausea, vomiting, abdominal discomfort, and anorexia from visceral edema. Ascites is a late sign.

*Hepatic abscess.* Hepatomegaly may accompany fever (a primary sign), nausea, vomiting, chills, weakness, diarrhea, anorexia, and right upper quadrant pain and tenderness.

*Hepatic neoplasms.* Primary tumors commonly cause hepatomegaly, with pain or tenderness in the right upper quadrant and a friction rub or bruit over the liver. Common related findings are weight loss, anorexia, nausea, and vomiting. Peripheral edema, ascites, jaundice, and a palpable right upper quadrant mass may also be present.

*Hepatitis.* In viral hepatitis, hepatomegaly occurs in the icteric phase and continues during the recovery phase. Also, during the icteric phase, early signs and symptoms (nausea, anorexia, vomiting, fatigue, photophobia, sore throat, cough, and headache) diminish and others appear: liver tenderness, weight loss, dark urine, clay-colored stools, jaundice, pruritus, right upper quadrant pain, splenomegaly, and cervical adenopathy.

*Pericarditis.* In chronic constrictive pericarditis, elevated systemic venous pressure produces marked congestive hepatomegaly. Distended neck veins (more prominent on inspiration) are common. Other clinical features include peripheral edema, ascites, and decreased muscle mass.

*Other causes.* Amyloidosis, diabetes mellitus, granulomatous disorders, infectious mononucleosis, leukemia, lymphomas, obesity, and pancreatic cancer.

## Nursing considerations
• Prepare the patient for liver function studies, X-rays, liver scan, and ultrasonography to confirm hepatomegaly.
• Remind the patient that bed rest, relief from stress, and adequate nutrition help protect liver cells from further damage and allow regeneration of functioning cells.

**H**

# Jaw pain

Jaw pain may arise from either or both of the bones that hold the teeth in the jaw—the maxilla (upper jaw) and the mandible (lower jaw)—and includes pain in the temporomandibular joint (TMJ), where the mandible meets the temporal bone. Gradual or abrupt, mild or excruciating, jaw pain usually results from disorders of the teeth, soft tissue, or glands of the mouth or throat, or from local trauma or infections. Systemic causes include musculoskeletal, neurologic, cardiovascular, endocrine, immunologic, metabolic, and infectious disorders.

## History
Ask when the patient first noticed the jaw pain. Have him describe the pain, its location, and frequency. Ask about joint or chest pain, fatigue, headache, anorexia, weight loss, intermittent claudication, diplopia, and hearing loss.

## Physical exam
Inspect the jaw area for redness, and palpate for edema or warmth. Look for facial asymmetry indicating swelling. Palpate the TMJ while the patient moves his jaw. Note any crepitus in the joint. Then ask the patient to open his mouth. Less than 3 cm or more than 6 cm between upper and lower teeth is abnormal. Next, palpate the parotid area for pain and swelling, and inspect and palpate the oral cavity for lesions, tongue elevation, or masses.

## Causes
**Angina pectoris.** This disorder may produce jaw pain and left arm pain, which usually subsides with rest and administration of nitroglycerin.

**Arthritis.** In *osteoarthritis*, jaw pain increases with activity and subsides with rest. Other features are crepitus at the TMJ, enlarged joints with a restricted range of motion, and stiffness on awakening. *Rheumatoid arthritis* causes symmetrical pain in all joints, including the jaw. Joints display limited range of motion and are tender, warm, swollen, and stiff after inactivity.

**Head and neck cancer.** Many types of head and neck cancer produce jaw pain of insidious onset. Other findings include leukoplakia; palpable masses in the jaw, mouth, and neck; dysphagia; bloody discharges; drooling; and lymphadenopathy.

**Hypocalcemic tetany.** Besides painful muscle contractions of the jaw and mouth, this life-threatening disorder produces paresthesia and carpopedal spasms. Other findings include weakness, fatigue, palpitations, hyperreflexia, Chvostek's and Trousseau's signs, muscle twitching and cramps, and choreiform movements.

**Suppurative parotitis.** Life-threatening bacterial infection of the parotid gland by *Staphylococcus aureus* may develop in debilitated patients with dry mouth or poor oral hygiene. Jaw pain begins abruptly. Other findings include high fever, chills, edematous overlying skin, a swollen gland, and pus at the parotid ducts.

**Temporal arteritis.** Sharp jaw pain occurs after chewing or talking. Vascular lesions produce jaw pain; throbbing headache in the frontotemporal region; swollen and nodular temporal arteries.

**TMJ syndrome.** Jaw pain occurs at the TMJ, along with spasm and pain of the masticating muscle, popping or crepitus of the TMJ, and restricted jaw movement.

**Trigeminal neuralgia.** This causes paroxysmal attacks of intense unilateral jaw pain or shooting pains in one of the divisions of the trigeminal nerve. It may last for 10 to 15 minutes.

**Other causes.** Dental or surgical procedures, myocardial infarction, osteomyelitis, phenothiazines, sialolithiasis, tetanus, and trauma.

## Nursing considerations
- If the patient is in severe pain, withhold food, liquids, and drugs until the diagnosis is confirmed. Administer pain medications, as ordered.
- Prepare the patient for diagnostic tests.
- Apply an ice pack if the jaw is swollen, and discourage the patient from moving his jaws.

# Hiccups

Hiccups occur as a two-stage process: an involuntary, spasmodic contraction of the diaphragm followed by sudden closure of the glottis. Their characteristic sound reflects the vibration of closed vocal cords as air suddenly rushes into the lungs.

Usually benign and transient, hiccups are common and most often subside spontaneously or with simple treatment. However, in a patient with a neurologic disorder, they may indicate increasing intracranial pressure or extension of a brain stem lesion. They may also occur after ingestion of hot or cold liquids or other irritants, after exposure to cold, or with irritation from a drainage tube. Persistent hiccups cause considerable distress and may lead to vomiting.

Increased serum levels of carbon dioxide may inhibit hiccups; decreased levels may exacerbate them.

## History

Find out when the patient's hiccups began. If he's also vomiting and unconscious, turn him on his side to prevent aspiration. Then notify the doctor.

If he's conscious, find out if the hiccups are tiring him. Ask if he's had hiccups before, what caused them, and what made them stop. Also note if he has a history of abdominal or thoracic disorders.

## Causes

*Abdominal distention.* The most common cause of hiccups, abdominal distention also causes a feeling of fullness and, depending on the cause, abdominal pain, nausea, and vomiting.

*Gastric dilatation.* Besides hiccups, possible clinical features include a sense of fullness, epigastric pain, and regurgitation or persistent vomiting.

*Gastritis.* This disorder can cause hiccups along with mild epigastric discomfort (sometimes the only symptom). The patient may have upper abdominal pain, eructation, fever, malaise, nausea, vomiting, hematemesis, and melena.

*Increased intracranial pressure.* Early findings may include hiccups, drowsiness, and headache. Classic later signs include changes in pupillary reaction and respiratory pattern, elevated systolic pressure, and bradycardia.

*Pancreatitis.* Hiccups, vomiting, and sudden and steady epigastric pain (often radiating to the back) may occur in this disorder. A severe attack may also cause persistent vomiting, extreme restlessness, fever, and abdominal tenderness and rigidity.

*Other causes.* Abdominal surgery, brain stem lesion, chronic renal failure, and pleural irritation.

## Nursing considerations

• Teach the patient simple methods of relieving hiccups, such as increasing his serum carbon dioxide level by holding his breath repeatedly or by rebreathing into a paper bag. Other treatments include gastric lavage or finger pressure on the closed eyelids.

• If hiccups persist, a phenothiazine (especially chlorpromazine) or nasogastric intubation may provide relief. (*Caution*: The tube may cause vomiting.) If simpler methods fail, treatment may include a phrenic nerve block.

**H**

# Jaundice

Also called icterus, jaundice is a yellow discoloration of the skin or mucous membranes, indicating excessive levels of conjugated or unconjugated bilirubin in the blood. It is commonly accompanied by pruritus, dark urine, and clay-colored stools.

## History

Ask the patient when he first noticed the jaundice. Ask about past episodes or a family history of jaundice. Does he have pruritus, clay-colored stools, or dark urine? Has he experienced fatigue, fever, or chills; anorexia, abdominal pain, nausea, or vomiting; or shortness of breath or palpitations? Ask the patient about alcohol use, any history of cancer or of liver or gallbladder disease, weight loss, and any medications he's taking.

## Physical exam

Examine the patient in a room with natural light. Inspect the skin for texture, dryness, and hyperpigmentation and xanthomas. Also look for spider angiomas or petechiae, clubbed fingers, or gynecomastia. If the patient has congestive heart failure (CHF), auscultate for arrhythmias, murmurs, and gallops. For all patients, auscultate for crackles and abnormal bowel sounds. Palpate the lymph nodes for swelling and the abdomen for tenderness, pain, or swelling. Palpate and percuss the liver and spleen for enlargement, and test for ascites with the shifting dullness and fluid wave techniques. Evaluate the patient's mental status.

## Causes

*Carcinoma.* Jaundice may result from carcinoma of the ampulla of Vater, of the liver, and of the pancreas. Many symptoms are nonspecific, including abdominal pain and tenderness, fever, nausea, diarrhea, peripheral edema, weight loss, pruritus, and back pain.

*Cirrhosis.* In *Laennec's cirrhosis,* mild to moderate jaundice with pruritus usually signals hepatocellular necrosis. Common early findings include ascites, weakness, leg edema, nausea, vomiting, diarrhea or constipation, anorexia, weight loss, and right upper quadrant pain. Gynecomastia, scanty chest and axillary hair, and testicular atrophy occur in the male patient, and menstrual irregularities in the female patient.

In *primary biliary cirrhosis,* fluctuating jaundice may appear years after the onset of other signs and symptoms, such as pruritus that worsens at bedtime, weakness, fatigue, weight loss, and abdominal pain.

*Hepatitis.* Dark urine and clay-colored stools usually develop before jaundice in late acute viral hepatitis. Early findings include fatigue, nausea, vomiting, malaise, arthralgias, myalgias, headache, anorexia, photophobia, pharyngitis, cough, diarrhea or constipation, and low-grade fever.

*Sickle cell anemia.* Hemolysis produces jaundice in this disorder. Other findings include impaired growth and development, increased susceptibility to infection, life-threatening thrombotic complications, leg ulcers, and painful, swollen joints with fever and chills.

*Other causes.* Abdominal surgery; acquired hemolytic anemia; acute pancreatitis; agnogenic myeloid metaplasia; cholangitis; CHF; cholecystitis; drugs, such as phenylbutazone, I.V. tetracycline, isoniazid, oral contraceptives, sulfonamides, mercaptopurine, erythromycin estolate, niacin, troleandomycin, androgenic steroids, and phenothiazines; Dubin-Johnson syndrome; glucose-6-phosphate dehydrogenase (G6PD) deficiency; hepatic abscess; leptospirosis; surgical shunts used to reduce portal hypertension; and Zieve syndrome.

## Nursing considerations

• Instruct the patient to eat less protein and more carbohydrates. If he has obstructive jaundice, encourage a balanced low-fat diet and frequent, small meals.
• Bathe the patient frequently, and apply an antipruritic lotion.
• Prepare the patient for any diagnostic tests.

Hirsutism is the excessive growth of dark, coarse body hair in females. Excessive androgen production stimulates hair growth on the pubic region, axilla, chin, upper lip, cheeks, anterior neck, sternum, linea alba, forearms, abdomen, back, and upper arms. In *mild hirsutism,* fine and pigmented hair appears on the sides of the face and the chin (but doesn't form a complete beard) and on the extremities, chest, abdomen, and perineum. In *moderate hirsutism,* coarse and pigmented hair appears on the same areas. In *severe hirsutism,* coarse hair also covers the whole beard area, the proximal interphalangeal joints, and the ears and nose.

Hirsutism may result from endocrine abnormalities and idiopathic causes. It may also occur in pregnancy from transient androgen production by the placenta or corpus luteum, and in menopause from increased androgen and decreased estrogen production.

## History

Where did the patient first notice growth of excessive hair? How old was she then? Where — and how quickly — did other hirsute areas develop? Ask what hair removal technique she uses (if any), how often she uses it, and when she used it last. Next, obtain a menstrual history.

Ask about medications, too. If the patient is taking a drug containing an androgen or progestin compound, or another drug that can cause hirsutism, find out its name, dosage, and therapeutic aim. Does she sometimes miss doses or take extra ones?

## Physical exam

Examine areas of excessive hair growth. Does it appear only on her upper lip or on other body parts as well? Is it mild but pigmented or dense and coarse? Is the patient obese? Observe for signs of virilization.

## Causes

*Cushing's disease.* Facial hirsutism is a common finding. This disorder also causes increased hair growth on the abdomen, breasts, chest, or upper thighs. Other findings: truncal obesity, buffalo hump, moon face, thin skin, purple striae, ecchymoses, petechiae, muscle wasting and weakness, poor wound healing, hypertension, fatigue, excessive diaphoresis, hyperpigmentation, menstrual irregularities, and personality changes.

*Drugs.* Hirsutism can result from drugs containing androgens or progestins, aminoglutethimide, glucocorticoids, metoclopramide, cyclosporine, and minoxidil.

*Idiopathic hirsutism.* In patients with normal-sized ovaries and no evidence of adrenal hyperplasia or adrenal or ovarian tumors, excess hair appears at puberty and increases into early adulthood. It's accompanied by thick, oily skin; acne; obesity; and infrequent or anovulatory menses. Idiopathic hirsutism with regular ovulation and no menstrual abnormalities may be hereditary or related to certain geographic areas and ethnic groups hypersensitive to androgens.

*Ovarian overproduction of androgens.* The most common cause of hirsutism, this condition is associated with anovulation progressing slowly over several years.

*Polycystic ovary disease.* Ovarian cysts — particularly chronic ones — can cause hirsutism. This usually occurs after the onset of menstrual irregularities, which may begin at puberty.

*Other causes.* Acromegaly, adrenocortical carcinoma, hyperprolactinemia, and ovarian tumor.

## Nursing considerations

• Prepare the patient for blood tests of luteinizing hormone, follicle-stimulating hormone, prolactin, and other hormones. Other tests may include computed tomography scan and ultrasonography.

• Help relieve the patient's anxiety by explaining the cause of excessive hair growth and by encouraging her to talk about her self-image problems or fears.

• At the patient's request, provide information on methods for eliminating excess hair.

Slightly raised, irregular, and nontender, Janeway's spots are small, erythematous lesions (1 to 4 mm in diameter) on the palms and soles. They blanch with pressure and with elevation of the affected extremity; rarely, they form a diffuse rash over the trunk and extremities. They disappear spontaneously.

Janeway's spots are a common finding in infective endocarditis and may reflect an immunologic reaction to an infecting organism. They're a telltale sign of this disorder if other lesions (such as petechiae and Osler's nodes) and signs and symptoms of infection (such as fever) are present.

### History

Note any history of valvular or rheumatic heart disease. If the patient has had valvular or rheumatic disease, ask about recent dental procedures or invasive diagnostic tests. Does he have a prosthetic replacement valve? Find out about recent meningitis and any skin, bone, or respiratory infections. Does the patient have renal disease requiring an arteriovenous shunt, or has he had recent long-term I.V. therapy, such as total parenteral nutrition?

If the patient has had rheumatic fever or valvular disease, find out if his doctor has advised him to take prophylactic antibiotics. Ask the patient to describe how he feels. Does he have weakness, fatigue, chills, anorexia, or night sweats, possibly indicating an infection? Does he have other complaints?

### Physical exam

Inspect the patient's skin for other lesions, such as petechiae on his trunk or mucous membranes or Osler's nodes on his palms, soles, finger pads, or toe pads. Inspect the fingers for clubbing and splinter hemorrhages.

Take the patient's vital signs, noting fever and tachycardia—which may indicate heart failure if it persists after fever disappears. Inspect and palpate his extremities for edema. Auscultate for gallops and murmurs. Assess other body systems for embolic complications of infective endocarditis, such as acute abdominal pain and hematuria. Examining his eyes with an ophthalmoscope may reveal Roth's spots.

### Causes

*Acute infective endocarditis.* Janeway's spots are a late sign. Early effects include sudden onset of shaking chills and fever, peripheral edema, dyspnea, petechiae, Osler's nodes, Roth's spots, and hematuria.

*Subacute infective endocarditis.* Janeway's spots may appear late in this disorder, which has an insidious onset. Early findings may include weakness, fatigue, weight loss, fever, night sweats, anorexia, and arthralgia. Other clinical features include elevated pulse, pale skin, Osler's nodes, splinter hemorrhages under the fingernails, petechiae, Roth's spots, clubbing of the fingers (in long-standing disease), splenomegaly, and murmurs. Embolization may produce acute signs and symptoms, such as chest, abdominal, and extremity pain; paralysis; hematuria; or blindness.

### Nursing considerations

• Tell the patient that the spots will disappear without damaging his skin. Treatment for infective endocarditis includes antibiotics and (with complications such as heart failure) diuretics and cardiac glycosides.

• Monitor the patient's intake, output, and cardiac status, and be alert for embolic complications. Notify the doctor immediately if the patient develops acute chest pain, abdominal pain, or paralysis.

# Hoarseness

A rough or harsh sound to the voice, hoarseness can result from infections or inflammatory lesions or exudates of the larynx, from laryngeal edema, and from compression or disruption of the vocal cords or recurrent laryngeal nerve. It's characteristically worsened by excessive alcohol intake, smoking, inhalation of noxious fumes, cheering, and shouting.

Hoarseness can be acute or chronic. For example, chronic hoarseness and laryngitis (an occupational hazard of clergymen and singers) result when irritating polyps form on the vocal cords. It may also result from progressive atrophy of the laryngeal muscles and mucosa from aging, leading to diminished control of the vocal cords.

### History

Consider the patient's age and sex; laryngeal cancer is most common in men between the ages of 50 and 70. Ask about the onset of hoarseness. Has the patient been overusing his voice? Has he experienced shortness of breath, a sore throat, dry mouth, a cough, or difficulty swallowing dry food? Explore associated symptoms. Does the patient have a history of cancer or other disorders? Does he regularly drink alcohol or smoke?

### Physical exam

Inspect the oral cavity and pharynx for redness or exudate, possibly indicating an upper respiratory infection. Palpate the neck for masses and the cervical lymph nodes and the thyroid for enlargement. Palpate the trachea — is it midline? Ask the patient to stick out his tongue: If he can't, he may have paralysis from cranial nerve involvement.

Take the patient's vital signs, noting especially fever and bradycardia. Inspect for asymmetrical chest expansion or signs of respiratory distress — nasal flaring, stridor, and intercostal retractions. Then auscultate for crackles, rhonchi, wheezes, or tubular sounds, and percuss for dullness.

### Causes

*Laryngeal cancer.* Hoarseness is an early sign of vocal cord cancer but may not occur until later in cancer of other laryngeal areas. Other common findings: a mild, dry cough and minor throat discomfort.

*Laryngitis.* Persistent hoarseness may be the only sign of *chronic laryngitis*. In *acute laryngitis*, hoarseness or a complete loss of voice develops suddenly. Related findings include pain (especially during swallowing or speaking), cough, fever, profuse diaphoresis, sore throat, and rhinorrhea.

*Tracheal trauma.* Torn tracheal mucosa may cause hoarseness, hemoptysis, dysphagia, neck pain, airway occlusion, and respiratory distress.

*Vocal cord paralysis.* Unilateral vocal cord paralysis causes hoarseness and vocal weakness. Paralysis may accompany signs of trauma, such as pain and swelling of the head and neck.

*Vocal cord polyps.* Raspy hoarseness, the chief complaint, accompanies a chronic cough and a crackling voice.

*Other causes.* Hypothyroidism, inhalation injury, prolonged intubation, pulmonary tuberculosis, rheumatoid arthritis, Sjögren's syndrome, surgical severing of the recurrent laryngeal nerve, thoracic aortic aneurysm, and tracheostomy.

### Nursing considerations

• Carefully observe the patient for stridor, which may indicate bilateral vocal cord paralysis.
• If the patient has laryngitis, advise him to use a humidifier. Stress the importance of resting his voice: Talking — even whispering — further traumatizes the vocal cords. Suggest other ways to communicate (such as using pen and paper or body language).
• Urge the patient to avoid alcohol, smoking, and the company of smokers.
• Tell the patient to report hoarseness that lasts more than 2 weeks. The doctor may perform indirect laryngoscopy, observing the larynx at rest and during phonation.

## 145

Most common in the legs, intermittent claudication is cramping limb pain brought on by exercise and relieved by 1 or 2 minutes of rest. It may be acute or chronic. When acute, it may signal acute arterial occlusion. In occlusive artery disease, it results from an inadequate blood supply.

Pain in the calf or foot indicates disease of the femoral or popliteal arteries; pain in the buttocks and upper thigh, disease of the aorta or iliac arteries. This symptom may also be caused by narrowing of the vertebral column at the level of the cauda equina, which creates painful pressure on the nerve roots to the legs.

▶ **Emergency interventions**

If the patient experiences *sudden* intermittent claudication along with severe or aching leg pain at rest, check the leg's temperature and palpate pulses. Also check the leg's color and ask about numbness and tingling. If pulses are absent and the leg is cool and pale, cyanotic, or mottled, with paresthesia and pain, suspect acute arterial occlusion. Notify the doctor immediately. Don't elevate the leg; instead, protect it and let nothing press on it. Prepare the patient for preoperative blood tests, urinalysis, electrocardiography, and chest X-rays. Start an I.V. line, and administer an anticoagulant and pain medication, as ordered.

## History

If the patient has *chronic* intermittent claudication, obtain a history first. Ask the patient how far he can walk before the pain occurs and how long he must rest before it subsides. Ask if the pain has worsened.

Ask about risk factors for atherosclerosis, about impotence (in men), paresthesia in the affected limb, and color changes in the patient's fingers when he smokes, is exposed to cold, or is under stress.

## Physical exam

Focus on the cardiovascular system. Palpate for femoral, popliteal, dorsalis pedis, and posterior tibial pulses. Listen for bruits over the major arteries. Note color and temperature differences between the legs or as compared with the arms; also note the leg level where changes in temperature and color occur. Elevate the affected leg for 2 minutes; if it becomes pale or white, blood flow is severely decreased. Inspect arms for color changes and palpate for changes in temperature, for muscle wasting, and for a pulsating subclavian mass. Palpate for and compare the radial, ulnar, brachial, axillary, and subclavian pulses. Examine the feet, toes, and fingers for ulceration, and inspect the hands and lower legs for tender nodules and erythema along blood vessels.

## Causes

*Acute arterial occlusion.* Sudden severe or aching leg pain is aggravated by exercise. A saddle embolus may affect both legs. Associated findings include paresthesia, paresis, cyanosis, and sensations of cold in the affected limb.

*Aortic arteriosclerotic occlusive disease.* Intermittent claudication occurs in the buttocks, hip, thigh, and calf along with absent or diminished femoral pulses. Bruits can be auscultated over the femoral and iliac arteries.

*Arteriosclerosis obliterans.* This disorder usually affects the femoral and popliteal arteries, causing intermittent claudication in the calf.

*Other causes.* Buerger's disease, Leriche's syndrome, neurospinal disease, and thoracic outlet syndrome.

## Nursing considerations

• Urge the patient to immediately report skin breakdown that doesn't heal as well as chest discomfort that may occur when circulation is restored to his legs. Advise him to exercise and to avoid prolonged sitting, standing, or crossing his legs at the knees. Also urge him to inspect his legs and feet for ulcers and to keep his extremities warm, clean, and dry. Counsel the patient about risk factors, and encourage him to stop smoking.

# Homans' sign

## 146

Homans' sign is positive when deep calf pain results from strong and abrupt dorsiflexion of the ankle. This pain results from venous thrombosis or inflammation of the calf muscles. However, because a positive Homans' sign appears in only 35% of patients with these conditions, it's an unreliable indicator. Even when accurate, a positive Homans' sign doesn't indicate the extent of venous disorder.

This elicited sign may be confused with continuous calf pain, which can result from strains, contusions, cellulitis, or arterial occlusion; or with pain in the posterior ankle or Achilles tendon (for example, in a woman with Achilles tendons shortened from wearing high heels).

## History
When you detect a positive Homans' sign, focus your history on signs and symptoms that can accompany deep vein thrombosis (DVT) or thrombophlebitis: throbbing, aching, heavy, or tight sensations in the calf and leg pain during or after exercise or routine activity. Ask about predisposing events, such as leg injury, recent surgery, pregnancy, and prolonged bed rest.

## Physical exam
Inspect and palpate the patient's calf for warmth, tenderness, redness, swelling, and the presence of a palpable vein. Measure the circumferences of both calves. The one with the positive Homans' sign may be larger from edema and swelling.

## Causes
***Deep vein thrombophlebitis.*** A positive Homans' sign and calf tenderness may be the only clinical features of this disorder. But the patient may also have severe pain, heaviness, warmth, and swelling of the affected leg; visible, engorged superficial veins or palpable, cordlike veins; and fever, chills, and malaise.

***Deep vein thrombosis.*** DVT causes a positive Homans' sign along with tenderness over the deep calf veins, slight edema of the calves and thighs, a low-grade fever, and tachycardia. If DVT affects the femoral and iliac veins, you'll notice marked local swelling and tenderness. If it's causing venous obstruction, you'll notice cyanosis and, possibly, cool skin in the affected leg.

## Nursing considerations
• If you detect a positive Homans' sign in a patient whose calf is tender and feels warm, notify the doctor. Place the patient on bed rest with the affected leg elevated above the heart level. Apply warm, moist compresses to the affected area, and administer mild oral analgesics, as ordered.
• For further assessment, you may be asked to slowly inflate a blood pressure cuff that's wrapped around each calf and then to compare the pressures at which the patient first reports pain. Pain occurring at a cuff pressure of under 180 mm Hg indicates DVT or thrombophlebitis. However, because this test may dislodge a clot, you'll need to closely monitor the patient for sudden onset of signs and symptoms of pulmonary embolism — dyspnea, cough, pleural pain, and tachycardia. If any of these occurs, notify the doctor immediately.
• Once the patient is ambulatory, advise him to wear elastic support stockings after his discomfort decreases (usually in 5 to 10 days) and to continue wearing them for at least 3 months. Instruct him to keep the affected leg elevated while sitting and to avoid crossing his legs at the knees.
• If the patient is put on long-term anticoagulant therapy with a coumadin compound such as warfarin, instruct him to report any signs of prolonged clotting time. These include brown or red urine, bleeding gums, bruises, and black, tarry stools. Stress the importance of keeping follow-up appointments so his prothrombin time can be monitored.

H

The inability to fall asleep, remain asleep, or feel refreshed by sleep, insomnia may be acute and transient during periods of stress. It may, however, become chronic, causing constant fatigue, extreme anxiety, and even psychiatric disorders. Insomnia occurs occasionally in about 25% of Americans and chronically in about 10%. It may be caused by jet lag, arguing, lack of exercise, medical and psychiatric disorders, pain, drug adverse effects, and idiopathic factors.

## History
Find out when the patient's insomnia began and the attending circumstances. Is he trying to stop using sedatives? Does he use stimulants or caffeine-containing drugs and beverages?

Find out if the patient has any chronic or acute sleep-disturbing conditions, or painful or pruritic conditions. Ask about drug or alcohol abuse. Note behavior that may indicate alcohol withdrawal. Ask about jet lag, daytime fatigue, regular exercise, periods of dyspnea or apnea, and frequent body repositioning. Also question the patient's spouse or sleep partner because the patient may not be aware of his behavior.

Assess the patient's emotional status, and try to estimate his level of self-esteem. Ask about personal and professional problems and psychological stress.

## Physical exam
After reviewing any complaints that suggest an undiagnosed disorder, perform a physical examination.

## Causes
*Affective disorders. Depression* commonly causes chronic insomnia with difficulty falling asleep, wakefulness, or waking early in the morning. Episodes of *mania* reduce the need for sleep and produce elevated mood and irritability.

*Alcohol withdrawal syndrome.* Abrupt cessation of alcohol after long-term use causes insomnia that may persist for up to 2 years. Other findings may include excessive diaphoresis, tachycardia, increased blood pressure, restlessness, headache, nausea, flushing, and nightmares.

*Generalized anxiety disorder.* Hyperattentiveness from anxiety can cause chronic insomnia. Other findings may include fatigue, restlessness, diaphoresis, dyspepsia, high resting pulse and respiratory rates, and apprehension.

*Pain.* Almost any condition that causes pain may cause insomnia. Related findings reflect the specific cause.

*Sleep apnea syndrome.* Apneic periods begin with the onset of sleep, continue for 10 to 90 seconds, then end with a series of gasps and arousal. In *central sleep apnea*, respiratory movement ceases for the apneic period; in *obstructive sleep apnea*, upper airway obstruction blocks incoming air, although breathing movements continue. Some patients display both types. Other findings include morning headache, daytime fatigue, hypertension, ankle edema, and personality changes.

*Other causes.* Nocturnal myoclonus; pheochromocytoma; pruritic conditions; thyrotoxicosis; and use of, abuse of, or withdrawal from such drugs as sedatives, hypnotics, or central nervous system stimulants.

## Nursing considerations
• Prepare the patient for tests to evaluate his insomnia, such as blood and urine studies for 17-hydroxycorticosteroids and catecholamines; sleep EEG; or other tests such as EEG, electro-oculography, and electrocardiography.
• Teach the patient comfort and relaxation techniques. Advise him to awaken and retire at the same time each day and to exercise regularly. Urge him to use his bed only for sleeping, not for relaxing.
• Advise him to use tranquilizers or sedatives for acute insomnia only when relaxation techniques fail. If appropriate, arrange for counseling, biofeedback training, or other interventions.

Excessive skin coloring, hyperpigmentation usually reflects overproduction, abnormal location, or maldistribution of melanin—the dominant brown or black pigment found in skin, hair, mucous membranes, and elsewhere. It can also reflect abnormalities of other pigments: carotenoids (yellow), oxyhemoglobin (red), and hemoglobin (blue).

Hyperpigmentation most commonly results from exposure to sunlight. However, it can also result from other causes. Typically asymptomatic and chronic, hyperpigmentation can have distressing psychosocial implications. It varies in location and intensity and may fade over time.

## History

Do any other family members have the same problem? Was the patient's hyperpigmentation present at birth? Did other signs, such as rash, accompany or precede it? Obtain a history of medical disorders and contact with or ingestion of chemicals, metals, plants, vegetables, or fruits. Was the onset of hyperpigmentation related to exposure to sunlight or season change? Is the patient pregnant or taking medication? Does the patient have other signs?

## Physical exam

Examine the skin. Note the color of hyperpigmented areas: Brown suggests excess melanin in the epidermis; slate gray or a bluish tone suggests excess pigment in the dermis. Inspect for other changes, too—thickening and leatherlike texture and changes in hair distribution. Check the skin and sclera for jaundice, and note any spider angiomas, palmar erythema, or purpura. Take vital signs and evaluate general appearance.

## Causes

*Adrenocortical insufficiency.* This disorder produces diffuse tan, brown, or bronze to black hyperpigmentation of exposed and unexposed areas—the face, knees, knuckles, elbows, beltline, palmar creases, lips, gums, tongue, and buccal mucosa. Normally pigmented areas, moles, and scars become darker. Early in the disorder, persistent tanning occurs after sun exposure.

*Biliary cirrhosis.* Hyperpigmentation is a classic feature. A widespread and accentuated brown hyperpigmentation appears on areas exposed to sunlight, but not on the mucosa. Pruritus may be the earliest symptom, followed by weakness, fatigue, weight loss, and vague abdominal pain.

*Drugs.* Hyperpigmentation can stem from use of barbiturates, salicylates, chemotherapeutic agents, chlorpromazine, antimalarial drugs, hydantoin, minocycline, metals (silver and gold), adrenocorticotropic hormone, and phenothiazines.

*Hemochromatosis.* Early and progressive hyperpigmentation results from melanin deposits in the skin. It develops as generalized bronzing and metallic-gray areas accentuated over sun-exposed areas, genitalia, and scars.

*Laënnec's cirrhosis.* After about 10 years of excessive alcohol ingestion, progressive liver dysfunction causes diffuse, generalized hyperpigmentation on sun-exposed areas.

*Scleroderma.* Localized or systemic scleroderma produces generalized dark brown hyperpigmentation unrelated to sun exposure. Areas of depigmentation and spider angiomas appear. Skin thickening progresses to taut, shiny, leathery skin over the hands and forearms, then over the arms, chest, abdomen, and back. Tight, inelastic facial skin becomes masklike, pinching the mouth.

*Other causes.* Acromegaly, arsenic poisoning, malignant melanoma, porphyria cutanea tarda, and thyrotoxicosis.

## Nursing considerations

• Hyperpigmentation may persist even after treatment. Bleaching creams may not be effective if most of the excess melanin lies in subepidermal layers.
• Advise patients to use corrective cosmetics, to avoid excessive sun exposure, and to apply a sunscreen or sun blocker. Advise those who stop using bleaching agents to keep using sun blockers.
• Advise consultation with the doctor if the lesion's size, shape, or color changes.

**H**

# Impotence

Impotence is the inability to achieve and maintain penile erection sufficient to complete satisfactory intercourse; ejaculation may or may not be affected. Impotence varies from occasional and minimal to permanent and complete. Occasional impotence occurs in about half of adult men.

Organic causes of impotence may include vascular disease, diabetes mellitus, hypogonadism, a spinal cord lesion, alcohol and drug abuse, and surgical complications. Psychogenic causes range from performance anxiety and marital discord to moral or religious conflicts.

## History

If the patient complains of impotence, let him describe his problem without interruption. Then begin with a psychosocial history. Is the patient married, single, or widowed? How long has he been married or had a sexual relationship? What's the age and health status of his sexual partner? Find out about past marriages, if any, and ask him why he thinks they ended. If you can do so discreetly, ask about sexual activity outside marriage or his primary sexual relationship.

Focus your medical history on the causes of erectile dysfunction. Does the patient have Type II diabetes mellitus, hypertension, or heart disease? Ask about its onset and treatment. Also ask about neurologic diseases. Get a surgical history.

Ask about intake of alcohol, drug use or abuse, smoking, diet, and exercise.

Ask when his impotence began. How did it progress? What's its current status? How often does the patient awaken in the morning or at night with an erection? Has his sexual drive changed? How often does he attempt intercourse with his partner? Can he ejaculate with or without an erection?

## Physical exam

Inspect and palpate the genitalia and prostate for structural abnormalities. Assess sensory function, concentrating on the perineal area. Next, test motor strength and deep tendon reflexes in all extremities, and note other neurologic deficits. Take vital signs and palpate pulses for quality. Note any signs of peripheral vascular disease, such as cyanosis and cool extremities. Auscultate for abdominal aortic, femoral, or iliac bruits, and palpate for thyroid enlargement.

## Causes

*Alcohol and drugs.* Alcohol and drug abuse are associated with impotence, as are many prescription drugs, especially antihypertensives.

*Central nervous system disorders.* Spinal cord lesions from trauma produce sudden impotence. A complete lesion above S2 (upper motor neuron lesion) causes loss of voluntary erectile control but not the reflexive ability for erection and ejaculation. But a complete lesion in the lumbosacral spinal cord (lower motor neuron lesions) causes loss of reflex ejaculation and reflex erection. Spinal cord tumors and degenerative diseases (such as multiple sclerosis) cause progressive impotence.

*Peripheral neuropathy.* Systemic diseases, such as diabetes mellitus, can cause progressive impotence if they progress to peripheral neuropathy. This occurs in about 50% of male diabetics.

*Psychological distress.* Impotence can result from diverse psychological causes, including depression, performance anxiety, memories of previous traumatic sexual experiences, moral or religious conflicts, and troubled relationships.

*Other causes.* Endocrine and penile disorders, trauma (including surgical), vascular disorders.

## Nursing considerations

• Prepare the patient for screening tests for hormonal irregularities and for Doppler readings of penile blood pressure to rule out vascular insufficiency. Other possible tests include voiding studies, nerve conduction tests, evaluation of nocturnal penile tumescence, and psychological screening.
• Treatment for psychogenic impotence may include counseling of both the patient and his sexual partner; treatment for organic impotence focuses on reversing the cause, if possible.